NURSING IMPLICATIONS OF LABORATORY TESTS

Third Edition

Mary Brambilla McFarland, R.N., Ed.D.

Associate Professor and Associate Dean

Oregon Health Sciences University School of Nursing, Portland, Oregon

Marcia Moeller Grant, R.N., D.N.Sc., FAAN

Director of Nursing Research and Education and Associate Research Scientist

City of Hope Medical Center, Duarte, California

Contributor

Jill L. Schumacher, R.N., M.S.N.

Assistant Professor

Oregon Health Sciences University School of Nursing, Portland, Oregon

Delmar Publishers Inc.

I(T)P™

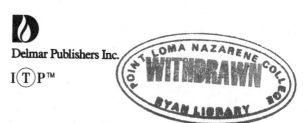

Notice to the Reader

Publisher does not warrant or guarantee any of the products described herein or perform any independent analysis in connection with any of the product information contained herein. Publisher does not assume, and expressly disclaims, any obligation to obtain and include information other than that provided to it by the manufacturer.

The reader is expressly warned to consider and adopt all safety precautions that might be indicated by the activities described herein and to avoid all potential hazards. By following the instructions contained herein, the reader willingly assumes all risks in connection with such instructions.

The publisher makes no representations or warranties of any kind, including but not limited to, the warranties of fitness for particular purpose or merchantability, nor are any such representations implied with respect to the material set forth herein, and the publisher takes no responsibility with respect to such material. The publisher shall not be liable for any special, consequential, or exemplary damages resulting, in whole or in part, from the reader's use of, or reliance upon, this material.

Cover design by Spiral Design

Delmar Staff
  Associate Editor: Elisabeth Williams
  Project Manager: Carol Micheli
  Production Coordinator: Mary Ellen Black
  Art Coordinators: Lisa L. Pauly and Mary Siener

For information, address Delmar Publishers Inc.
3 Columbia Circle, Box 15-015
Albany, New York 12212

Printed in the United States of America
published simultaneously in Canada
by Nelson Canada,
a division of the Thomson Corporation

3 4 5 6 7 8 9 10 XXX 00 99 98 97 96 95

Library of Congress Cataloging-in-Publication Data

McFarland, Mary Brambilla.
    Nursing implications of laboratory tests / Mary Brambilla
McFarland, Marcia Moeller Grant : contributor, Jill L. Schumacher.—
3rd ed.
        p.   cm.
    Includes bibliographical references and index.
    ISBN 0-8273-5135-6
    1. Diagnosis, Laboratory.   2. Nursing.   I. Grant, Marcia Moeller.
II. Schumacher, Jill L.   III. Title.
    [DNLM: 1. Diagnosis, Laboratory—nurses' instruction.
2. Diagnostic Tests, Routine—nurses' instruction.   3. Patient
Education.   QY 4 M478n 1994]
RT48.5.M34   1994
616.07'56—dc20
DNLM/DLC
for Library of Congress   93-23603
                                                                     CIP

Preface

This third edition of *Nursing Implications of Laboratory Tests*, like the two previous editions, is written for nurses, nursing students and other health professionals. Undergraduate nursing students in both associate degree and baccalaureate degree programs will find this an accessible reference. It is also meant to be used as a quick clinical guide for nurses practicing in hospitals, clinics, nursing homes, and community health agencies including home care.

This third edition includes several changes, some of which have been added in response to suggestions from readers. Obsolete studies have been removed, new studies added and all chapters updated. Normal ranges include adult, newborn and pediatric values.

Chapter 1 contains information that will help the nurse prepare patients for laboratory tests done on blood, urine, sputum, stool, bone marrow, and cerebrospinal fluid. It also describes in detail the methods used for collection of specimens. Updated information about Universal Precautions has been added and is also summarized in Appendix B. Chapters 2 through 10 are organized according to body systems. This approach allows the reader to understand the relationships among tests performed to determine the presence of pathological conditions within a body system. It also provides a clinically oriented focus. A new chapter, *Laboratory Tests of Reproductive System*, was developed to cluster well established tests with new tests in this expanded area of health care. Tests that can be used to determine deviations in more than one body system are included in each corresponding chapter. The chapter entitled *Laboratory Tests of Infectious Diseases and Allergic Reactions* has been expanded to include additional information about microorganisms responsible for the increased incidence of infectious diseases.

Chapter 13, entitled *Diagnostic Tests*, is organized by general categories of diagnostic studies, including angiography, diagnostic studies, endoscopy, nuclear scans, radiography, magnetic resonance imaging, computer tomography, and ultrasound. Specific studies are presented to address special considerations.

Patient education is emphasized throughout the text. The importance of informing patients about the type of test being done and how the specimen is to be collected is discussed in Chapter 1. In addition, patient education is included among nursing interventions when abnormal test results will require further nursing or medical treatment or result in a change in the patient's lifestyle. Teaching is also an important part of the section on diagnostic tests. Patient education is especially important in the current climate of health care, where information on the purpose and need for laboratory tests is a critical part of patient teaching. The clinical nurse is in the important position of helping patients and families understand the purpose of laboratory tests and how they relate to one's own health care.

Contents

Note to the Reader

When looking at deviations from normal, it is important to remember that laboratory tests are not always positive in the presence of disease or negative in its absence. The discussions in this text should be used to guide the nurse when making decisions about nursing care. The reader will see that the results of many tests may be affected by non-disease-associated influences such as diet, physical activity, drugs, and genetic factors. Therefore, the nurse must be aware of the fact that it is often difficult to make the transition from a test result to a clinical picture of the patient and related nursing care. We warn the user of this book not to have a "knee jerk" reaction to a test result, be it positive or negative, but to look at the result with reference to the total patient.

The discussions of causes of deviation from normal and nursing implications vary depending on the condition causing the abnormal test result. Normal ranges included for each test are the normal values seen in 95% of normal, healthy subjects. It is important to remember that 5% of the population of healthy people can be expected to have values outside the normal range. This may be the reason for an abnormal test result for a person in whom all else is normal. The sections describing causes of deviation from normal and nursing implications of abnormal findings provide the link between the abnormal laboratory tests and related nursing care. Because it is a nursing responsibility to assess patients whose laboratory results deviate from normal, nurses must understand what the deviations mean when they plan nursing interventions. The implications for nursing care contain only specific areas for assessment and interventions. They do not include all of the details of nursing care for the specific physiological problems that cause abnormal test results. The reader should consult current nursing texts and journals for that information as well as the bibliography at the end of each chapter.

Collection of Specimens

When diagnostic tests are done, there are many variables that may alter test results. The nurse should take care to avoid extrinsic variables and to report those factors that cannot be controlled. Ensuring the accuracy of laboratory test results begins with the collection of the specimen. The procedure for collection can become routine, and accuracy is essential to avoid making mistakes. Specimen containers should be labeled with the patient's name and hospital number before collection begins. The patient's identification band should be used to identify the patient before collecting the specimen. Verbal identification alone should not be relied on, since patients who are confused, hard of hearing, or joking may answer to an incorrect name.

Prolonged application of a tourniquet may cause elevations of macromolecular and cellular constituents of blood because of ultrafiltration across the vessel. This problem is compounded when dehydration is present. When venipuncture is difficult, a note on the laboratory slip will be helpful in interpreting the results.

Laboratory reports are sometimes filed in the wrong patient's record, particularly when two patients on the same unit have the same or similar names. Patients have been given medication and other therapy based on laboratory reports erroneously filed in their records. Safeguards against this error should be made.

The circadian or diurnal variations of some biochemical substances result in variation among test results taken at different times of the day. This can be avoided by collecting all routine specimens at the same time each day. The time of day that the specimen was collected should be noted on the laboratory slip. This also avoids conflicts with mealtimes, medical treatments, medications, and other diagnostic tests.

Posture can also affect test results. A change in position from lying to standing may result in an elevation of nonfilterable blood constituents within 15 minutes. Reverse changes may also occur. Collection of specimens in the early morning, before patients begin moving about, helps minimize this effect.

The results of many blood tests are affected by drugs. Whenever a patient is taking medications that may interfere with the results of the test being done, a note should be made on the laboratory slip and the physician who ordered the test notified.

Changes may occur in biochemical measurements as a result of aging. Table 1.1 gives an example of how serum albumin levels fall as a person ages. Mechanisms of production of pain and fever may be impaired and homeostatic mechanisms may also be affected by aging. For example, defective osmoregulation may occur in older people who are ill and cause severe disturbances in serum osmolality. Multiple diseases and drug regimens common to the elderly also make it difficult to interpret test results.

Food and fluid restrictions necessary before a specimen is collected must be explained to patients and enforced by the nursing staff. Precautions for the hos-

Table 1.1. Decreases in Serum Albumin With Age

| Age | Serum Albumin g/l | |
	Mean	Standard Deviation
20–29	40.03	2.94
30–39	39.25	2.95
40–49	38.47	2.95
50–59	37.68	2.94
60–69	36.90	2.94
70+	36.12	2.94

pitalized patient may include removing all food and fluid from the bedside, placing a sign on the patient's door, or withholding meals when a fasting specimen is required. Proper labeling and preparation, plus notification of the laboratory of potential causes for variation increase the reliability of the test results. The specimen should be sent to the laboratory as soon as possible as fresh specimens provide the most accurate test results.

In 1987 (MMWR, 1987), the Centers for Disease Control (CDC) recommended that blood and body fluid precautions be consistently used for all patients regardless of bloodborne infection status. This recommendation is referred to as Universal Precautions. In 1988 (MMWR, 1988), the CDC clarified the recommendation; Universal Precautions apply to blood and other body fluids containing visible blood, semen, and vaginal secretions. Universal Precautions do not apply to feces, nasal secretions, sputum, sweat, tears, urine, or vomitus unless they contain visible blood; the risk of transmission of the human immunodeficiency virus (HIV) and hepatitis B virus (HBV) from these fluids and materials is extremely low or nonexistent. The CDC has noted that gloves reduce the incidence of blood contaminating the hands during phlebotomy, but cannot prevent penetrating injuries caused by needles or other sharp instruments.

Universal Precautions are recommended because all blood is assumed to be potentially infective for bloodborne pathogens. However, in settings where the prevalence of infections is low, there has been a relaxation of the recommendations for using gloves for phlebotomy. The CDC has indicated that gloves should be available to health-care workers who wish to use them. They have also published the following guidelines (MMWR, 1988):

1. Use gloves for performing phlebotomy when the health-care worker has cuts, scratches and/or other breaks in the skin.
2. Use gloves in situations where the health-care worker judges that hand contamination with blood may occur; for example, when performing phlebotomy on an uncooperative patient.
3. Use gloves for performing finger and/or heel sticks on infants and children.
4. Use gloves when persons are receiving training in phlebotomy.

BLOOD EXAMINATION

Preparation of the Patient

The patient should be informed of the reasons the specimen was ordered, how it is to be collected, the equipment needed, and the stinging sensation that may be felt. The patient should also be told to remain still and to hold the arm extended, either resting flat on the bed or supported firmly. A brief explanation should be given to comatose patients as well.

Method For Specimen Collection
VENIPUNCTURE

Venipuncture may be performed using either a syringe or a Vacutainer system. Collecting tubes have colored stoppers indicating what additive, if any, is in the tube. The color-coding is as follows:

- *Red*—No additive
- *Lavender*—EDTA (Ethylenediaminotetraacetate)
- *Light blue*—Sodium Citrate
- *Green*—Sodium Heparin
- *Gray*—Potassium Oxalate
- *Black*—Sodium Oxalate

All collecting tubes should be labeled with the patient's name and medical record number before the specimen is drawn. Gloves should be worn during the collection procedure. The characteristics of some patient's veins make venipuncture difficult. The skin of infants and babies may be thin and the veins fragile and rolling. The skin of older children is often thick and strong. Their veins may also resist puncture due to vasospasm or vasoconstriction. In elderly patients, the veins tend to roll away from the needle or yield poor blood return once punctured due to thickening and hardening which occurs with aging. In all patients larger, non-scarred, visible veins should be used first, proceeding from the antecubital space to the arm and then to the hand. The legs and feet should not be used, due to the increase in complications associated with skin punctures in these areas. Blood should not be drawn from the same extremity that is being used for intravenous (IV) fluid infusions or medications or for blood administration. However, if there is no other venipuncture site, a sample may be drawn by slowing the IV to a drip rate that will maintain patency, waiting 3–5 minutes, then drawing blood below the IV site. The first 5 cc's should be discarded and a note should be sent to the laboratory stating the blood was drawn below an IV site.

Procedure for Venipuncture.

1. Put on gloves.

2. Apply a tourniquet or blood-pressure cuff until a pressure between the systolic and diastolic readings is obtained.

    - The tourniquet should occlude venous blood flow causing the vein to swell, but should not occlude arterial flow.
    - The tourniquet should not be left on for more than one minute prior to venipuncture or for more than 2–3 minutes after the vein is entered.

3. Instruct the patient to open and close the fist several times and to keep the fist closed while the vein is being located.

■ If it is difficult to find a distended vein, the hand may be wrapped in a warm compress to promote peripheral distention. Care should be taken not to apply a compress that is too hot.

4. Cleanse the site with a disinfectant such as povidone-iodine (Betadine) or 70% alcohol and dry with a sterile gauze pad. Once cleansed, the site should not be palpated again.

■ For some tests, such as blood alcohol, some cleansing solutions are contraindicated. See specific tests for those exceptions.

5. Select an appropriate gauge needle.

■ A 20 or 21 gauge needle should be selected for veins in the antecubital space or forearm and a 25 gauge needle for veins in the wrist or hand.

6. Stabilize the vein by placing the thumb below the point of entry and hold the needle bevel side up at a 15° angle to the patient's arm, and pointed in the direction of the vein path.

■ If a Vacutainer system is used, the Vacutainer tube is pushed into the holder until the rubber stopper is punctured and blood flows into the tube. If more than one tube of blood is being drawn, each tube is removed as soon as it is filled and another inserted until the specimen collection is complete.

■ If a syringe is used, the tourniquet is removed once blood flow begins. Gentle suction is placed on the plunger until the desired amount of blood is obtained. The blood is then transferred to the appropriate Vacutainer tubes by inserting the needle into the stopper and allowing the vacuum to draw the blood from the syringe into the tube. An alternate method is to remove the needle from the syringe and the stopper from the tube and slowly inject the blood into the tube.

■ When there is an additive in the collecting tube, mix the specimen gently before sending it to the laboratory.

7. After the specimen is obtained, withdraw the needle and apply pressure to the venipuncture site instructing the patient to hold the arm over the head. If bleeding occurs from the area, apply a pressure dressing, keep the arm elevated, and stay with the patient until it stops.

SKIN PUNCTURE

Skin puncture is used for tests performed on capillary blood. Sites that may be used are the earlobe, palmar fingertip, and plantar heel surface. The earlobe is less sensitive and is useful for patients who are in shock or have edematous limbs. The finger is used for small children and people with poor veins. It is often convenient to use the finger method on patients confined to bed rest, but the finger is difficult to clean adequately and therefore susceptible to infection. In infants, the plantar heel is the most commonly used site.

Procedure for Skin Puncture.

1. Put on gloves.
2. Select the site to be used.
3. Cleanse the site with a disinfectant such as povidone-iodine (Betadine) or 70% alcohol and allow to dry.
   - If the patient has a low white cell count, the site should be cleansed for several minutes.
4. Puncture the site 2 mm deep with a firm, quick stab using a sterile lancet.
   - When possible, the side surface of the fingertip or heel should be used to avoid irritation of or damage to nerve endings.
5. Wipe away the first drop of blood containing tissue fluids with a sterile gauze pad.
6. Allow the next blood drops to flow without squeezing.
   - Gentle pressure may be applied to the area adjacent to the site.
   - The hand may be placed in a dependent position or warmed to encourage blood flow.
7. Collect the blood in microhematocrit tubes or in micropipettes.
8. Expel the blood into tubes containing the appropriate reagents or dilutents.
   - When blood is being collected for several tests, including a platelet count; blood for the latter should be collected first, because platelets aggregate at the puncture site.
9. Apply pressure to the puncture site with a sterile pad once blood collection is complete.

BLOOD CULTURE

When a blood culture is ordered, it is collected in a sterile closed system. It should be collected before antibiotic therapy is instituted. A series of three cultures is generally taken at intervals of 30 minutes or more. The person collecting the specimen should wear gloves and use aseptic technique. The proposed puncture site should be cleansed with an antiseptic solution, such as providone-iodine (Betadine). Once the site is cleansed the vein should not be palpated again. Caution should be carried out to prevent contamination of the collecting bottle. After the specimen is obtained, the needle should be changed and a new, sterile needle used to inject the culture bottles. Venipuncture should be done as described above. The specimen should be transported to the laboratory immediately.

SERIAL BLOOD SAMPLING

1

Serial blood sampling is being used in some institutions for patients who require large amounts of blood to be drawn for laboratory studies. The advantage of this system is it reduces patient discomfort from multiple venipunctures. Patients who are scheduled to have this procedure should be informed of its purpose. The advantages and disadvantages of having an indwelling catheter compared to a series of venipunctures should also be discussed.

The procedure involves starting an IV infusion with an 18-gauge venous catheter. Two stopcocks are attached to an adapter at the end of the catheter, with the capped sections of both stopcocks pointing upward. When blood is to be drawn, a 10-ml syringe is inserted into the stopcock closest (proximal) to the insertion site and a 3-ml syringe is attached to the stopcock furthest (distal) from the insertion site. When blood is to be drawn, the following steps should be taken:

1. Stop the IV flow by turning the distal stopcock valve off.
2. Remove saline from the IV catheter and stopcock by aspirating 2–3 ml of fluid into the 3-ml syringe.
3. Turn the valve of the proximal stopcock off.
4. Draw the amount of blood needed into the 10-ml syringe.
5. Return the stopcock valves to their original positions.
6. Remove the syringes and replace the sterile caps on the stopcocks.
7. Adjust the IV rate as needed.

Before using the system, the nurse should be familiar with the use of in-line stopcocks. To prevent the chances of clots forming in the stopcocks, the IV should be kept running slowly. If a serial blood-sampling system is in place for 24 hours or longer, stopcocks, intravenous tubing, and dressings should be changed.

ARTERIAL BLOOD GAS SAMPLING

Preparation of the Patient

Explain the procedure while the patient is alert and responsive. A brief explanation should also be given to a comatose patient. Ask the patient to breathe normally. Breath holding and tachypnea can cause abnormal results. The patient should be warned that an arterial puncture usually causes a momentary deep throbbing or cramping pain.

Method for Puncture of the Radial Artery

On hospital units where arterial puncture is a nursing responsibility, nurses should be specifically prepared to perform this procedure safely. An easily palpable artery should be selected. The most accessible arteries are the brachial, radial, and femoral. In most settings, the radial artery is chosen for routine specimens. The following procedure should be used:

1. Select the site to be used and examine it for the presence of arterial occlusive disease.
   - The pulse should be easily palpable and of good quality.
2. Perform the Allen test.
   - Ask the patient to clench the fist tightly.
   - Apply digital pressure to occlude both the radial and ulnar arteries.
   - Ask the patient to unclench the fist while digital pressure is maintained and observe the palm for blanching.
   - Release the ulnar artery while maintaining occlusion of the radial artery. Observe the palm for immediate blushing. If the blush is delayed beyond 10 seconds, inadequate ulnar flow or an incompetent palmar arch is indicated. In this situation, radial artery puncture is contraindicated.
3. Position the hand by placing the wrist in slight to moderate extension.
   - A roll of gauze or a small towel may be used to support and angle the dorsum of the wrist.
4. Moisten the barrel of a 3–5 ml glass syringe with 0.1 ml of heparin if disposable syringes specifically prepared for arterial blood gas sampling are not available.
5. Remove all air bubbles from the syringe and attach a 20–21 gauge needle.
6. Palpate the artery is just proximal to the site of puncture.
7. Put on gloves.
8. Cleanse the skin with an antiseptic agent such as povidone-iodine (Betadine) and allow it to dry.
9. Pass the needle through the skin and direct it across the axis of the artery toward the point of maximal pulsation felt by the tip of the palpating finger. Either a 45° or 90° angle may be used for the puncture.
   - When approaching the artery at a 45° angle, enter slowly, from the side.
   - When approaching the artery at a 90° (vertical) angle, pierce the artery and withdraw the needle until blood flashes back into the syringe.
   - It is obvious that the artery has been pierced when pulsations of blood flow into the syringe.
10. Allow the syringe to be filled by the pulsating artery; the aspiration of air may occur if the plunger is pulled back manually.

11. After the sample has been obtained, remove the needle from the artery.

12. Expel any air or air bubbles from the syringe and cap it tightly.

13. Place the syringe in a container of ice and send to the laboratory for analysis.

14. Apply direct pressure to the site for a minimum of 3–5 minutes as a pre-caution against bleeding.

   ■ If the patient is taking an anticoagulant, pressure should be main-tained until no bleeding is present.

Following arterial puncture, watch for the clinical manifestations of arterial occlusion which can be caused by clot formation or by raising an intimal flap with the needle. These signs include numbness and tingling of the hand, dusky color, and absence of a peripheral pulse, which can lead to gangrene of the extremity. Laceration of the artery can also occur if poor technique is used.

   Indwelling arterial (A) lines may be used for arterial blood gas sampling. Since the heparin solution used to keep A lines patent distorts lab results, the first milliliters of blood drawn must be discarded. The amounts suggested range from 2–6 mls. Recent nursing research has shown that 2 ml may be the optimal discard amount thus preventing unnecessary blood loss in critically ill patients (Preusser et al., 1989).

BONE MARROW EXAMINATION

Preparation of the Patient

Many patients who must have a bone marrow examination are frightened and anxious. Fear of the procedure itself may cause these feelings as well as concern about the results of the examination. The nurse should describe common physi-cal sensations such as pain during aspiration, pressure and cold during prepara-tion of the skin, and numbness following the anesthetic. A description of the purpose, duration, and location of the bone marrow examination should also be included.

   The patient undergoing bone marrow examination must sign a special con-sent form for the procedure. If the patient is very apprehensive, a sedative may be administered after the consent form is signed. If the sternum is to be used, the patient should be placed in a supine position with a small pillow under the thoracic spine. If the iliac crest is used, a side position is maintained. The patient should be told that the area will be anesthetized and that a small sting-ing sensation may be felt at the onset. A feeling of pressure may also be experi-enced as the specimen is withdrawn. The patient should remain still during the procedure. Relaxation methods that the patient has successfully used in the past may be identified and, if appropriate, encouraged. Rest in bed is required for 30 minutes after the procedure; usual activity can then be resumed. After the needle or biopsy instrument is removed, direct pressure and a sterile dressing is applied. Tenderness over the puncture site can be expected for 3–4 days.

Method of Bone Marrow Collection

The physician usually collects the bone marrow specimen with the assistance of the nurse. Aseptic technique is used throughout the procedure to prevent the introduction of infectious material into the bone marrow. The skin is cleansed with an antiseptic solution, and a sterile drape is used. After local anesthesia is injected, a short rigid needle with a stylet is introduced into the marrow cavity, and approximately 0.2–0.5 ml of marrow fluid is aspirated. The specimen may be placed in collection tubes, culture tubes, or directly onto slides, depending on the kind of analysis desired. All specimens should be clearly marked with the patient's name, medical record number, date, and the doctor's name, and should be accompanied by a filled-in laboratory request slip. The whole procedure should not take longer than 5 to 10 minutes. After the needle is removed, direct pressure should be placed over the area and a sterile bandage applied.

BONE MARROW SMEAR

When a bone marrow smear for cell identification and classification is being done, the slides are likely to be prepared at the patient's bedside. The nurse should make sure that these slides are identified with the patient's name and medical record number.

BONE MARROW CULTURE

When a bone marrow examination is being conducted for the identification of microorganisms, the specimen should be aseptically collected in a sterile tube and transported to the laboratory immediately.

BONE MARROW BIOPSY

If a biopsy of tissue of the bone marrow is needed, a needle biopsy is carried out after aspiration of the bone marrow sample.

URINE EXAMINATION

Preparation of the Patient

The patient should be told the type of specimen needed and the best time of day to collect it. The first morning specimen is best for routine urinalysis, because it is most concentrated, unaffected by diet, and more likely to reveal abnormalities. Postprandial specimens are obtained 2 hours after a meal. This is when they are most likely to contain protein and glucose.

1

When a twenty-four-hour urine specimen is needed, the patient should be instructed to empty the bladder at the beginning of the twenty-four-hour period (e.g., ten AM) and discard the specimen. All urine should be saved for twenty-four hours. Inform the patient if the sample is to be refrigerated. The patient should then be instructed to void again at the end of the twenty-four-hour period (e.g., ten AM) and to add that final specimen to the total collection. If the patient does not void at the specific time the test is to end, the exact time of last voiding should be noted on the bottle. One large container should be used to collect the entire specimen. It should be labeled with the patient's name, date, type of specimen, and the time the collection was started and ended. When patients collect twenty-four-hour specimens at home, these instructions should be given to the patient with a specimen bottle for collection. Hospitalized patients using bedpans should be reminded to void before having a bowel movement to prevent contamination of the specimen. Toilet paper should not be placed in the bedpan as it absorbs urine and decreases the amount saved.

If a clean-voided midstream specimen (clean-catch) is needed, the method for collecting the specimen described below should be explained to the patient. If the patient is able to collect the specimen alone, materials and instructions to obtain the specimen should be provided.

Method for Urine Collection

Routine Analysis. The patient is asked to void into a clean bedpan or urinal or directly into the specimen container. The specimen is then sent to the laboratory. If the patient has a large amount of vaginal discharge, menstrual bleeding, or frequent diarrhea, a clean-voided (clean-catch) specimen should be obtained (see below). Whenever blood is present, gloves should be used.

Clean-Voided Specimen. A clean-voided midstream specimen is obtained when a bacteriological culture is ordered or if a random (routine) specimen may be contaminated by vaginal discharge or feces.

Procedure for Specimen Collection.

1. Three or four sterile cotton balls saturated with an antiseptic solution, or sterile, presaturated towelettes are provided for cleaning.

2. If a patient is being taught to collect a clean midstream specimen, the importance of keeping the specimen container and the cover sterile should be stressed. A bathroom or private area should be provided that has a clean area on which the container cover can be placed with the outer portion down.

3. The foreskin of the male patient is retracted or the labia of the female patient spread apart.

4. The saturated cotton balls or towelettes are used to clean the area. Each one is used only once. The area around the meatus in the male patient is cleansed using a circular motion. The meatus in the female patient is cleansed from front to back using a downward stroke.

5. With the meatus still exposed, the patient begins to void, passing the first portion of urine into the toilet bowl, urinal, or bedpan. The remaining urine should be voided into the specimen container until the container is almost full. The rim and the inside of the container should not be touched with fingers. Males should be told not to touch the container with the penis.

6. The container should be covered tightly and sent to the laboratory immediately. If the urine cannot be analyzed promptly, the specimen should be refrigerated.

Procedure for Specimen Collection—Infants and Young Children.

1. Place the child in a supine position with the hips externally rotated and abducted with the knees flexed.

2. Clean the perineal area with cotton balls saturated in an antiseptic solution or use sterile, presaturated towelettes. If the perineum is soiled with fecal material and/or old urine, clean the area with soap and water.

3. Apply the collection bag. For boys, apply the urine collection bag over the penis and scrotum pressing the flaps of the bag against the perineum to prevent leakage. For girls, tape the collection bag to the perineum starting at the mid-posterior point and working toward the front.

4. Place a diaper over the collection bag to keep it in place.

5. Remove the bag immediately after collection.

6. Transfer the urine to a properly labeled urine specimen container and send to the laboratory.

Note. Catherization should not be used when collecting urine specimens. This procedure increases the risk of genitourinary tract infections by introducing a foreign body into the bladder.

SPECIMENS OBTAINED FROM A CLOSED URINARY DRAINAGE SYSTEM

If urine is needed for bacteriological culture or for glucose and acetone testing, the side of the catheter or collecting port should be cleansed with an antiseptic solution, and a small-gauge needle should be inserted to obtain the specimen.

When a specimen is needed for routine analysis, urine may be collected from the catheter or the drainage tube by clamping it off until enough urine for the specimen is produced. The specimen is then obtained by separating the catheter and the drainage tube and allowing the urine to flow directly from the catheter into the specimen container. A specimen should never be obtained from a collection bag.

CEREBROSPINAL FLUID EXAMINATION

Preparation of the Patient

Before the performance of a lumbar puncture to obtain cerebrospinal fluid for examination, the patient needs to sign an informed consent statement. The nurse should inform the patient of the sensations that may occur during the procedure. For example, the patient may feel discomfort because of position, pain from the needle insertion, and pain and tingling in the legs during the procedure. Before the procedure, the patient should be asked to empty his bladder and bowel. Once the procedure has begun, the patient should be encouraged to maintain the flexed body position required and to relax. Breathing slowly through the mouth may be helpful.

Method for Cerebrospinal Fluid Collection

The physician collects cerebrospinal fluid under sterile conditions. The patient is placed in a side-lying position with the knees flexed up to the abdomen and the head flexed down to the chest. The nurse may assist the patient in maintaining this position by keeping his head flexed with one arm and looping her other arm through the patient's knees to maintain knee flexion. After selection of the puncture site, the skin is cleansed with an antiseptic solution. A sterile drape is used to protect the puncture site. A local anesthetic is injected slowly, and the spinal needle is inserted. Once the needle is in place, the stylet is removed and the manometer is attached to measure the opening pressure. The nurse should be prepared to record the time and reading of this pressure. If a Queckenstedt test is done, pressure is recorded when both jugular veins are occluded and again when they are released. Three specimen tubes are filled with a total of 5–10 ml of cerebral spinal fluid. These tubes should be labeled with the patient's name, medical record number, date, doctor's name, and whether they were collected in tube #1, #2, or #3. The manometer is again attached to the needle and the closing pressure is read and recorded by the nurse. The spinal needle is removed and a small pressure dressing or a bandage is applied. Specimens should be taken to the laboratory for immediate analysis. The patient should remain lying flat for 4 to 8 hours after the procedure in order to prevent headache. Fluids should be encouraged, as they may prevent or alleviate a headache. The nurse should observe the patient for any untoward effects, such as changes in neurological status, increased blood pressure, numbness and tingling, or paralysis of the lower extremities. The puncture site should also be checked for leakage. These symptoms should be compared with symptoms present before the test.

Conditions that contraindicate doing a lumbar puncture for cerebrospinal fluid examination include:

1. Increased intracranial pressure, especially with papilledema

2. Serious spinal deformity

3. Extreme age

4. Dermatological disease or infection in the lumbar area.

SPUTUM EXAMINATION

Preparation of the Patient

When a sputum specimen is needed, the patient should be taught to cough deeply and to expectorate material brought up from the tracheobronchial tree. The nurse should explain that sputum is *not* saliva or secretions from the postnasal area. A heated aerosol spray of a hypertonic solution may be used if the patient is unable to produce an adequate amount of sputum. The patient should be instructed to collect the specimen early in the day soon after arising and before brushing his teeth. Care should be taken not to contaminate the outside of the container with sputum. The specimens are usually ordered to be collected on three separate days.

Method for Sputum Collection

Sputum should be collected in sterile containers with tight-fitting caps. A 1–3-ml specimen is sufficient for all testing except cultures for tuberculosis organisms, which require 5–10 ml of sputum. A specimen should be labeled with the patient's name, the date, and organism suspected and sent to the laboratory as soon as it is collected.

FECAL STUDIES

Preparation of the Patient

Patients should be told the reason for the stool collection and how the results of the test will be used in the diagnosis or treatment of medical problems. The hospitalized patient should be instructed to defecate into a clean bedpan. If the specimen is to be collected at home or in an outpatient clinic, the stool should be passed directly into a wide-mouthed container. The patient should also be told that toilet paper should not be placed in the bedpan or container, since it might interfere with the examination results. Under no circumstances should the stool be collected from a toilet bowl, because water can obscure the consistency of the specimen, destroy some of the parasites, or contain organisms that might contaminate the specimen. Urine should not be mixed with the specimen.

Method for Stool Collection

All stool specimen containers should be labeled with the patient's name, date, and type of examination to be done. This information should also be marked on the laboratory slip. Specimens from patients with hepatitis should be clearly marked so that laboratory personnel can take special precautions when handling the specimens.

Stool Culture. When bacterial infection is suspected, a freshly passed stool should be sent for immediate examination. It should be collected as soon as a bacterial disease is suspected and before antimicrobial therapy is begun. A small amount of the stool collected can be transferred to a sterile container. A tongue blade may be used for this purpose. If there has been a diarrheal stool, a large swab can be used to transfer the specimen to a sterile test tube. Any purulent-appearing patches should be collected on the swab. Although rectal swabbing for stool collection is not as valuable for diagnosis as direct collection of specimens, it can be used when a diarrheal disease is present, an institutional outbreak is suspected, or a specimen is not easily obtained. To obtain a rectal swab specimen, the anus is thoroughly cleansed and a swab designed for this purpose inserted into the rectum. Visible fecal material must be present on the swab. Gloves should be worn when collecting a stool specimen which contains blood.

A specimen collected for examination for viruses must be examined immediately or frozen. When a rectal swab is used, it should be placed in a culture tube containing antibiotics.

Stools for Parasites. When a stool is collected for examination for parasites, the patient should not be given an enema or a purgative medication containing oil or bismuth. These substances, like barium, interfere with the stool examination. Any mucus or blood that is present with the stool should be included in the specimen, since parasites can be found in this material.

Stools for Occult Blood. A small amount of stool is adequate for examination for occult blood. Whenever a false-positive result is suspected, the patient should be given meat-free meals for 3 days before the specimen is collected.

Stools for 24-, 48-, and 72-Hour Examination. When stools are collected over a prolonged period of time, the entire amount of stool passed should be placed in a container and refrigerated. Multiple specimens should be labeled consecutively.

THROAT CULTURES

Preparation of the Patient

The patient should be told the reason for the throat culture and how the specimen will be obtained. It is important to explain to children that the procedure will be uncomfortable but that it will be done quickly.

Method for Throat Culture

The patient is either placed in a good light or a flashlight is used to visualize the area of the throat to be swabbed. The patient's tongue is depressed with a tongue blade and a sterile swab rubbed over the back of the throat, both tonsils or fossae, and areas of inflammation, using a rotating motion. White patches, exudates, or areas of ulceration should also be swabbed. The swab should not touch the tongue or lips. It is immediately placed in a test tube or kit with a culture medium and sent to the laboratory.

Note. The nurse should wear a mask or stand to the side of the patient since most patients gag or cough during this procedure.

AMNIOCENTESIS

Preparation of the Patient

Patients who must have an amniocentesis are often anxious about the procedure and its potentially harmful effect on the fetus. The nurse should explain the procedure to the patient and assure her that injury to her or the fetus is extremely rare. The patient can also be taught relaxation techniques to use prior to and during amniocentesis. She should also be told that she may experience nausea, dizziness and mild cramps during the procedure. She should be assured that even though the needle is long, only a small portion of it actually passes into the uterus. An informed consent form must be signed prior to the test.

Method for Amniocentesis

An ultrasound is usually performed prior to amniocentesis to determine the position of the placenta, to detect the possible presense of a multiple pregnancy, and to determine gestational age of the fetus.

1. Inform the patient that the procedure will be performed by the physician and will 20–30 minutes.

2. Place the patient in a supine position with the head and/or legs slightly raised for comfort. The patient may be asked to place her arms behind

her head to prevent her from touching the sterile field during the procedure.

3. Prepare the skin with an antiseptic solution and protect the area with sterile drapes.

4. The physician gives the patient a local anesthetic and then inserts a 5-inch, 22-gauge needle through the abdomen and uterine wall.

5. The physician attaches a plastic syringe to the needle after the stylet is removed and withdraws a sample of 10–20 ml of amniotic fluid.

6. The needle is removed and slight pressure applied to the site. When there is no evidence of bleeding or oozing, an adhesive bandage is placed over the site.

7. Amniotic fluid samples are taken or sent to the laboratory immediately.

Note. The nurse should tell the patient to call her physician if she has abdominal pain, vaginal bleeding, fever, chills, loss of amniotic fluid, uterine contractions, or changes in fetal activity.

BIBLIOGRAPHY

Baer, D.M., and R.E. Belsey. *Bedside Testing: New Requirements from the JCAHO.* **RN,** 54:19–20 (June 1991).

Brennan, J.M. *Sharpening Your Skills for Arterial Sticks.* **RN,** 47:59–61 (April 1984).

Bease, P.G., and J.L. Myers. **Principles and Practice of Adult Health Nursing.** St. Louis: The C.V. Mosby Company, 1990.

Byrne, C.J., D.F. Saxton, P.K. Pelikan, and P.M. Nugent. **Laboratory Tests: Implications for Nursing Care.** Menlo Park: Addison-Wesley, 1986.

Collecting a 24-Hour Urine Sample. **Patient Care,** 24:17 (October 30, 1990).

Comella C., and T.P. Bleck. *The Technique of Lumbar Procedure.* **Journal of Critical Illness,** 3:61–66 (September 1988).

Centers for Disease Control. *Recommendations for Preventing Transmission of Infection with Human T-Lymphotropic Virus Type III/Lymphadenopathy-Associated Virus in the Workplace.* **Morbidity and Mortality Weekly Report,** 34:681–686, 691–695 (November 15, 1985).

Centers for Disease Control. *Recommendations for Prevention of HIV Transmission in Health-Care Settings.* **Morbidity and Mortality Weekly Report,** 36:1–17 (Supplement No. 2S) (August 21, 1987).

Centers for Disease Control. *Update: Universal Precautions for Prevention of Transmission of Human Immunodeficiency Virus, Hepatitis-B Virus, and Other Bloodborne Pathogens in Health-Care Settings.* **Morbidity and Mortality Weekly Report,** 37:377–382, 387–388 (June 24, 1988).

Centers for Disease Control. *Guidelines for Prevention of Transmission of Human Immunodeficiency Virus and Hepatitis-B Virus to Health-Care and Public Safety Workers.* **Morbidity and Mortality Weekly Report,** 38:1–37 (Supplement No. S-6) (February 1989).

Centers for Disease Control. *Recommendations for Preventing Transmission of Human Immunodeficiency Virus and Hepatitis-B Virus to Patients During Exposure-Prone Invasive Procedures.* **Morbidity and Mortality Weekly Report,** 40:1–9 (Recommendations and Reports) (July 12, 1991).

Fahey, V.A., and B.A. Finkelmeier. *Iatrogenic Arterial Injuries.* **AJN,** 84:448–451 (April 1984).

Focus on Urinalysis-Part 2. **Nursing Times (Supplement),** 1–5 (May 14, 1986).

Gelman, G.R. *The Predictive Value of Diagnostic Procedures.* **Nurse Practitioner,** 10:27–41 (April 1985).

Gurevich, I. *Appropriate Collection of Specimens for Culture and Sensitivity.* **American Journal of Infection Control,** 8:113–119 (November 1980).

Ignatavicius, D.D., and M.V. Bayne. **Medical-Surgical Nursing: A Nursing Process Approach.** Philadelphia: W.B. Saunders, 1991.

Kee, J.L., and E.R. Hays. *Assessment of Patient Laboratory Data in the Acutely Ill.* **Nursing Clinics of North America,** 25:751–759 (December 1990).

Lewis, S.M., and I.C. Collier. **Medical-Surgical Nursing: Assessment and Management of Clinical Problems.** St. Louis: Mosby Yearbook, 1992.

Luckman, J., and K.C. Sorensen. **Medical-Surgical Nursing: A Psychophysiological Approach.** Philadelphia: Saunders, 1987.

Markus, S. *Taking the Fear Out of Bone Marrow Examinations.* **Nursing 81,** 11:64–67 (April 1981).

Millam, D. *Hard to Get into Hard to Stick Veins.* **RN,** 48:34–35 (April 1985).

O'Rourke, A. *Bone Marrow Procedure Guide.* **Oncology Nursing Forum,** 13:66–67 (January–February 1986).

Phipps, W.S., B.C. Long, N.F. Woods, and V. Cossmeyer. **Medical-Surgical Nursing.** St. Louis: Mosby Yearbook, 1991.

Preusser, B.A., J. Lash, K.S. Stone, M.L. Winningham, D. Gonyon, and J.T. Nickel. *Quantifying the Minimum Discard Sample Required for Accurate Arterial Blood Gases.* **Nursing Research,** 38:276–279 (September and October 1989).

Ravel, R. **Clinical Laboratory Medicine.** Chicago: Year Book Medical Publishers, 1989.

Reker, D., and E. Webb. *Multiple Blood Samples Without Multiple Sticks.* **RN,** 49:39–41 (April, 1986).

Relleva, R.J. *Performing an Arterial Puncture for Blood Gas Analysis.* **Nursing Life,** 5:50 (November–December 1985).

Sacher, R.A., and R.A. McPherson. **Widmann's Clinical Interpretation of Laboratory Tests.** Philadelphia: F.A. Davis, 1991.

1

Smetzer, S.C., and B.G. Ball. *Brunner and Sudarth's Medical-Surgical Nursing.* New York: J.B. Lippincott, 1992.

Wilson, J.D. et al. *Harrison's Principles of Internal Medicine,* New York: McGraw-Hill, 1991.

York, K., and G. Moddeman, *Arterial Blood Gases.* **AORN,** 49:1308–1329 (May 1989).

CHAPTER

2

Laboratory Tests of Hematological Function

Complete Blood Count

Hematocrit and Hemoglobin

Red Cell Count

White Cell Count

Leukocyte Count

Differential White
Cell Count

Red Cell Indices

Mean Corpuscular Volume

Mean Corpuscular
Hemoglobin

Mean Corpuscular
Hemoglobin
Concentration

Stained Red Cell
Examination
(Peripheral Blood Smear)

Platelet Count

Erythrocyte
Sedimentation Rate

Glucose-6-Phosphate
Dehydrogenase (G-6-D)

Erythrocyte Fragility
(Osmotic Fragility)

Hemoglobin Electrophoresis

Haptoglobin

Blood Volume Studies

Sickle Cell Test (Sickledex)

Reticulocyte Count

Leukocyte Alkaline
Phosphatase Stain

Serum Iron

Total Iron-Binding Capacity

Blood Typing

ABO Blood Groups

RH Factor

Crossmatch

RH Antibody Titer

Human Leukocyte
Antigen (HLA)

Bone Marrow
Examination

COMPLETE BLOOD COUNT

The complete blood count (CBC), a screening test, is one of the most fre-quently ordered laboratory procedures. It is a group of tests that usually includes the hematocrit, hemoglobin, red blood cell (RBC) count, white blood cell (WBC) count, differential white cell count, red cell indices, and stained red cell examination (peripheral blood smear). A platelet count may also be included in the CBC. These tests are discussed separately on the following pages.

HEMATOCRIT AND HEMOGLOBIN

Description
HEMATOCRIT

The *hematocrit* is a measurement of the concentration of red cells in the total volume of blood. It is expressed as the percentage of red cells in the total blood volume. The hematocrit reading is obtained by filling a capillary hematocrit tube with venous blood to which an anticoagulant has been added. The tube is centrifuged and a reading is taken of the height of the packed cells in the tube.

NORMAL RANGE *	
Adults	
Women	37–47%
Men	45–54%
Newborns	44–64%
Children	31–43%
Infants	30–40%

*People living at high altitudes will have increased values.

Specimen Required

A specimen of venous blood is collected in a tube containing disodium edetate (EDTA). The tube must be filled. A microhematocrit may be done on a small amount of blood collected in a capillary tube, usually from a finger stick. If the tourniquet is left on for 2 minutes or longer, the prolonged hemostasis caused by vasoconstriction may cause an elevated hematocrit.

Preparation of the Patient
There are no food or fluid restrictions before collection of the specimen.

Description
HEMOGLOBIN

Hemoglobin is the main component of red blood cells. Its main function is to carry oxygen from the lungs to the body tissues and to transport carbon dioxide, the product of cellular metabolism, back to the lungs. One molecule of hemoglobin contains two pairs of polypeptide chains, called globin, and four heme groups, each containing one ferrous iron atom. Each gram of fully saturated hemoglobin holds 1.34 ml of oxygen. Fully saturated arterial blood is bright red in color. Venous blood, which transports carbon dioxide, is dark red. Hemoglobin acts as a buffer to help maintain acid-base balance.

N O R M A L R A N G E *	
Adults	
Women	12–16 g/dl
Men	14–18 g/dl
Children	11–16 g/dl
Infants	10–15 g/dl
Newborns	14–24 g/dl

*People living at high altitudes will have increased values.

Specimen Required
A 2-ml sample of venous blood is collected in a tube containing EDTA. A hemoglobin test may be done on a small amount of blood collected in a pipette or Unopette capillary tube, usually from a finger stick.

Preparation of the Patient
There are no food or fluid restrictions before collection of the specimen. If a tourniquet is left on for 1 minute or longer, the prolonged hemostasis caused by vasoconstriction may cause an elevated hemoglobin.

Causes of Deviation from Normal
Hematocrit. A decrease in hematocrit level is seen in (1) massive or prolonged blood loss, (2) anemia, (3) leukemia, and (4) excessive rapid intravenous fluid administration. There may also be a decrease during the last trimester of preg-

nancy. Hematocrit levels are elevated in conditions that cause an increase in the percentage of red cells in the blood. These include hemoconcentration caused by severe burns, surgery, or shock; severe dehydration caused by abnormally low fluid intake, persistent vomiting, severe diarrhea, or copious sweating; loss of plasma into the interstitial fluid; polycythemia vera; or chronic obstructive pulmonary disease.

Hemoglobin. When the hemoglobin level falls below 10 g/dl in women or 12 g/dl in men, an anemia is present. The anemia can be caused by (1) an iron deficiency, (2) increased blood destruction, (3) decreased blood production, or (4) massive or prolonged blood loss. Hemolytic reactions that can also decrease hemoglobin levels include (1) transfusions of incompatible blood, (2) reactions to chemicals, drugs, or infectious agents, (3) artificial heart valves, and (4) other diseases, such as cirrhosis, systemic lupus erythematosus, Hodgkin's disease, lymphoma, leukemia, and most other cancers. There may be a normal drop during the last trimester of pregnancy due to the expanded plasma volume. The causes of an increase in the hemoglobin levels are the same as those for increase in hematocrit.

When red cells are normal in size and have normal hemoglobin content, a predictable relationship exists between the hematocrit and hemoglobin. The hematocrit level should be three times the hemoglobin reading $\pm 3\%$. For example, when the hemoglobin is 15 g/dl the hematocrit will be $15 \times 3 = 45\% \pm 3\%$, or between 42% and 48%.

Nursing Implications of Abnormal Findings
HEMATOCRIT AND HEMOGLOBIN

Assessment and Interventions. Abnormal hematocrit and hemoglobin values indicate to the nurse specific areas that should be included in the data-gathering process. Although they are not helpful in identifying a specific problem area, these values may confirm a nursing judgment about the patient's health status. For example, when the information gathered indicates that severe dehydration may be present, an increase in the hematocrit and hemoglobin will help the nurse make a final diagnosis. When a decrease in the hematocrit and hemoglobin values is seen in a patient who has been diagnosed as having peptic ulcer disease, the nurse should be alerted that bleeding from the ulcer may have begun. Specific interventions depend on the underlying problem. General medical-surgical textbooks discuss the specific nursing care for the many disorders that cause alterations in the hematocrit and hemoglobin.

The hematocrit and hemoglobin may not be abnormal following a moderate to massive blood loss because both plasma and red blood cells have been lost in equal proportions. During recovery, however, the hematocrit and hemoglobin will decrease.

RED CELL COUNT

Description

The *red cell* (erythrocyte) *count* is a determination of the number of red cells found in each cubic millimeter of whole blood. In the adult, red cells are formed in the marrow of the bones in the chest, base of the skull, and upper arms and legs. The main characteristic of erythrocytes is the presence of hemoglobin, an iron-containing protein that binds oxygen. The life span of a mature RBC is 120 days. As they age, RBCs become more fragile and disintegrate. RBCs are destroyed by a group of phagocytes called macrophages, which are found in the liver, spleen, bone marrow, and lymph nodes. The number of RBCs destroyed every day is equal to the number that are released into the circulatory system.

NORMAL RANGE	
Adults	
Men	4.6–6.2 million/mm^3 or 10^{12}/L
Women	4.2–5.4 million/mm^3 or 10^{12}/L
Children	3.9–5.2 million/mm^3 or 10^{12}/L
Infants (6 mos)	3.5–5.5 million/mm^3 or 10^{12}/L
Newborns	4.8–1.0 million/mm^3 or 10^{12}/L

Specimen Required

A 5–10-ml sample of venous blood should be collected in a tube containing EDTA. Note on a laboratory slip whether the patient was sitting or recumbent when sample was obtained. The count will be lower than normal if blood is obtained from a recumbent person.

Preparation of the Patient

There are no food or fluid restrictions before venipuncture.

Causes of Deviation From Normal

There are many causes for a decrease in the RBC count. These include the anemias (Table 2.1), hemorrhage, diseases of the bone marrow, endocrine disorders, lupus erythematosus, and rheumatic fever. Polycythemia vera and secondary polycythemia are the major causes of an increase in the erythrocyte count. Secondary polycythemia is often due to a chronic lung disease. It is also

TABLE 2.1. Types of Anemias

2

Classification	Type of Anemia
Anemias caused by decreased red cell production	
Microcytic hypochromic	Iron deficiency anemia
	Sideroblastic anemia
	Thalassemias
Macrocytic megaloblastic	Vitamin B_{12} deficiency (pernicious anemia)
	Folic acid deficiency anemia
	Drug-induced anemia
Normocytic-normochromic	Aplastic anemia
	Myelophthisic anemias
	Secondary anemias of chronic inflammation, uremia, chronic liver disease
Anemias caused by red cell destruction (hemolytic)	Acquired from mechanical trauma, direct toxic effect, antibody production
	Hereditary, as in spherocytosis, enzyme defects, hemoglobinopathies (including sickle cell anemia), glucose-6-phosphate dehydrogenase deficiency
Anemias caused by excessive blood loss	Acute posthemorrhagic anemia
	Chronic hemorrhagic anemia

seen in children with congenital heart defects and patients with severe diarrhea.

Nursing Implications of Abnormal Findings

Assessment. The nursing care described here is general and does not include specifics related to each type of anemia. The reader is referred to a general medical-surgical nursing textbook for additional information.

There are general areas to assess for any patient with an anemia. These include the clinical manifestations: fatigue, dizziness, headache, and sensations of numbness in the extremities, especially fingers and toes. The patient's diet and exercise tolerance should also be included. The nurse should note any medications the patient has been taking or any exposure to toxic substances. Signs of bleeding should be recorded, such as tarry stools, dark smoky stools, or bright red drainage coming from any part of the body. A family history should be included, because some anemias are hereditary.

If there is an increase in the RBC count because of polycythemia, the nurse should gather data about the onset of symptoms, the presence of chronic obstructive pulmonary disease, and whether the patient has been living or working for a prolonged time at a high altitude. The severity of symptoms such as hypertension, shortness of breath, and thrombus formation should be assessed so that appropriate nursing interventions can be planned.

Interventions. The goals of care include controlling causative factors when possible, relieving symptoms, preventing complications, and developing a teaching plan for self-care. Plans should be made to provide frequent rest periods to avoid fatigue, good skin and mouth care to prevent breakdown or ulcerations, and protection from chills due to poor circulation.

Patient teaching should include information about nutrition and diet, depending on the type of anemia present. Eating six small meals a day may be helpful for patients who are anorexic, and avoiding hot, spicy meals will help the patient with a sore mouth, tongue, or esophagus. General diet instruction about planning well-balanced meals containing an adequate amount of iron may be needed by the patient with an iron deficiency.

When an increase in the RBC count is caused by polycythemia, the most important aspect of nursing care is patient teaching. Patients should be taught to avoid foods high in iron, particularly if a phlebotomy has been performed, since these foods counteract some of its therapeutic effect. They should be encouraged to walk to prevent the development of thrombi. Teaching patients to maintain a high fluid intake will also prevent thrombus formation by reducing the viscosity of the blood. If the polycythemia is secondary to the hypoxia that results from exposure to high altitudes, patients should be reminded that it will reverse itself if they return to lower altitudes and resume their usual eating and drinking patterns.

WHITE CELL COUNT

Description
LEUKOCYTE COUNT

The total *white blood count* (WBC) is the absolute number of white blood cells (leukocytes) circulating in a cubic millimeter of blood. White cells are produced in the red bone marrow and lymphatic tissue. After they are formed they enter the blood, which transports them to the parts of the body where they are needed to (1) defend against invading organisms through phagocytosis and (2) produce or transport and distribute antibodies to help maintain immunity.

2

NORMAL RANGE

Adults	5,000–10,000/mm³
Children	5,000–10,000/mm³
Newborns	9,000–30,000/mm³

Description

DIFFERENTIAL WHITE CELL COUNT

There are five types of normal white cells, divided into two main groups: *granulocytes* (polymorphonuclear leukocytes) and *agranulocytes* (mononuclear leukocytes) (Table 2.2). The differential white cell count is done to identify the five types of leukocyte cells on a stained slide of peripheral blood. It helps the clinician make a final decision about the patient's status, to follow the patient's progress, or to determine the relative numbers of each type of leukocyte. The cells are counted and the differential count is expressed in relative percentage values, which are mathematically correlated to their absolute values. The total of the relative percentage values is 100%.

NORMAL RANGE

Adults
Note: Normal values vary slightly depending on laboratory equipment.

Cell Type	Relative Value %	Absolute Value μL (mm³)
Granulocytes		
Neutrophils (Total)	50–70	2500–7000
Segments	50–65	2500–6500
Bands	0–05	0–500
Eosinophils	1–4	100–300
Basophils	0.5–1.0	50–100
Agranulocytes		
Lymphocytes	25–45	1500–4000
Monocytes	2–6	100–500

Children	Consult laboratory for differential values at different ages.

TABLE 2.2. White Cells

Granulocytes	Comprise half or more of the white cells. Granules are present in their cytoplasm, arising from the bone marrow.
Neutrophils	Also called polymorphonuclear leukocytes (PMNs, polys) they are the first line of defense against infection. Their name reflects the lobular nucleus bound in the mature cell which progresses through the following stages: (1) myeloblast; (2) promyelocyte; (3) myelocyte; (4) metamyelocyte; (5) band neutrophil; (6) segmented neutrophil. The protective function of the neutrophils includes phagocytosis. Foreign particles are degraded and pyrogens are released, producing fever by acting on the hypothalamus to set the body's thermostat at a higher level.
Eosinophils	Their protective function is not fully understood. They play a role in allergic reactions, possibly inactivating histamine.
Basophils	Their protective function is not fully understood. They contain histamine and heparin and appear to be involved in immediate hypersensitivity reactions.
Agranulocytes	Also called mononuclear leukocytes; they comprise the rest of the white cells. Their cytoplasm does not contain granules, and they originate in bone marrow and lymphoid tissue.
Lymphocytes	Their protective function is in antibody production and immunological reactions. In a humoral response, B-lymphocytes produce antibodies that react against foreign antigens. T-lymphocytes are involved in cell-mediated immune responses by attacking and destroying specific foreign cells.
Monocytes	Their protective function is phagocytosis against bacteria and large protozoa such as fungi and parasites. They are the second line of defense against bacterial and viral disease.

Specimen Required

A 5–10-ml specimen is collected in a tube that contains EDTA. If the patient is taking any drugs that affect the CBC a note should be made on the laboratory slip identifying the drug involved (Table 2.5).

2

Preparation of the Patient

There are no food or fluid restrictions before venipuncture.

Causes of Deviation from Normal

General changes in the white cells indicate the presence of disease. A rise in the WBC above 10,000 mm³ (leukocytosis) is usually caused by conditions that stimulate the bone marrow to produce white blood cells to fight off invading organisms. Many conditions can increase the WBC (Table 2.3). A fall in the white cell count below 4,000 mm³ (leukopenia) usually indicates bone marrow depression is occurring because of increases of toxic chemicals (Table 2.4). The following descriptions form a guide to help in the differentiation of possible causes of illness.

Neutrophils. An increase in the number of *neutrophils* indicates the presence of a bacterial or parasitic infectious process. If the infection is prolonged and severe, the bone marrow may release immature band cells. Chemotherapeutic drugs and disorders of cell production such as leukemia may also cause the release of immature neutrophils.

The increase in neutrophils is related to the total white blood count. When the white cell (leukocyte) count increases proportionately to the neutrophils, the patient's resistance is good and the body is fighting the infection. If the increase in neutrophils is much greater than the total leukocyte count, the infectious process may be so severe that the body's resistance is lowered.

A decrease in neutrophils may be caused by hematological diseases such as acute lymphoblastic leukemia, agranulocytosis, or aplastic and pernicious anemias. An acute viral infection may also be the cause. A "shift to the left" means that many band cells and their precursors are present. It is an indication of an acute bacterial infection. A "shift to the right" is said to be present when there is an increase in mature cells. It occurs in hepatic disease and pernicious anemia.

Eosinophils. An increase in the *eosinophil* count may be caused by a hyper-immune or allergic reaction where there is an antigen–antibody response. Some cancers, such as Hodgkin's disease, myelogenous leukemia, and lung and

TABLE 2.3. Conditions that Increase the WBC

Acute infection	Malignant disease
Circulatory disease	Necrosis
Drugs	Toxins
Hemorrhage	Trauma
Leukemia	Serum sickness
Surgery	

TABLE 2.4. Conditions that Decrease the WBC

Acute leukemia	Malaria
Agranulocytosis	Multiple myeloma
Alcoholism	Radiation
Aplastic and pernicious anemia	Rheumatoid arthritis
Diabetes	Systemic lupus erythematosis (SLE)
Heavy metals	Viral infections
Hypersplenism	

bone cancer, cause a rise in eosinophils. Parasitic infections also cause eosinophilia.

A decrease in eosinophils may be associated with congestive heart failure, infectious mononucleosis, Cushing's syndrome, and aplastic and pernicious anemias. Bodily stress, which results in increased adrenal steroid production, also causes a decrease in eosinophils. There is a diurnal variation in the production of eosinophils. The count is lowest in the morning and rises from noon until after midnight. This rhythm is reversed in people who work at night and in asthmatics.

Basophils. *Basophils* are not as well understood as other white cells. They appear to play a role in allergic and anaphylactic reactions, since their number decreases when these conditions are present. There may also be a decrease during stress reactions associated with some disease states and after prolonged steroid therapy. Increases are most often associated with blood dyscrasias such as granulocytic and basophilic leukemia and myeloid metaplasia.

Lymphocytes. Viral infections are the primary cause of an increase in the *lymphocyte* count. However, bacterial infections, such as infectious mononucleosis, cytomegalovirus infection, mumps, rubella and infectious hepatitis in addition to hormonal disorders, such as hypothyroidism and hypoadrenalism, lymphocytic leukemia, lymphosarcoma, and acquired immune deficiency syndrome (AIDS) may also effect an increase.

Decreases in lymphocytes are associated with Hodgkin's disease, lupus erythematosus, burns, trauma, and the administration of corticosteroids.

Monocytes. Since *monocytes* act as scavenger cells to dispose of noninfectious foreign substances, they are not as diagnostically significant as other white cells. They may be increased in viral, bacterial, and parasitic infections, collagen diseases, and some malignant hematological disorders. Decreases have no significance in relation to disease.

Nursing Implications of Abnormal Findings

Assessment and Interventions. The WBC and differential, if performed, must be monitored by the nurse and assessed along with other data collected.

When the WBC is elevated, signs and symptoms of both local and systemic infections must be explored. Abnormalities that have been found should be followed closely and report of progress or resolution should be made. Nursing interventions depend on the data collected. For example, if a patient with a recently elevated white cell count is on twice daily temperatures, the nurse may decide to take the temperature more often to watch for any upward trends. When there is a diurnal variation in the WBC, as with eosinophils, nursing interventions should not be changed until the patient's normal diurnal variation has been established. When there is a decrease in the white blood count, measures should be taken to prevent infection. Meticulous hand washing should be practiced and staff members and visitors with colds, sore throats, or other infections should not come into close contact with the patient. The reason for these and other precautions outlined by the hospital should be explained to the patient. Medical-surgical nursing textbooks should be consulted for more detailed discussion of the nursing care of specific disease entities.

TABLE 2.5. Drugs that Affect the WBC

Drugs that Increase the WBC	Drugs that Decrease the WBC
Allopurinol	Acetomenophen
Antibiotics	Antibiotics
Ampicillin	Cephalothins
Erythromycin	Penicillins
Kanamycin	Antihistamines
Methicillin	Antimetabolites
Tetracycline	Barbiturates
Streptomycin	Benzine
Vancomycin	Cancer Chemotherapy
Aspirin (acetylsalicilic acid)	Chlordiazepoxide
Digitalis	Chloramphenocol
Epinephrine	Diazepam
Gold compounds	Ethacrynic Acid
Heparin	Furosemide
Histamine	Indomethacin
Hydantoin derivatives	Methyldopa
Lithium	Oral Hypoglycemics
Potassium Iodide	Phenothiazine
Procainamide	Propylthiouracil
Quinine	Rifampin
Sulfonamides (long acting)	
Triamterene	

RED CELL INDICES

Red cell indices are a group of hematology studies that include three values calculated from the RBC count, the hemoglobin (Hgb), and the hematocrit (Hct). These are:

Mean corpuscular volume (MCV)

Mean corpuscular hemoglobin (MCH)

Mean corpuscular hemoglobin concentration (MCHC)

These values provide information about the exact size, weight, and hemoglobin concentration of an average red cell and are the best way to describe red cell changes in anemias and some other diseases. They are useful in classifying types of anemias but are not enough to establish a definite medical diagnosis.

Description
MEAN CORPUSCULAR VOLUME

The MCV describes individual red cell size. It is the ratio of the volume of packed cells to the red cell count.

$$MCV = \frac{Hct \times 10}{RBC \text{ count}}$$

NORMAL RANGE	
Adults	80–98 μm^3
Children	82–92 μm^3
Newborns	98–108 μm^3

Specimen Required
A 7-ml sample of venous blood is collected in a collecting tube or syringe containing EDTA. A capillary blood sample may also be used. This test is usually done when a complete blood count is requested.

Preparation of the Patient
There are no food or fluid restrictions before venipuncture.

Causes of Deviation from Normal
Decreases in the MCV are present in the following anemias: pernicious anemia, iron deficiency anemia, thalassemia, and the anemias associated with chronic

blood loss. Increases are associated with liver diseases, alcoholism, folate or vitamin B_{12} deficiencies, or sprue.

A wide variety of red cells in the blood may be represented in a normal MCV, because the MCV represents an average of many cells.

2

Nursing Implications of Abnormal Findings

Assessment and Intervention. When there is a decrease in MCV, indicating the presence of an anemia, the nurse should refer to the nursing implications discussed under red cell count. Because an increase in MCV may occur in several pathophysiological problems, the abnormal value should be assessed with all other data gathered. General medical-surgical texts should be consulted for specific nursing care.

Description
MEAN CORPUSCULAR HEMOGLOBIN

The MCH measures the weight of hemoglobin in an average red cell. It is related to the MCV because the weight of a red cell increases when its amount of hemoglobin, thus its size, increases.

$$MCH = \frac{Hb \times 10}{RBC \text{ count}}$$

N O R M A L R A N G E	
Adults	27–31 pg
Children	27–31 pg
Newborns	32–34 pg

Specimen Required

A 7-ml sample of venous blood is collected in a collecting tube or syringe containing EDTA. A capillary blood sample may also be used. This test is usually done when a complete blood count is requested.

Preparation of the Patient

There are no food or fluid restrictions before venipuncture.

Causes of Deviation from Normal

Abnormal values are related to severe anemic conditions. An increase occurs with macrocytic anemia and a decrease with microcytic anemia.

Nursing Implications of Abnormal Findings

Refer to the nursing implications for patients with anemias discussed under red cell count.

Description

MEAN CORPUSCULAR HEMOGLOBIN CONCENTRATION

The MCHC measures the proportion of hemoglobin in each red blood cell. It is the ratio of the weight of hemoglobin to the volume of red blood cells.

$$MCHC = \frac{Hb \times 100}{Htc}$$

N O R M A L R A N G E	
Adults	32–36% or 0.32–0.36 g/dl RBC
Children	32–36% or 0.32–0.36 g/dl RBC
Newborns	32–33% or 0.32–0.33 g/dl RBC

Specimen Required

A 7-ml sample of venous blood is collected in a collecting tube or syringe containing EDTA. A capillary blood sample may also be used. This test is usually done when a complete blood count is requested.

Preparation of the Patient

There are no food or fluid restrictions before venipuncture.

Causes of Deviation from Normal

Decreases in MCHC occur with the following anemias: iron deficiency anemia, thalassemia, and macrocytic anemia. An increase usually indicates that spherocytosis is present.

Nursing Implications of Abnormal Findings

Refer to the nursing implications for patients with anemias discussed under Red Cell Count.

STAINED RED CELL EXAMINATION (PERIPHERAL BLOOD SMEAR)

Description

A *stained red cell examination* is done to inspect the morphology of erythrocytes. The size, shape, color, structure, and content of the cells are examined, as well as cell origin and maturity.

Note. See Table 2.6 for variations from normal of stained red cells.

NORMAL RANGE

Size: Erythrocytes range in size from 6 to 8μ in diameter. Red cells of normal size are called normocytic.

Shape: Red cells are biconcave discs. They have a donut-shaped appearance because the outer portions of the cells have a greater depth of hemoglobin and stain more deeply than the center.

Color: Erythrocytes have a reddish-orange appearance when stained. They have a central pallor and deeper coloring around the perimeter. Red cells of normal color are called normochromic.

Structure: Normal mature red cells do not contain nuclei, nuclear remnants, or any cellular inclusions.

Specimen Required

A 5-ml specimen of venous blood is collected in a tube containing EDTA.

Preparation of the Patient

There are no food or fluid restrictions before venipuncture.

Causes of Deviation from Normal

See Table 2.7.

Nursing Implications of Abnormal Findings

Assessment and Interventions. When a peripheral blood smear has been done, the results should be considered along with all other data collected. This can help the nurse plan care related to the medical diagnosis; however, there are no specific interventions, since there are several disease conditions in which the normal peripheral smear can be altered.

PLATELET COUNT

Description

Platelets, also called thrombocytes, are large, non-nucleated cells derived from the megakaryocytes produced in the bone marrow. Two-thirds are found in the blood and one-third in the spleen. One-tenth of the platelets found in the blood maintain endothelial integrity and the rest are available for hemostasis. The adhesive or sticky quality of platelets allows them to clump together or aggregate and adhere to injured surfaces. They release a substance that begins the coagulation process. Platelet plugs form and occlude breaks in the integrity of small vessels. Along with fibrin, they form the network for a clot to form.

TABLE 2.6. Variations of Stained Red Cells

Size	
Microcytes	Mature red cells that are abnormally small (6μ or less) and often contain amounts of hemoglobin.
Macrocytes	Mature red cells that are abnormally large (8μ or more).
Anisocytosis	Variations in the normal cell dimensions.
Shape	
Poikilocytosis	Any variation or irregularity in cell shape.
Elliptocytes	Mature red cells that have become elliptic or oval.
Spherocytes	Red cells that are thicker and smaller than normal. They are round and lack the central pallor of normal RBC's.
Target cells (leptocytes; Mexican hat cells)	Thin red cells with an enlarged central area resembling a bullseye.
Schistocytes	Rough, bizarre-shaped red cells that appear distorted and irregularly shaped.
Acanthocytes	Abnormally created red cells that appear thorny on a stained smear.
Color	
Hypochromic	Red cells that have a large central area of pallor caused by a decreased amount of hemoglobin.
Hyperchromic	Red cells that have an area of central pallor smaller than normal or non-existent.
Structure	
Basophilic stippling	An aggregation of irregular basophilic granules within the red cells.
Howell-Jolly bodies	Smooth round remnants of nuclear chromatin within the red cells.
Cabot rings	Ring-shaped, figure-eight, or loop-shaped structures within the red cells.
Malarial stippling	The fine granular appearance of red cells that harbor the parasites of tertiary malaria.
Siderotic granules	Particles of iron that appear as bluish-purple specks on the stained red cells.
Heinz bodies	Particles of denatured hemoglobin with mature red cells.

TABLE 2.7. Causes of Deviation From Normal Size, Shape, Color, and Structure of Erythrocytes

2

Abnormal Stain	Cause of Deviation
Size	
Amniocytosis	Present in newborns
	Anemia
Microcytes	Iron Deficiency Anemia
	Thalassemia Major
	Spherocytic Anemia
	Anemia secondary to chronic hemorrhage
Macrocytes	Pernicious Anemia
	Folic Acid Deficiency Anemia
	Thalassemia
	Hypothyroidism
Shape	
Poikilocytosis	Defective formation and maturation of erythrocytes
Elliptocytes	Hereditary Elliptocytosis
	Iron Deficiency Anemia
	Megaloblastic Anemias
	Sickle Cell Anemia
Spherocytes	Hereditary Spherocytosis
	Acquired Hemolytic Anemia
	Thermal injury to cells
Target cells	Thalassemia
	Hemoglobin C disease
	Liver disease
	Splenectomy
Schistocytes	Microangiopathic Hemolytic Anemia
	Burns
	Valvular stenosis
	Prosthetic heart valves
	Disseminated Intravascular Coagulation (DIC)
Acanthocytes	Hereditary or acquired abetalipoproteinemia
	Liver disease
Color	
Hypochromic	Conditions associated with abnormal or decreased hemoglobin, including most anemias and leukemia
Hyperchromic	Severe, prolonged dehydration

(Continued)

TABLE 2.7. *(Continued)*

Abnormal Stain	Cause of Deviation
Structure	
Basophilic stippling	Heavy metal intoxication (lead, silver, bismuth, and mercury)
Howell-Jolly bodies	Splenectomy
	Splenic atrophy or congenital absence of a spleen
	Leukemia
	Various anemias
Cabot rings	Severe anemias, particularly pernicious anemia
Malarial stippling	Tertiary malaria
Siderotic granules	Primary Acquired Sideroblastic Anemia
Heinz bodies	Hemolytic Anemia
	Drug-induced erythrocyte injury

NORMAL RANGE

Adults	150,000–450,000/mm³
Infants and children	200,000–473,000/mm³
Newborns	140,000–300,000/mm³

Specimen Required

A 5–10-ml sample of venous blood is collected in a tube containing EDTA. If the tourniquet is on longer than 1 minute, fragile platelets could be damaged, causing false results. If the patient is taking any drugs that affect the platelet count, a note should be made on the lab slip identifying the drug involved (Table 2.8).

Preparation of the Patient

There are no food or fluid restrictions before venipuncture.

Causes of Deviation from Normal

It should be noted that an abnormal platelet count does not necessarily indicate a pathological condition. Decreased platelet counts may be seen in newborns during the first few days of life or in women during the two weeks prior to

TABLE 2.8.   Drugs That Cause a Decrease in Platelets

Acetazolamide	Methyldopa
Acetohexamide	Novobiocin
Antineoplastic agents	Oxyphenbutazone
Arsenicals	Penicillamine
Benzene	Phenindione
Bismuth	Phenothiazines
Carbamazepine	Phenylbutazone
Cardiotonic glycosides	Potassium perchlorate
Chloramphenicol	Prednisone
Chloroquine	Procainamide
Chlorothiazide	Propranolol
Chlorpropamide	Pyrazinamide
Colchicine	Rifampin
DDT	Ristocetin
Diazoxide	Salicylates
Diethylstilbestrol	Stilbesterol
Diphenylhydantoin	Streptomycin
Gentamicin	Sulfonamides
Gold salts	Sulfonylureas
Heparin	Thioridazine
Isoniazid	Thiourea
Lincomycin	Tolbutamide
Meprobamate	

the onset of menstruation. Increases may be seen in individuals living at high altitudes or following intense physical exercise. Platelet counts may also be higher in winter than in summer. Aspirin can also alter platelet function for up to a week by interfering with the enzyme activity that gives platelets their "stickiness."

Disorders in the platelet count may result in a decrease or increase in the number of circulating platelets. A decrease in the number of platelets to below 100,000/cu mm is called thrombocytopenia, a disorder that can have several causes. These include idiopathic thrombocytopenic purpura; bone marrow injury or failure; lesions involving the bone marrow, such as carcinoma, leukemia, or lymphoma; deficiencies of vitamin B_{12} or folic acid; infection; hemorrhage and massive blood transfusion; and destruction caused by systemic lupus erythematosus, hemolytic anemias, or the toxic effects of drugs (Table 2.8).

Platelets may be temporarily elevated, a condition called thrombocytosis. This may occur as a result of hemorrhage, surgery, splenectomy, iron deficiency, or chronic inflammatory disorders. Thrombocytosis may also be associated with carcinoma and Hodgkin's disease. A sustained elevation of the platelet count is called thrombocythemia. It may occur alone or be associated with polycythemia vera, chronic myelogenous leukemia, or myelosclerosis.

Nursing Implications of Abnormal Findings

Assessment and Interventions. The nursing care of a patient with an abnormal platelet count should focus on the possibility of spontaneous and prolonged bleeding, which can occur with either thrombocytopenia or thrombocytosis. (See the section on prothrombin time in Chapter 3 for a detailed discussion of related nursing care.) In addition, patients with an increased platelet count may have venous or arterial thrombosis. Because a detailed discussion of these complications is not within the scope of this text, refer to a general medical-surgical textbook for this information.

ERYTHROCYTE SEDIMENTATION RATE

Description

The *erythrocyte sedimentation rate* (ESR or sed rate) is a test to determine the rate at which erythrocytes settle out of unclotted blood in a 1-hour period. This rate increases as cell weight increases and decreases as cell surfaces enlarge. Small cells settle more slowly than clumped cells. In normal blood, very little settling occurs because the gravitational pull of individual red cells is almost balanced by the upward current generated by the displacement of plasma. The composition of plasma, particularly the physical state of plasma proteins, is an important part of the ESR. Alterations in these proteins result in aggregation of red cells, making them heavier and more likely to settle out of unclotted blood more rapidly. High levels of fibrinogen have a similar effect.

NORMAL RANGE			
	Westergren	**Wintrobe**	**Cutler**
Men			
<50 yrs	0–15 mm/hr	0–7 mm/hr	0–8 mm/hr
>50 yrs	0–20 mm/hr	5–7 mm/hr	0–8 mm/hr
Women			
<50 yrs	0–20 mm/hr	0–15 mm/hr	0–10 mm/hr
>50 yrs	0–30 mm/hr	25–30 mm/hr	0–10 mm/hr

Children	0–10 mm/hr	0–13 mm/hr	
	Landau (micro)		**Smith (micro)**
Children			
<2 yrs	1–6 mm/hr		0–1 mm/hr
2–14 yrs	1–9 mm/hr		3–13 mm/hr

2

Specimen Required

At least 4 ml of venous blood should be collected in a tube containing EDTA. The blood sample should be sent to the laboratory as soon as possible after collection. ESR will increase if the sample is allowed to stand. If a patient is taking any drugs that affect ESR, a note should be made on the laboratory slip identifying the drugs involved (Table 2.9).

Preparation of the Patient

There are no food or fluid restrictions before collection of the specimen.

Causes of Deviation from Normal

This test is nonspecific and cannot be used to confirm the presence of a specific disease process. Results may be affected by physiological factors (see Table 2.10).

The sedimentation rate may be useful in following the progress of diagnosed inflammatory diseases, such as rheumatoid arthritis, rheumatic fever, respiratory

TABLE 2.9. Drugs That Affect the Erythrocyte Sedimentation Rate

Drugs That Increase ESR	Drugs That Decrease ESR
Dextran	ACTH
Methyldopa	Cortisone
Methysergide	Ethambutol
Oral contraceptives	Quinine
Penicillamine	Salicylates
Procainamide	
Theophylline	
Trifluperidol	
Vitamin A	

TABLE 2.10. Physiological Factors that Affect the Erythrocyte Sedimentation Rate

High blood sugar
High albumin level
High cholesterol levels
Menstruation

infections, and acute myocardial infarction. An elevated ESR may be used as a rough index that a disease process is present.

Multiple myeloma, macroglobulinemias, and hyperfibrinogenemias tend to cause very high ESRs. Moderate increases are seen with active inflammatory diseases such as rheumatoid arthritis, chronic infections, collagen diseases, and neoplastic disease. There is also a moderate increase from the tenth to the twelfth week of pregnancy, continuing until about 1 month postpartum.

Nursing Implications of Abnormal Findings

Assessment and Interventions. Although ESR lacks specificity, the test results may be helpful to the nurse in assessing a patient with a known inflammatory process. A decrease in ESR indicates some improvement in the disease process. An increase may mean that the inflammatory disease is becoming worse or that a new inflammatory process has begun. The ESR must be considered with all other data gathered but may be misleading if more than one inflammatory disease is present.

Specific interventions are not planned as a result of this test alone but may be initiated based on additional data collected regarding the patient's general condition. ESR data can also be helpful to the nurse caring for a patient whose medical diagnosis has not been established. When a patient with chest pain has an elevated ESR, nursing care should be planned based on the assumption that a myocardial infarction (MI) has occurred. On the other hand, a normal ESR level in the same patient can mean that angina pectoris is the source of the pain, since the ESR rises with an MI but remains normal with angina. The ESR is also helpful when the patient's diagnosis is uncertain and the ESR is specific for one disease but not another. For example, the ESR increases when there are metastases from stomach cancer yet is normal in peptic ulcer disease.

GLUCOSE-6-PHOSPHATE DEHYDROGENASE (G-6-PD)

Description

Glucose-6-phosphate dehydrogenase is an enzyme present in erythrocytes. It protects erythrocytes from injury and assists in glucose metabolism by erythrocytes. It uses oxidative substances and protects erythrocytes from injury.

N O R M A L R A N G E	
Adults and children	
Screen test	negative
Quantitative test	8–18.6 U/g of hemoglobin

Specimen Required

A 5-ml sample of venous blood is collected in a tube containing disodium edetate (EDTA).

Preparation of the Patient

Food and fluids are not restricted before venipuncture.

Causes of Deviation from Normal

A decrease in the level of G-6-PD is caused by a sex-linked recessive trait carried on the X chromosome. It is inherited by males from their mothers, who are usually asymptomatic. Some individuals may have continuous problems with hemolysis while others have no detectable abnormality. However, hemolytic episodes may be triggered by normal doses of drugs (Table 2.11), infections, acidotic states, or the ingestion of fava beans. There are two types of G-6-PD deficiencies. Type A, which is found in the Black population, and the Mediterranean type, found in Orientals and whites, particularly Greeks, Sardinians, and Sephardic Jews. G-6-PD may be increased in patients with pernicious anemia, hyperthyroidism, myocardial infarction, hepatic coma, chronic blood loss and other megaloblastic anemias.

TABLE 2.11. Drugs that Cause Hemolysis in Patients with Glucose-6-Phosphate Dehydrogenase Deficiency

Acetanilid	Pentaquine
Acetylphenylhydrazine	Phenacetin
Antipyrine	Phenylhydrazine
Ascorbic Acid	Primaquine
Aspirin	Probenecid
Aspirin compounds	Quinacrine
Chloramphenicol	Quinidine
Nalidizic Acid	Quinine
Naphthalene	Sulfonamides
Nitrofurantoin	Vitamin K
Nitrofuran	

Nursing Implications of Abnormal Findings

Assessment and Interventions. The nurse should help patients who have had episodes of hemolysis identify precipitating factors such as drugs or infections. Drugs that cause hemolysis should be identified and avoided. If infection is the precipitating factor, patients should be encouraged to seek medical treatment as soon as the infection occurs. Patients with a mild asymptomatic deficiency should be given a list of drugs that may precipitate hemolysis and be encouraged to share it with physicians, nurses, and dentists.

ERYTHROCYTE FRAGILITY (OSMOTIC FRAGILITY)

Description

The *erythrocyte fragility* (osmotic fragility and autohemolysis) *test* is done to determine the ability of red cells to resist hemolysis in a hypotonic solution. This test is done to determine if RBC's are unusually fragile and easily destroyed. Those that have an increased osmotic fragility will hemolyze in relatively high concentrations of saline. Cells that are spherical in shape hemolyze in relatively high concentrations of saline that is barely hypotonic. Those that are flat hemolyze in lower concentrations of saline that is greatly hypotonic.

NORMAL RANGE

Adults and children
Normal fragility demonstrates:
  Initial hemolysis at 0.40–0.45% saline solution
  Complete hemolysis at 0.30–0.35% saline solution

Specimen Required

A 5–10-ml sample of venous blood is collected in a heparinized tube or syringe.

Preparation of the Patient

There are no food or fluid restrictions before venipuncture.

Causes of Deviation from Normal

An increase in the erythrocyte osmotic fragility test is useful in establishing the diagnosis of hereditary spherocytosis. Other conditions that cause an increase in osmotic fragility are autoimmune hemolytic disease due to ABO or Rh incompatibility, pernicious anemia, acquired hemolytic anemia, hemolytic jaundice, burns, chemical poisoning, and drugs. Decreases in osmotic fragility may be caused by sickle cell anemia, iron deficiency anemia, polycythemia vera, hemoglobin C disease, thalassemia major, liver disease, obstructive jaundice, or splenectomy. An increase in the sed rate is a normal occurrence during pregnancy.

Nursing Implications of Abnormal Findings

Assessment and Interventions. When an erythrocyte fragility test has been done, its results should be considered along with all other data collected. The results can help the nurse plan care related to the medical diagnosis. There are no specific interventions because there are several disease conditions in which erythrocyte fragility can be altered.

2

HEMOGLOBIN ELECTROPHORESIS

Description

Hemoglobin electrophoresis is a specialized technique that separates different types of hemoglobin according to mobility in an electric field. Hemolyzed red cell material is matched against standard bands for the various known hemoglobins. This method aids in the diagnosis of hemolytic anemias that cannot be identified by ordinary laboratory tests.

This method of examination is particularly helpful in distinguishing between the genetically transmitted homozygous and heterozygous hemoglobin S. When both genes carry hemoglobin S, the person is homozygous and has sickle cell disease. Sickle cell trait, a less serious condition, is present in people who are heterozygous, having inherited one normal gene, which carries hemoglobin A, and one that carries the abnormal variant hemoglobin S.

Fetal hemoglobin (HgbF) is manufactured by the fetal RBC's and is the major hemoglobin of the fetus. The amount of HgbF drops during the first two years of life, reaching adult levels after age three. An alkali denaturation test is performed when increased concentrations are detected during routine hemoglobin electrophoresis or when thalassemia is suspected.

N O R M A L   R A N G E

The types of normal hemoglobin identified by electrophoresis are:

HgbA$_1$	The major component of normal adult blood.	95%–98%
HgbA$_2$	The minor component of normal adult blood.	2%–3%
Hgb F	The most common hemoglobin molecules present during fetal life.	.08–2%
	Newborn	60–90%
	After age 2	0–2%
HgbS	The hemoglobin responsible for sickle cell anemia.	0%
HgbC	The hemoglobin that may result in a mild hemolytic anemia.	0%

The most common abnormal hemoglobin seen during electrophoresis is hemoglobin S. This occurs in approximately 10% of African Americans. Other variants include HbC, HbH, HbD, aned HbE.

Specimen Required

A specimen of venous blood should be collected in a tube containing EDTA. The tube should be filled completely and delivered to the laboratory promptly.

Note. If a blood transfusion has been given during the preceding 4 months this should be noted on the laboratory slip, as the presence of donor cells may affect test results.

Preparation of the Patient

There are no food or fluid restrictions before venipuncture.

Causes of Deviation from Normal and Nursing Implications of Abnormal Findings

Hemoglobin electrophoresis is done to distinguish different types of hemoglobin and to help establish abnormal hemoglobin variations. The reader is referred to the section on the Sickle Cell Test for further information about sickle cell disease, and to the section on the Red Cell Count for further information about hemolytic anemias. If thalassemia is diagnosed, a medical-surgical textbook should be consulted for related nursing care.

HAPTOGLOBIN

Description

Haptoglobins are alpha-2 globulins produced in the liver. They bind with free hemoglobin released from lysed erythrocytes (red blood cells). This binding capacity preserves iron that would otherwise be lost in the urine. Serum haptoglobin is depleted when hemolysis of red blood cells is extensive.

NORMAL RANGE	
Adults	60–265 mg/dl or 0.6–2.65 g/L
Children	after 6 months, gradually increased to adult levels
Infants	0–30 mg/dl or 0.03 g/L
Newborns	0–10 mg/dl or 0–0.1 g/L

Specimen Required

A 5-ml sample of venous blood is obtained in a plain collecting tube or syringe. The specimen should be handled carefully to avoid RBC lysis that could alter test results.

Preparation of the Patient

Food and fluids are not restricted before venipuncture.

Causes of Deviation from Normal

Any condition causing hemolysis of red blood cells, such as hemolytic anemias, sickle cell disease, thalassemia, liver disease, transfusion reactions, systemic lupus erythematosis and prosthetic heart valve implantation will result in a decrease in haptoglobin. Increased levels are seen in a variety of disorders including acute and chronic infections and inflammation, malignancies, steroid therapy, rheumatoid arthritis, ulcerative colitis, peptic ulcer, oral contraception, and pregnancy.

Nursing Implications of Abnormal Findings

Assessment. When haptoglobin levels are below normal, the patient's vital signs, particularly respirations, should be assessed. When the oxygen-carrying capacity of hemoglobin is diminished, breathing may be altered. Urinary output should also be assessed, since extensive hemolysis could result in free hemoglobin which could cause renal damage.

Interventions. Nursing interventions are related to the specific disease or cause of the abnormal haptoglobin. A medical-surgical nursing textbook should be consulted for specific care. The physician should be notified if signs and symptoms indicate that tissue damage may be occurring as a result of extensive red blood cell hemolysis.

BLOOD VOLUME STUDIES (DETERMINATION)

Description

Blood volume studies are done to determine the total amount of circulating blood volume. This test is used when a patient has significant uterine or gastrointestinal bleeding, hemorrhage or other potential causes of hypovolemia. It may also be done when an elevated total volume is suspected. Blood volume studies may be done to determine the blood component (RBC's and/or plasma) required for replacement therapy following blood loss during surgery.

N O R M A L R A N G E	
Adult	
Total Blood Volume:	55–80 ml/kg of body weight
Red Cell Volume:	Males 25–35 ml/kg body weight
	Females 20–30 ml/kg body weight
Plasma Volume:	Males 32–45 ml/kg body weight
	Females 30–45 ml/kg body weight
Children	
	Consult laboratory for reference values for the height and weight of the child being tested.

Specimen Required

A 5–10-ml sample of venous blood is obtained in a plain collecting tube or syringe. The nuclear medicine laboratory will mix a radioisotope with the blood sample. After 15–30 minutes the blood containing the radioisotope is re-injected into the patient. Fifteen minutes later another blood sample is collected.

Preparation of the Patient

The height and weight of the patient should be obtained and recorded in the chart and on the laboratory slip immediately before the procedure. The whole procedure should be explained including a description of how often the blood will be drawn and the reason for re-injecting a sample into the patient. The patient should also be told that the radioactive material to be used is a small amount and is not harmful. Since intravenous fluids can affect test results, blood volume studies should be done before starting an IV.

Causes of Deviation from Normal

Decreases in total blood volume and plasma volume are caused by massive bleeding that occurs with uterine or gastrointestinal bleeding or hemorrhaging from other parts of the body, dehydration, or hypovolemic shock. Blood loss during surgery can also be a cause. An increase in the RBC volume is caused by polycythemia vera and dehydration. If over hydration is present, the total volume may be increased.

Nursing Implications of Abnormal Findings

Assessment. The reason a blood volume study is ordered will guide the nurse's assessment and interventions. If the patient has hemorrhaged or had massive blood loss during surgery, signs and symptoms of shock and dehydration should be noted. These include tachycardia, rapid, shallow respirations and pale, cold, clammy skin. Hypotension will occur when blood loss is 15–25% of blood volume. Signs of dehydration such as poor skin turgor and dry mucous membranes should also be assessed. If there is an increase due to polycythemia vera, the patient should be observed for increased blood pressure, dizziness, tinnitus, joint pain, and the development of peripheral thrombophlebitis.

Interventions. Nursing interventions for patients who have experienced massive blood loss relate to the type of therapy they are receiving. Medical-surgical nursing texts should be consulted for specific nursing care for hypovolemia, decreased tissue perfusion, decreases in cardiac output, and other related problems. Mechanical assistance and monitoring devices may be used when blood volume deficit has led to hypovolemic shock. If polycythemia has caused an increase in the blood volume, patients should be encouraged to exercise to prevent peripheral venous thrombosis. Fluids may also be recommended to reduce blood viscosity. If phlebotomy is scheduled to reduce blood volume, the procedure should be explained and the patient observed for signs of hypo-volemia, since rapid withdrawal of blood could lead to hemodynamic changes.

SICKLE CELL TEST (SICKLEDEX)

2

Description

The *sickle cell test* (Sickledex) is performed to determine if hemoglobin S (an abnormal form of hemoglobin) is present in red cells. Under normal conditions, red cells maintain their normal shape when oxygen tension is adequate. It is only when available oxygen is reduced that those red cells containing hemoglo-bin S assume a distorted crescent- or sickle-shaped form. When the sickle cell test is performed in the laboratory, all oxygen is removed from the erythrocytes and their shape is examined.

Sickling is rapid and complete if hemoglobin S is the only hemoglobin present. Positive results also occur when there are large amounts of hemoglobin A or other non-S hemoglobins. Therefore, this procedure cannot differentiate between sickle cell trait and sickle cell disease. Electrophoresis must be done to distinguish hemoglobin patterns completely.

NORMAL RANGE

Normal red cells in both adults and children do not contain hemoglobin S and do not acquire a sickle shape when deprived of oxygen.

Specimen Required

A 3-ml sample of venous blood is collected in a tube containing EDTA or dou-ble oxalate anticoagulants.

Preparation of the Patient

There are no food or fluid restrictions before collection of the specimen. If the patient has received a blood transfusion within 4 months before the test this should be noted on the laboratory slip; test results may be altered by the pres-ence of the donor's red cells.

Causes of Deviation from Normal

A positive sickle cell test occurs when a person has a genetically transmitted sickle cell disorder. When hemoglobin electrophoresis reveals a heterozygous pattern, a sickle cell trait is present. This means that the person has inherited a normal hemoglobin A gene from one parent and an abnormal hemoglobin S gene from the other. When sickle cell trait is present, the person will have few or no clinical manifestations. If two people with sickle cell trait marry, their children may inherit sickle cell anemia. Sickle cell anemia is present when hemoglobin electrophoresis reveals a homozygous pattern. This occurs when the hemoglobin S gene has been inherited from both parents. All of the clinical manifestations of the disease will be exhibited in people with this pattern.

Nursing Implications of Abnormal Findings

Assessment. When sickle cell trait is first diagnosed, the nurse must determine the amount of knowledge the patient has about sickle cell disease. An assessment should also be made of the patient's attitude and emotional acceptance of the diagnosis. During the assessment period, the nurse must determine when the patient is ready to accept genetic counseling and teaching about sickle cell disease. If sickle cell anemia is present, the nursing assessment should also include an evaluation of the patient's physical status to determine the presence of clinical manifestations that occur as a result of the destruction of the sickled red blood cells, thrombosis, and infarction from the occlusion of the microcirculation by the sickled cells, and an elevated bilirubin caused by the release of hemoglobin. The nurse should also assess the patient for the presence of medical conditions that may cause hypoxia such as cardiopulmonary disease, shock, and hypothermia.

Intervention. The primary focus of nursing care for people with sickle cell disease is counseling and education. Black people should be encouraged to be tested for the presence of hemoglobin S. Parents should also be counseled to have their children tested. Young black people who are carriers of sickle cell trait should be encouraged to seek genetic counseling before marrying and having children. People who have only the trait should be told that they may become symptomatic if they are exposed to low oxygen tension or do strenuous exercise or work extremely hard. The stress of pregnancy may also produce symptoms. People with sickle cell disease should avoid becoming hypoxic. Situations in which hypoxia may occur include traveling in high-altitude areas or in unpressurized aircraft. They should also be told that hypoxia may occur during strenuous exercise.

For people with sickle cell anemia, nursing care is mainly supportive, since the sickled erythrocytes can collect and lodge in the circulatory system of all organs. Specific interventions depend on the part of the body involved. The nursing care plan should focus on the prevention and treatment of infection and complications such as leg ulcers, cholelithiasis, pathological fractures, and cardiac arrhythmias. Pregnant women also risk development of pulmonary or renal complications.

Note. Patients should be told *not* to take aspirin or aspirin-containing products as they can cause cells to sickle more easily. Acetaminophen can be used instead.

RETICULOCYTE COUNT

Description

Reticulocytes are immature, non-nucleated erythrocytes found in the bone marrow. They contain nuclear material that stains in the laboratory and appears as dark blue dots under the microscope. The reticulocyte count is an index of the bone marrow production of mature red cells. This test is done to differentiate anemias caused by bone marrow failure from those caused by hemorrhage or hemolysis.

N O R M A L R A N G E	
Adults	0.5–2.0% of total erythrocytes
Children	0.5–2.0% of total erythrocytes
Infants	0.5–3.5% of total erythrocytes
Newborns	2.5–6.0% of total erythrocytes

Specimen Required

A 7-ml sample of venous blood is collected in a tube containing EDTA. Capillary blood may be drawn into a pipette containing an equal volume of new methylene blue solution and is to be used for the reticulocyte count.

Preparation of the Patient

There are no food or fluid restrictions before venipuncture.

Causes of Deviation from Normal

An increase in the reticulocyte count occurs when there are diseases present that cause an increase in erythrocyte production by the bone marrow. The degree of elevation (reticulocytosis) is proportional to the severity of the disease. Elevations are caused by hemolytic anemia, hereditary spherocytosis, sickle cell anemia, posthemorrhagic anemia, and treatment of iron deficiency anemia and B_{12} and folic acid deficiency. An increase in the reticulocyte count after an acute blood loss or treatment for anemias from iron, vitamin B_{12}, or folic acid deficiencies indicates that the bone marrow is functioning normally.

Decreases in the reticulocyte count may occur in aplastic anemia, iron deficiency anemia, untreated pernicious anemia, chronic infection, and radiation therapy.

Nursing Implications of Abnormal Findings

Refer to the section on the red cell count test for a description of the general areas for nursing care of patients with anemias. General medical-surgical nursing texts should be consulted for additional information.

LEUKOCYTE ALKALINE PHOSPHATASE STAIN

Description

The *leukocyte alkaline phosphatase* (LAP) *stain test* is done to determine the activity of alkaline phosphatase in neutrophils. It shows the intercellular metabolic activity represented by granulation in the cytoplasm within these cells.

NORMAL RANGE

Each laboratory must be consulted to determine the normal range it has established. These values generally range from 15 to 130.

Specimen Required

A 7-ml sample of venous blood is collected in a plain collecting tube or syringe.

Preparation of the Patient

There are no food or fluid restrictions before venipuncture.

Causes of Deviation from Normal

The LAP test is done to differentiate chronic granulocytic leukemia from neutrophilic leukemoid reactions. A value below normal is seen in acute and chronic granulocytic leukemia; a value above normal is present in leukemoid reactions that present a blood picture that looks like leukemia. The LAP may also be used to differentiate polycythemia vera from secondary erythrocytosis. Above-normal reactions may also be seen in polycythemia vera.

Nursing Implications of Abnormal Findings

Assessment and Interventions. The most important aspect of nursing care for patients who undergo this test is to assess the patient's emotional status, particularly if the diagnosis of leukemia versus a leukemoid reaction is still pending. Providing emotional support to the patient and his family during this period of uncertainty is the primary nursing activity. The nurse should be careful not to provide false hope but to help the patient understand the reasons for diagnostic tests and for the physician's reluctance to make a final diagnosis until all the data about the patient's physical status have been evaluated.

SERUM IRON

Description

Iron travels in the bloodstream bound to the plasma protein transferrin. It is absorbed into the bloodstream from the small intestine and becomes bound to transferrin in the bone marrow. Iron is used for hemoglobin formation and for the production of bone cellular enzymes.

2

N O R M A L R A N G E	
Adults	
Men	60–150 µg/dl
Women	50–130 µg/dl
Children	50–120 µg/dl
Infants	40–100 µg/dl
Newborns	100–250 µg/dl

Note. There are diurnal variations; the highest levels occur in the morning, and levels decrease as the day progresses.

Specimen Required

A 5-ml sample of venous blood is collected in a plain collecting tube or syringe.

Preparation of the Patient

There are no food or fluid restrictions before venipuncture.

Causes of Deviation from Normal

Increases in serum iron levels usually occur in the following conditions: excessive red cell destruction, as in hemolytic disorders or mechanical hemolysis of red blood cells; excessive release of stored iron, as in hemochromatosis; and a conditions in which the body is unable to incorporate iron into hemoglobin, as in a sideroblastic anemia.

The serum iron is low in anemias associated with chronic illness, chronic infections, malignant neoplasm, acute or chronic blood loss, chronic renal disease, extensive burns, and iron deficiency anemias associated with poor dietary intake of iron and pregnancy. A decrease may also be seen during periods of rapid growth (e.g., ages 6 months to 2 years), or in people at any age who have a decrease in iron intake for 2–3 months or longer. See Table 2.12 for a list of substances that affect serum iron levels.

TABLE 2.12. Drugs that Affect Serum Iron Values

Drugs that cause an increase
Chloramphenicol
Iron dextran complex
Progestin–estrogen
Combinations in oral contraceptives
Drugs that cause a decrease
ACTH
Hydroxyurea
Steroids
Drugs that can cause either an increase or a decrease
Fluorides
Oxalate
Tungstate

Nursing Implications of Abnormal Findings

Assessment. When there is an abnormally high serum iron level, nursing care depends on the specific cause of the abnormal value. When the serum iron is low, nursing assessment depends on the cause of the blood loss. The patient should be observed for pallor, weakness, fatigue, dizziness, and sensitivity to cold as well as for signs of acute or chronic bleeding. When the low serum iron is attributable to nutritional deficiencies, a diet history should be taken that includes an assessment of the patient's knowledge of a well-balanced diet as well as the ability and willingness to follow such a diet.

Interventions. Nursing interventions are related to the correction of the iron deficit by the administration of iron preparations and the recommendation of a diet high in iron. Oral iron preparations should be given with meals or snacks and patients should be taught to take their iron with food after they are discharged from the hospital.

A teaching plan should be established to help the patient understand the importance of eating a well-balanced diet. The nurse should make use of the dietary referral system while the patient is in the hospital and should make plans for home visits by a dietitian or nurse if needed. The patient should also be referred to community resources such as Meals on Wheels when appropriate.

TOTAL IRON-BINDING CAPACITY

Description

The *total iron-binding capacity* is a measurement of the amount of iron present in the body after transferrin is exposed to excess iron. It represents the amount of iron that could be carried if all the transferrin were completely saturated. Normally, the binding sites of transferrin are capable of transporting more iron than is present in the serum.

N O R M A L R A N G E	
Adults	250–450 μg/dl
Children	100–350 μg/dl
Infants	100–400 μg/dl
Newborns	60–175 μg/dl

Specimen Required

A 5-ml sample of venous blood is collected in a plain collecting tube or syringe.

Preparation of the Patient

There are no food or fluid restrictions before venipuncture.

Causes of Deviation from Normal

An elevated iron-binding capacity may occur in some of the same conditions that cause a low serum iron level. These include acute and chronic blood loss, iron deficiency anemia, hepatitis, and pregnancy.

Decreases in the iron-binding capacity occur in acute and chronic infections, hemochromatosis, malignancy, starvation, chronic liver disease, renal failure, chronic hemolytic anemias, sickle cell anemia, and thalassemia.

Nursing Implications of Abnormal Findings

Assessment and Interventions. Nursing care of a patient with an abnormal iron-binding capacity depends on the cause of the abnormality. The patient's clinical manifestations will help the nurse assess the patient's status and plan appropriate interventions. When iron deficiency anemia is the cause, the nursing care discussed for low serum iron should be followed.

BLOOD TYPING

Descriptions

ABO BLOOD GROUPS

ABO *blood groups* are inherited characteristics that consist of the presence or absence of either A or B antigens, usually referred to as agglutinogens. There are four main blood types: A, or presence of A antigen only; B, or presence of B antigen only; AB, or presence of both A and B antigens; and O, absence of

TABLE 2.13. Homozygous and Heterozygous Blood Types

Parental Phenotypes	Homozygous Phenotype in Offspring	Heterozygous Phenotype in Offspring
AB + A	A	AB
AB + AB	A or B	AB

both A and B antigens. The four combinations of the A and B antigens depend upon genetic inheritance. A person may inherit the same gene from each parent and be homozygous or may inherit different genes from each parent and be heterozygous (Table 2.13).

Blood typing may be done for a variety of reasons including when a person plans to donate blood, needs a blood transfusion, or is pregnant. In blood transfusion, compatibility must be established between the donor's and recipient's blood to prevent a transfusion reaction caused by the agglutination (clumping) of red cells. Each person has agglutinins (antibodies) in the serum that will react with foreign agglutinogens (antigens). For example, a person with blood type A has anti-B agglutinins. If given blood from a donor with blood type B, this person would have agglutination of the red blood cells, which could result in death. The reverse would be true for a person with blood type B receiving a transfusion of type A blood. When O is the blood type, both anti-A and anti-B agglutinins are present.

Rh FACTOR

The *Rh factor* is an antigen found on the red cells. The term "Rh factor" is designated by the symbol Rh_O, and Rh positive is designated by Rh_O (D). Most people have an Rh antigen and are designated Rh positive. Those who do not have the antigen are Rh negative. Because the Rh factor is found in conjunction with the ABO blood groups, a person may be any combination of the two groups, such as A Rh positive, B Rh positive, O Rh negative, AB Rh negative, and so forth. The serum of an Rh-negative person does not contain anti-Rh agglutinins unless there has been a previous exposure to Rh-positive blood from a blood transfusion or a pregnancy with an Rh-positive child. This results in a gradual build-up of anti-Rh agglutinins. No harm results unless a second exposure occurs. During a second transfusion, agglutination of the red cells occurs. When a woman who has anti-Rh agglutinins becomes pregnant with a child with Rh-positive blood, intravascular hemolysis of the infant's cells occurs during pregnancy, resulting in hemolytic disease of the newborn (HDN), also called erythroblastosis fetalis. Rh-negative blood does not harm an Rh-positive person.

2

NORMAL RANGE

Possible blood types are:

O Rh-positive	B Rh-positive
O Rh-negative	B Rh-negative
A Rh-positive	AB Rh-positive
A Rh-negative	AB Rh-negative

Specimen Required

A 5-ml sample of venous blood is obtained in a plain collecting tube or syringe.

Preparation of the Patient

There are no food or fluid restrictions before venipuncture.

Causes of Deviation from Normal

A person's blood type generally does not change. However, some bone marrow transplant patients undergo blood-type changes when the donor's blood type is different.

Nursing Implications of Abnormal Findings

Not applicable.

CROSSMATCH

Description

The *crossmatch* is a test done before blood transfusion to determine compatibility between the patient's (recipient's) and donor's blood. When there is no hemolysis (clumping) after donor and recipient serum and cells are mixed and incubated, the two blood samples are compatible. A *major crossmatch* is done between the recipient's serum and the donor's cells to determine if the recipient's serum has antibodies that will damage or destroy the donor's cells. A *minor crossmatch* is done between the donor's serum and the recipient's cells to determine if the donor's serum has antibodies against the recipient's cells.

NORMAL RANGE

If two blood samples are compatible, there is no hemolysis (clumping) when the serum and cells are mixed.

Specimen Required

A 10-ml sample of venous blood is obtained in a plain collecting tube or syringe.

Preparation of the Patient

There are no food or fluid restrictions before venipuncture.

Causes of Deviation from Normal

Incompatibility occurs when antibodies are present that cause hemolysis of either the donor's or recipient's blood.

Nursing Implications of Abnormal Findings

Assessment and Interventions. Any patient who receives a blood transfusion must be assessed for the signs and symptoms of a transfusion reaction because there may be undetected sources of incompatibility. Clinical manifestations include tachycardia, chest pain, cyanosis or pallor, dyspnea and/or tachypnea, headache, chills, hematuria, oliguria, bleeding from wounds, and generalized oozing of blood.

When a blood transfusion is started, precautions should be taken to prevent administering the wrong blood, which is the most common cause of hemolytic transfusion reaction. Before the blood transfusion is begun, two professionals must compare the blood type and identifying number on the donor blood with those of the recipient. If the patient is comatose, the person administering the blood must be sure of the patient's identity. The flow rate should be slow for the first fifteen minutes and then increased to the proper level if there are no signs of a transfusion reaction. If a reaction does occur, the transfusion must be stopped and the needle removed. The protocol used to examine and discard the blood remaining after the transfusion varies with each institution. The blood bank should be consulted about the method of disposal.

Rh ANTIBODY TITER

Description

This test is performed when it appears that a person with Rh-negative blood may be producing antibodies against the Rh factor. It should be noted that there are several Rh haplotypes and a person's antibodies may demonstrate specificity to more than one.

NORMAL RANGE

Normally there are no antibodies present in the serum.

Specimen Required

A 10-ml sample of venous blood is obtained in a plain collecting tube or syringe.

Preparation of the Patient

There are no food or fluid restrictions before venipuncture.

Causes of Deviation from Normal

A person with Rh-negative blood will have a positive antibody titer if an incompatible transfusion of whole blood, packed cells, platelets, or granulocytes has been given, or a child has been conceived whose father is Rh-positive and a fetal-maternal hemorrhage has occurred.

Nursing Implications of Abnormal Findings

Assessment. There are no clinical manifestations the first time a person with Rh-negative blood receives Rh-positive antigens. However, subsequent exposures result in prompt destruction of red cells. Although all patients receiving blood transfusions should be observed for the signs and symptoms of a transfusion reaction, the person with Rh-negative blood must receive special attention, since previous exposure to the Rh-positive antigen might have gone unnoticed. A pregnant woman who has already had one Rh-positive baby or has aborted or miscarried a pregnancy conceived with an Rh-positive partner may have a rising antibody titer that should be noted.

Interventions. When a transfusion reaction occurs, the transfusion should be stopped, the physician and blood bank notified, and the remaining blood saved and returned to the blood bank. If a pregnant woman has rising antibody titers, the physician should be informed as soon as possible so that a decision can be made about the need for intrauterine transfusion of the fetus. Nonjudgmental emotional support should be provided for the mother, particularly if she neglected to be protected with Rh_O immune globulin. When the mother's antibody titer indicates the need for a transfusion of the fetus, nursing care should focus on assisting the mother during the transfusion and providing supportive care during and after the procedure.

Note. When an Rh-negative woman gives birth to a baby with Rh-positive blood or has had an abortion, miscarriage, or ectopic pregnancy, she should be given Rh immune globulin (Rhogram) seventy-two hours after delivery or termination of the pregnancy. This immune globulin suppresses the development of antibodies, based on the principle of passive immunity.

HUMAN LEUKOCYTE ANTIGEN (HLA)

Description

Human leukocyte antigens are present on all nucleated cells except red blood cells. They are classified into five series designated as A, B, C, D, and DR

(D-related). Each series contains several distinct antigens which can be HLA phenotyped to determine histocompatibility.

N O R M A L   R A N G E

Not applicable. HLA testing is done to determine histocompatibility between individuals.

Specimen Required
A 10-ml sample of venous blood is collected in a tube containing heparin. Care should be taken to avoid hemolysis. The specimen should be sent to the laboratory immediately after it is obtained.

Preparation of the Patient
There are no food or fluid restrictions before venipuncture.

Causes of Deviation from Normal
Not applicable. HLA testing is done to determine: (1) tissue compatibility between recipients and donors for organ transplants; (2) if recipients of multiple platelet transfusions have developed antibodies to HLA antigens; (3) genetic factors associated with the development of ankylosing spondylitis, myasthenia gravis, Addison's disease and insulin dependent (Type I) diabetes; and (4) paternity.

Nursing Implications of Abnormal Findings
Assessment and Interventions. There are no abnormal findings for HLA testing. Nurses may assist patients who are having HLA testing by describing the test and the reason it is being done. A plan for emotional support should be developed for patients who are hopeful that they will be compatible with a donor for organ transplant. The nurse should be prepared to answer patients' questions about genetic factors related to inherited disease and concerns expressed by men who are having testing related to paternity issues.

BONE MARROW EXAMINATION

Description
Bone marrow examination involves evaluation and classification of the material obtained from bone marrow tissue by aspiration or biopsy. The bone marrow is the major site of the formation of blood cells; it produces millions of blood cells

each day. After examination and classification, the kind and number of each cell obtained by biopsy or aspiration are compared with a normal distribution of cell types in order to identify abnormal cells in kind or distribution. Bone marrow is a rust-red-colored thick fluid with visible amounts of fatty material and white fragments.

2

N O R M A L   R A N G E

Terminology for the types of cells found during bone marrow examination varies from one area and laboratory to another. The following is one such classification.

Mean Values*

Cell Type	Adults Mean %	Newborns Mean %	Children Mean %
Normoblasts, total	25.6	14.5	23.1
Pronormoblasts	0.5	0.02	0.5
Basophilic	1.6	0.24	1.7
Polychromatophilic	10.4	13.1	18.2
Orthochromatic	0.0	0.69	2.7
Neutrophils, total	53.6	60.4	57.1
Myeloblasts	2.0	0.31	1.2
Promyelocytes	5.0	0.79	1.4
Myelocytes	12.0	3.9	18.3
Metamyelocytes	17.1	19.4	23.3
Bands	12.4	28.4	n/a
Segmented	9.0	7.4	12.9
Eosinophils	3.1	2.7	3.6
Basophils	0.1	0.12	0.06
Lymphocytes, total	16.2	15.6	16.0
Transitional	—	1.2	—
Small (mature)	—	14.4	—
Plasma cells	1.3	0.00	0.4
Monocytes	0.3	0.88	n/a
Megakaryocytes	0.1	0.06	n/a
Reticulum cells	0.3	—	—
Myeloid/erythroid ratio	2.3	4.4	2.9

*Values are expressed as percent of nucleated cells present.

Specimen Required

A sample of 9.2–9.5 ml of marrow fluid is obtained by means of bone marrow aspiration or biopsy.

Preparation of the Patient

Food and fluids are not restricted before the procedure. See Chapter 1 for preparation of the patient for a bone marrow examination.

Causes of Deviation from Normal

Increases and decreases of numbers of white and red cells are associated with specific pathologies. Increased or decreased numbers of white cells may indicate leukemia. Decreased numbers of red cells can occur during iron deficiency anemia. Cancerous invasion of the bone from a primary or metastatic cancer can be demonstrated by the appearance of abnormal cancerous cells. Bone marrow depression is also associated with radiation therapy and drugs used in cancer therapy. Marrow examination at regular intervals is done to evaluate a patient's response to therapy. For example, bone marrow examination is done regularly in patients with leukemia to determine whether remission or relapse has occurred.

Nursing Implications of Abnormal Findings

Assessment and Interventions. When a patient has an abnormal bone marrow examination revealing a leukemic condition, the nurse should assess the patient's emotional state and provide support if needed while the patient adapts to the diagnosis. Test results change during treatment, and tests are administered at regular intervals to evaluate the patient's response to therapy. Since these tests may give the first indication of a remission or relapse, the nurse must always be prepared to assist the patient in adapting to the disease stage. If an anemia is present, the nurse should alternate the patient's periods of activity and rest. If therapy for anemia is to be continued after discharge, the nurse should formulate a teaching plan for the patient to ensure regular and complete follow-up.

BIBLIOGRAPHY

Brown, S.J. "Behind the Numbers on the CBC." *RN*, 53:46–49; 50–51 (February 1990).

Byrne, C.J., D.F. Saxton, P.K. Pelikan, and P.M. Nugent. *Laboratory Tests: Implications for Nursing Care*. Menlo Park: Addison-Wesley, 1986.

Friedman, E.W. "Reticulocyte Counts: How to Use Them, What They Mean." *Diagnostic Medicine*, 6:29–33 (July 1984).

Henry, J.B. *Clinical Diagnosis and Management by Laboratory Methods*. Philadelphia: W.B. Saunders Co., 1991.

Gaedeke-Norris, M.K. "Lab test tips—How to Evaluate Platelet Values." *Nursing 91*, 21:20 (February 1991).

Herring, W.B., V.R. Sundaram, and R.E. Reed. "When the Hematocrit Rises." *Patient Care*, 23:176–180, 185–188, 191 (August 15, 1989).

Ignatavicius, D.D., and M.V. Bayne. *Medical-Surgical Nursing: A Nursing Process Approach*. Philadelphia: W.B. Saunders, 1991.

Koch, P.M. "Thrombocytopenia." *Nursing 84*, 14:55–57 (October 1984).

Lamb, C. "Why Is That Hematocrit High?" *Patient Care*, 20:46–48, 50, 55 (January 1986).

Lewis, S.M., and I.C. Collier, *Medical-Surgical Nursing: Assessment and Management of Clinical Problems*. St. Louis: Mosby Yearbook, 1992.

Luckman, J., and K.C. Sorensen. *Medical-Surgical Nursing: A Psychological Approach*. Philadelphia: Saunders, 1987.

Mansen, T.J. "Does That CBC Spell Trouble?" *RN*, 47:48–49 (July 1984).

McConnell, E.A. "Leucocyte Studies: What the Counts Can Tell You." *Nursing 86*, 16:42–43 (March 1986).

Phipps, W.S., B.C. Long, N.F. Woods, and V. Cossmeyer. *Medical-Surgical Nursing*. St. Louis: Mosby Yearbook, 1991.

Ravel, R. *Clinical Laboratory Medicine*. Chicago: Year Book Medical Publishers, 1989.

Sacher, R.A., and R.A. McPherson. *Widmann's Clinical Interpretation of Laboratory Tests*. Philadelphia: F.A. Davis, 1991.

Sheehy, S.B. "Laboratory Tests in Trauma." *Journal of Emergency Nursing*, 11:99–104 (March–April 1985).

Smetzer, C.C., and B.G. Ball. *Brunner and Sudarth's Medical-Surgical Nursing*. New York: J.B. Lippincott, 1992.

Wheby, M.S. "Interpreting the 'Message' of an Elevated Hematocrit." *Consultant*, 24:124–125, 128–129, 132, 137, 141–144 (December 1984).

Williams, W.J., E. Beutler, and A.J. Erslen. *Hematology*. New York: McGraw-Hill Inc., 1990.

Wilson, J., et al. *Harrison's Principles of Internal Medicine*. New York: McGraw-Hill, Inc., 1991.

CHAPTER

3

Laboratory Tests of Coagulation

HEMOSTASIS AND COAGULATION

HEMOSTATIC EVENTS

Hemostasis is a mechanism that minimizes blood loss from severed or ruptured blood vessels. The mechanisms included in this process are:

1. Vasoconstriction of the damaged vessel.
   Spasm of the smooth muscle is a result of vessel trauma, sympathetic reflexes caused by pain associated with the trauma, and the release of chemicals that cause vasoconstriction. This mechanism prevents massive blood loss during the initial stage of injury.

2. Clumping of platelets to form a platelet plug.

When the endothelium of the injured vessel is disrupted, platelets begin to adhere to the underlying connective tissue. These platelets become sticky, allowing new platelets to adhere to the old ones until a plug of platelets is built up at the site of injury.

3. Formation of a fibrin clot.

The clotting process is initiated by activator substances from both the traumatized vascular wall and the platelets. The clot that forms fills the end of the injured vessel within 3–6 minutes.

4. Fibrous organization of the blood clot.

After the clot has formed, fibroblasts invade the area, resulting in complete organization of the clot in 7–10 days.

MECHANISM OF BLOOD COAGULATION

Coagulation consists of a series of reactions that result in the formation of a clot (Fig. 3.1). This blood clotting mechanism is triggered by either an intrinsic or extrinsic mechanism. When the blood itself is traumatized, the intrinsic mechanism initiates clotting. This involves a more complex series of reactions than in the extrinsic mechanism. If a blood vessel is damaged, the extrinsic mechanism causes clotting to occur because of the release of tissue thromboplastin by the wall of the vessel. Once the clot has formed it begins to contract, and most of the plasma is expressed from it. The clot becomes denser and stronger and pulls the vessel walls adhering to the clot closer together. This clot retraction is caused by the platelets, which become attached to fibrin threads and band them together. The mechanism of clot retraction contributes to hemostasis.

Several blood studies are done to assess all parts of the blood clotting mechanism and help determine the cause of hemorrhagic disorders. The results of these laboratory tests are used in conjunction with the patient's clinical manifestations and history, as well as any family history of hemorrhagic disrders or bleeding tendencies. The tests described in the following sections are those most commonly performed when a hemorrhagic disorder is being evalu-ated.

It is important to remember that bleeding disorders can be very complex. Causes of deviation from normal and related nursing care must be correlated with the clinical history and related assessment data.

FACTOR ASSAY (COAGULATION FACTORS ASSAY)

Description

Factor assays are done to determine defects in the coagulation process. They are used to determine if inherited deficiencies are mild, moderate, or severe, and to follow the course of acquired bleeding disorders. The function of each factor during stages of coagulation is seen in Table 3.1.

NORMAL RANGE

Factor	Minimum Level for Hemostasis (mg/dl)
I	60–100
II	10–15
III	5–10
VII	10–20
VIII	30–35
IX	30–35
X	7–10
XI	20–30

Normal values may vary among laboratories.

Specimen Required

A 5–10 ml sample of venous blood is collected in a tube or syringe containing sodium citrate.

Preparation of the Patient

There are no food or fluid restrictions before venipuncture.

Causes of Deviation from Normal

Coagulation deficiencies associated with each factor are outlined on Table 3.2.

TABLE 3.1. Functions of Coagulation Factors

	Factor Name	Function during Stages of Coagulation
I	Fibrinogen	An essential plasma protein split by thrombin during stage III to form a clot.
II	Prothrombin	An inactive plasma protein converted to thrombin by the action of extrinsic and intrinsic thromboplastin during Stage II.
III	Thromboplastin	An enzyme-like protein that converts prothrombin to thrombin during Stage II.

TABLE 3.1. (Continued)

Factor Name	Function during Stages of Coagulation
IV	Calcium	An inorganic ion necessary for several stages of coagulation. At least 2.5 ml/dl must be present for coagulation to occur.
V	Proaccelerin (Labile factor)	A protein essential for accelerating the conversion of prothrombin to thrombin during stage II.
VI	Not Used	
VII	Proconvertin (Stable Factor)	Helps accelerate the conversion of prothrombin to thrombin during stage II. It is the first factor to be compressed following administration of oral anticoagulants.
VIII	Antihemophilic Factor (AHF)	A large molecule required for the generation of intrinsic plasma thromboplastin during stage I.
IX	Plasma Thromboplastin Component (PTC, Christmas factor, Antihemophilic Factor B)	Essential for the generation of intrinsic plasma thromboplastin in Stage I. It influences the amount of thromboplastin available to convert prothrombin to thrombin but not the rate at which it is produced.
X	Stuart Factor (Stuart-Prower Factor)	A protein essential for the conversion of prothrombin to thrombin in Stage II. Required for generation of intrinsic thromboplastin.
XI	Plasma Thromboplastin Antecedent (PTA, Anti-hemophilic Factor C)	Essential for plasma thromboplastin formation in Stage I coagulation.
XII	Hageman Factor	Essential for generation of intrinsic plasma thromboplastin in stage I. Converts plasminogen to plasmin in fibrinolysis.
XIII	Fibrin Stabilizing Factor (Fibrinase)	An enzyme necessary to stabilize the cross linkage of fibrin strands to form a firm clot.

3

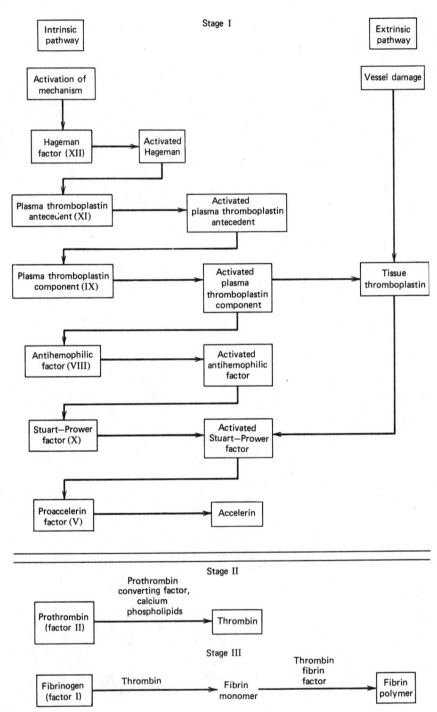

FIGURE 3.1. Stages of the blood clotting mechanism.

TABLE 3.2. Coagulation Factor Deficiencies

	Factor Name	Deficiency	Assessment
I	Fibrinogen	Afibrinogenemia, hypofibrinogenemia, liver disease, cachexia.	Easy bruising, ecchymoses, epistaxis, hematuria, gingival bleeding.
II	Prothrombin	Hypoprothrombinemia, Vitamin K deficiency, liver disease.	Easy bruising, ecchymoses, epistaxis, hematuria, gingival bleeding.
III	Thromboplastin	Thrombocytopenia.	Easy bruising, ecchymoses.
IV	Calcium	Decreased absorption caused by sprue, pancreatitis, Crohn's disease; primary hypoparathyroidism; excessive transfusions of citrated blood; malnutrition.	Clotting mechanism unaffected. Cardiac arrest would occur before coagulation affected.
V	Proaccelerin	Liver disease, parahemophilia.	Easy bruising, epistaxis menorrhagia.
VI		—Not Used—	
VII	Proconvertin (Stable Factor)	Hepatic carcinoma, hepatitis, Vitamin K deficiency, hemorrhagic disease of the newborn.	Easy bruising, epistaxis, menorrhagia.
VIII	Antihemophilic Factor (Hemophilic Factor A)	Hemophilia A (classic hemophilia) von Willebrand's syndrome, disseminated intravascular coagulation (DIC), multiple myeloma, rheumatoid arthritis, lupus erythematosis.	Spontaneous hemorrhagic eccymoses, hemarthrosis, post surgical and post trauma bleeding, muscle hemorrhage. Bleeding from mucous membranes.

3

(Continued)

TABLE 3.2. *(Continued)*

Factor Name	Deficiency	Assessment
IX Plasma Thromboplastin Component (PTC, Christmas Factor, Antihemophilic Factor B)	Hemophilia B (Christmas Disease), liver disease, Vitamin K deficiency, hemorrhagic disease of the newborn.	Spontaneous hemorrhage eccymoses, hemarthrosis, post-surgical and post-trauma bleeding. Muscle hemorrhage.
X Stuart Factor (Stuart-Prower Factor)	Liver disease, Vitamin K deficiency, hemorrhagic disease of the newborn.	Menorrhagia, eccymosis, CNS bleeding, excessive bleeding after childbirth.
XI Plasma Thromboplastin Antecedent (Antihemophilic Factor C)	Hemophilia C, liver disease, Vitamin K malabsorption, congenital heart disease.	Mild bleeding, bruising, epistaxis, retinal hemorrhage.
XII Hageman Factor	Rare congenital disorders.	Asymptomatic.
XIII Fibrin Stabilizing Factor	Agammaglobulinemia, myeloma, pernicious anemia, severe liver disease, rare congenital deficiency.	Poor wound healing, prolonged post-traumatic bleeding.

Nursing Implications of Abnormal Findings

Assessment and Interventions. Areas to assess for deficiencies relate to each factor outlined in Table 3.2. Interventions are similar to those planned for any patient with a bleeding disorder. (See section on prothrombin time in this chapter).

BLEEDING TIME

Description

The test for *bleeding time* measures the amount of time bleeding occurs from a small incision in the skin. It is a test of hemostatic efficiency that is done to determine the presence of coagulation disorders. It provides information about the platelet function of aggregation and the ability of blood vessels to constrict. The interaction of these factors affects the duration and degree of bleeding. The accuracy of the results of this test depends upon the method used.

3

NORMAL RANGE	
Adults	
Ivy method	1–7 minutes
Duke method	1–3 minutes
Standardized template	3–7 minutes
Children (Ivy method)	1–6 minutes
Newborns (Ivy method)	1–5 minutes

Note. Laboratory results may be inaccurate if (1) the puncture is not of standard depth and width, or (2) the incision area is touched during the test, breaking off fibrin particles and prolonging the bleeding time.

Specimen Required

There are several methods of determining bleeding time. The three most common are the *Ivy*, *Duke*, and *Standardized Template* methods. When the Ivy method is used, a blood-pressure cuff is placed on the arm and the pressure is maintained at forty mm Hg. A small, clean incision is then made on the volar surface of the forearm 5 mm deep and 1 mm wide. The blood produced is gently removed with filter paper every 30 seconds until bleeding stops.

In the Duke method, the dependent position of the earlobe is punctured 1–2 mm deep. The blood produced is gently removed with filter paper every 30 seconds until bleeding stops. This method is less satisfactory than the Ivy method because the capillary supply is variable and a uniform increase in hydrostatic pressure cannot be maintained.

The standardized template bleeding time is the most sensitive method used. A blood-pressure cuff is placed around the upper arm and inflated to forty mm Hg. Two incisions nine mm long and one mm deep are made on the forearm. The blood is blotted every thirty seconds with filter paper until bleeding stops. An average of the two sites is recorded as the bleeding time.

Preparation of the Patient

There are no food or fluid restrictions before this test is performed. Patients should be advised not to drink alcoholic beverages or take aspirin for 5 days prior to the test. A note should be made on the laboratory slip if the patient is a diagnosed alcoholic or has taken the following drugs which may cause an increase in the bleeding time:

Sulfonamides	Chlorothiazide compounds
Dextran	Pantothenyl alcohol
Mithramycin	Streptokinase-streptodornase
Acetylsalicylic acid (aspirin)	Anticoagulants

Causes of Deviation from Normal

The bleeding time may be prolonged in diseases that are associated with low platelet count, such as thrombocytopenia. Prolonged bleeding time can also occur in patients with von Willebrand's disease, especially following the ingestion of aspirin. Several vascular disorders including leukemia, aplastic anemia, disseminated intravascular coagulation, hypothyroidism, multiple myeloma, pernicious anemia, and prolonged oral anticoagulant therapy are also associated with prolonged bleeding time.

Nursing Implications of Abnormal Findings

Assessment. When a patient has a prolonged bleeding time, the nurse should ask about incidents of bleeding, their frequency and length, and the association of the bleeding with any specific event or procedure. The patient should also be asked about recent anticoagulation therapy or the taking of drugs that may cause a prolonged bleeding time. In addition, the patient should be observed continuously for signs of bleeding. This should include examination of the skin and the interior of the mouth for signs of petechiae and ecchymoses, and observation of the stools and urine for signs of bleeding. The subtle signs of internal hemorrhage (fainting, tachycardia, hypotension, confusion) as well as overt signs of bleeding, such as a nosebleed, should also be part of the assessment.

Interventions. Nursing care is similar to that planned for any patient with a bleeding disorder (see the section on prothrombin time in this chapter). The patient should be protected from trauma while in bed or ambulating. An electric razor should be used for shaving and a soft toothbrush used to prevent bleeding gums. Constipation should also be prevented to avoid trauma to the anal and rectal mucosa. Intramuscular injections should be given with a small needle, pressure should be applied to the injection site for several minutes, and the site should be examined frequently for signs of bleeding. The patient should also be taught to carry an identification card that states his blood disorder and blood type. Patients with von Willebrand's disease should be told not to take aspirin or any over-the-counter medications that contain aspirin.

CLOT RETRACTION

Description

Clot retraction is a simple test that involves allowing blood to clot in a test tube without an anticoagulant. Since platelets are needed for clot retraction to occur, the speed and extent of clot retraction are used to determine the degree of platelet adequacy. The quantity and utilization of fibrinogen also influence clot retraction.

NORMAL RANGE

3

Adults and Children
It takes 1 hour for a normal clot to separate from the sides of the tube and shrink to one-half its original size by expressing forty to sixty percent of its serum. Complete retraction occurs within twenty-four hours.

Specimen Required
A 5-ml sample of venous blood is collected in a plain collecting tube or syringe.

Preparation of the Patient
There are no food or fluid restrictions before venipuncture.

Causes of Deviation from Normal
The degree of clot retraction and the quality of the clot are directly related to the number of platelets and their ability to function. When the platelet count is less than 100,000/cu mm, the clot will retract slowly and appear soft. See the section on platelet count for further discussion.

Clot retraction is increased in severe anemia and hypofibrinogenemia. It is decreased in thrombocytopenia, von Willebrand's disease, and in disorders in which there is an increase in erythrocyte concentration such as polycythemia.

Nursing Implications of Abnormal Findings
Assessment and Interventions. See the section on platelet count for a discussion of nursing care for patients who have prolonged clot retraction as a result of a decreased platelet count. If an anemia or polycythemia is the cause of an abnormal value, see the section on red cell count (Chapter 2) for a discussion of related nursing care.

COAGULATION TIME

Description
The *coagulation time tests* (Lee–White Clotting Time, Whole Blood Clotting Time) assess the overall ability of the blood to form a solid clot and measure the time it takes for this to occur. Coagulation time involves every factor in the coagulation process. Therefore, it is the least sensitive test for detecting

hemorrhagic disorders. Although a prolonged clotting time may indicate a serious disorder, mild or moderate hemorrhagic problems can go undetected. This test has been replaced by the Partial Thromboplastin Time in many settings, but may still be used for monitoring and regulating heparin therapy.

N O R M A L   R A N G E

Adults and Children
The normal range is 5 to 15 minutes when plain glass tubes are used and 24 to 35 minutes when the tubes are siliconized or plastic. The techniques and normal ranges for individual laboratories may vary from the normal values cited here.

Note. A normal clotting time does not rule out a clotting defect.

Specimen Required

A sample of venous blood is collected in a plain collecting tube or syringe and exactly 1 ml is put into each of three or four small test tubes. A note should be made on the laboratory slip if the patient is taking a drug that either increases or decreased the coagulation time (Table 3.3).

Preparation of the Patient

There are no food or fluid restrictions before venipuncture.

Causes of Deviation from Normal

Since the coagulation time measures the time it takes for the interaction of all factors in the coagulation process, it may be prolonged in any coagulation dis-

TABLE 3.3. Drugs that Affect Coagulation Time

Drugs that Cause an Increase	Drugs that Cause a Decrease
Azathioprine	Corticosteroids
Carbenicillin	Epinephrine
Heparin	
Mithramycin	
Tetracyclines	

order. Usually a severe deficiency must be present before coagulation time is prolonged.

The coagulation time is also affected by heparin therapy and may be used to determine the amount of anticoagulant present. When the test is used for this purpose, the coagulation time is measured before therapy is started, then again 1 hour before each succeeding dose is administered. If the patient shows signs of bleeding during heparin therapy, an additional measurement may be taken.

Nursing Implications of Abnormal Findings

Assessment and Interventions. The nursing care for a patient with a pro-longed coagulation time is similar to that for any patient with coagulation problems (see the sections on prothrombin time and bleeding time in this chapter). When a patient is on heparin therapy, the nurse should be aware of the possibility of a sudden massive hemorrhage and should be continually alert to signs and symptoms of sudden hemorrhage. Protamine sulfate, the antidote for heparin overdose and hemorrhage, should be readily available.

EUGLOBIN LYSIS TIME

Description

The *euglobin lysis time* is done to assess fibrinolytic activity. Euglobins are pro-teins that precipitate from acidified dilute plasma. The euglobin fraction con-tains fibrinogen, plasminogen, and plasminogen activator. Since there is very little antiplasmin activity, the euglobin fraction does not inhibit fibrinolysis. Therefore, a shortened euglobin lysis time indicates an increase in fi-brinolytic activity.

N O R M A L   R A N G E
Venous blood is acidified and mixed with calcium to form a clot. The euglobin lysis time is the time it takes for the formed clot to lyse. Adults and children

Normal lysis	2–6 hours
Increased fibrinolysis	less than 2 hours

Specimen Required

A 5-ml sample of venous blood is collected in a collecting tube contain-ing sodium citrate. The puncture site should not be rubbed vigorously, nor should there be excessive pumping of the fist. Pressure should be applied to the puncture site for 3–5 minutes. The tourniquet should be released as soon as the vein is entered.

Preparation of the Patient
Food and fluids are not restricted before venipuncture.

Causes of Deviation from Normal
An increase in fibrinolysis resulting in a shortened euglobin lysis time occurs in primary hyperfibrinolysis, cancer of the prostate or pancreas, incompatible blood transfusions, liver disease, and in fibrinolytic therapy with streptokinase. It may also be increased for several days following surgery.

Nursing Implications of Abnormal Findings
Assessment. When a patient has a decreased euglobin lysis time, the nurse should observe the patient for signs of bleeding. This includes examination of the skin and interior of the mouth for petechiae and eccymoses. Stools and urine should also be observed for signs of bleeding.

Interventions. Nursing care is similar to that planned for any patient with a bleeding disorder. The patient should be protected from trauma, advised to use a soft toothbrush to prevent trauma to the oral cavity, and use an electric razor to prevent cuts while shaving. Parenteral injections should be given with a small gauge needle and pressure applied to the site for 3–5 minutes after administration.

FIBRINOGEN

Description
Fibrinogen (clotting factor I) is a large protein molecule that is synthesized by the liver and present in soluble form in the plasma. It is an essential component of the blood clotting mechanism and is converted to fibrin strands by the splitting action of thrombin during the coagulation process.

NORMAL RANGE	
Adults and children	200–400 mg/dl
Newborns	160–300 mg/dl

Specimen Required
Venous blood should be collected in a tube that contains the anticoagulant required by the laboratory performing the test. Sodium oxalate is the most com-

monly used anticoagulant, although in some instances sodium citrate may be used. The entire tube should be filled with blood.

Preparation of the Patient

Food and fluids are usually not restricted before venipuncture. Digital pressure should be maintained over the puncture site for 2–3 minutes after the procedure. The venipuncture site should also be checked for further bleeding.

3

Causes of Deviation from Normal

Decreases in fibrinogen levels can be caused by congenital deficiencies in which (1) no fibrinogen is present (afibrinogenemia), (2) the amount of fibrinogen is less than 100 mg/dl (hypofibrinogenemia), and (3) fibrinogen is present in normal amounts but becomes decreased when thrombin is added during clot formation (dysfibrinogenemia). Hepatic disorders may also cause decreases in fibrinogen levels, since fibrinogen is synthesized by the liver; however, fibrinogen deficiency is not a common complication, since several procoagulants are also synthesized there. Hemorrhage and disseminated intravascular coagulation (DIC) may also cause hypofibrinogenemia. There is a normal increase in fibrinogen during pregnancy. Fibrinogen levels may also increase during inflammatory diseases, multiple myeloma, cancer, uremia, and hepatitis.

Nursing Implications of Abnormal Findings

Assessment and Interventions. When assessing a patient with a low fibrinogen level, it is important to find out if the abnormality causing the decrease is a long-standing congenital process or an acquired deficiency. If it is congenital, nursing interventions are related to the specific inherited defect. When hypofibrinogenemia (fibrinogenopenia) is caused by liver disease, hepatic damage is probably severe and a poor prognosis can be anticipated. Nursing interventions include continual evaluation of the clinical state of the patient in anticipation of a massive bleeding episode. The nurse should be ready to act quickly if one should occur, and should plan for the possibility that the patient may not recover. Plans should be made to assist the patient and family members who are aware of the poor prognosis. The nurse should also prepare for the possible psychological effect hemorrhage may have on the patient. See Fibrinogen Degradation Products for nursing care of patients with DIC.

FIBRINOGEN DEGRADATION PRODUCTS

Description

Fibrinogen degradation products (FDP's) or fibrinogen split products (FSP's) are the partially digested fragments that result from the lysis of fibrin by plasmin. They may also be released by the digestion of fibrinogen. FDP's have an anticoagulant effect that inhibits blood clotting when they circulate in large quantities.

N O R M A L   R A N G E

Adults	The normal FDP serum level is less than 10 μg/ml.
Children	Consult laboratory for reference values.

Specimen Required

A 5-ml sample of venous blood is obtained in a plain collecting tube or syringe. This test is performed on serum. The FDP's remain after fibrinogen is removed by means of clotting. Because this test may be done in conjunction with other tests of coagulation, the individual laboratory should be consulted about the type of specimen required.

Preparation of the Patient

There are no food or fluid restrictions before venipuncture.

Causes of Deviation from Normal

Fibrinogen degradation products accumulate in the blood in pathologic conditions associated with extensive intravascular clotting. DIC is the most common, although FDP's may also be high in thromboembolic disorders and in renal diseases. Increases may also be seen in venous thrombosis, pulmonary embolism, burns, infections, acute leukemia, hypoxia, and incompatible blood transfusions. In DIC the FDP's inhibit blood clotting by acting as anticoagulants, prolonging the thrombin clotting time by delaying polymerization of fibrin.

Nursing Implications of Abnormal Findings

Assessment. The nurse is often the first person to identify the signs and symptoms of DIC. When an increase in FDP's is the only clue that DIC may be present, the patient must be assessed frequently and carefully for any early manifestations, such as petechiae, ecchymoses, hemoptysis, hematuria, epistaxis, bloody stools, or oozing of blood from injection sites or other puncture wounds. Unexplained hypotension, particularly in the presence of hemorrhagic manifestations, may also indicate the presence of DIC. The following abnormal hematologic studies should be reported as soon as the data is received: (1) prolonged prothrombin time, (2) prolonged partial thromboplastin time, (3) prolonged thrombin clotting time, and/or (4) fibrinogen deficiency.

Interventions. The primary nursing interventions for patients with DIC are related to the nursing assessment of the patient and the medical treatment. Once any sign or symptom of obvious or occult bleeding is noted, steps should be taken to prevent further bleeding, such as protecting the skin and mucous membranes from trauma, giving medications through existing IV lines when possible, and cleaning the mouth and teeth with cotton swabs and a soft water spray to prevent gingival bleeding. Blood loss should be measured accurately when possible, and blood products should be administered with precautions taken to avoid side effects. A more detailed discussion of DIC can be found in medical-surgical nursing texts.

3

PARTIAL THROMBOPLASTIN TIME: ACTIVATED PARTIAL THROMBOPLASTIN TIME

Description

The *partial thromboplastin time* (PTT) is a screening test used to detect deficiencies in all plasma clotting factors except factors VII and XIII and platelets. The test is most helpful in detecting deficiencies in the formation of intrinsic thromboplastin. PTT is most likely to be prolonged by deficits in stage I of blood coagulation (Fig. 3.1). This test is not sensitive enough to identify mild deficiencies and will only be prolonged when factors in this stage fall below 25% of normal. PTT is more specific than the coagulation time and is often used to monitor heparin therapy. The activated partial thromboplastin time (APTT) is a modification of the PTT and can also be used to monitor heparin therapy and be used to detect coagulation deficiencies.

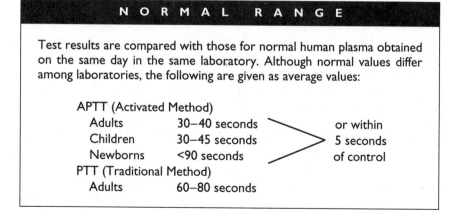

NORMAL RANGE

Test results are compared with those for normal human plasma obtained on the same day in the same laboratory. Although normal values differ among laboratories, the following are given as average values:

APTT (Activated Method)
Adults   30–40 seconds
Children   30–45 seconds   or within
Newborns   <90 seconds   5 seconds
                                    of control
PTT (Traditional Method)
Adults   60–80 seconds

Specimen Required

A 5-ml sample of venous blood should be collected in a collecting tube containing sodium oxalate or sodium citrate. The tube must be filled to capacity and delivered to the laboratory immediately. If the patient is receiving heparin, note the time and route of the last dose.

Preparation of the Patient

There are no food or fluid restrictions before venipuncture.

Causes of Deviation from Normal

One of the most common causes of a prolonged PTT is the presence in the blood of medically prescribed heparin. The PTT is used to monitor the effects of heparin, and dosage is adjusted depending on the test results. In general, it is maintained between two–three times the baseline PTT when there is a continuous heparin infusion.

The PTT may also be prolonged in patients with liver disease (cirrhosis and obstructive jaundice), DIC, salicylate therapy, vitamin K deficiency, and deficiencies of any factors necessary for stage I of blood coagulation.

A decrease in the PTT is not common but may be seen in extensive cancer without liver involvement, after acute hemorrhage, or in the early stages of DIC.

Nursing Implications of Abnormal Findings

Assessment. When the PTT is prolonged, the patient should be assessed for any signs of bleeding. The skin and mucous membranes should be examined for petechiae, ecchymoses, or hematomas. Stools should be checked for bright red bleeding or for the black, tarry appearance that occurs with the passage of old blood. The urine should be examined for hematuria and the patient observed for any signs of nosebleed. The nurse should also observe for signs of internal hemorrhage, such as tachycardia, hypotension, confusion, disorientation, air hunger, and faintness. When the PTT is abnormal because of liver disease, the nurse should be aware of the poor prognosis that accompanies this sign and should observe the patient closely for evidence of a worsening condition or sudden onset of a massive hemorrhage.

Interventions. When a patient's PTT is prolonged in response to heparin therapy, the nurse must know what the therapeutic level for the patient is and report any significant alterations in either direction as soon as they occur. The medication should be held and the physician consulted if the PTT is prolonged far beyond the therapeutic range. The patient should also be protected from trauma, particularly when on bedrest. Any person with a prolonged PTT should be advised to use a soft toothbrush to prevent trauma to the oral cavity, to use an electric razor to prevent cuts while shaving, and to avoid situations that may result in bruising of tissue. Parenteral injections should be given with caution, using a small-gauge needle and applying pressure to the injection site for several minutes following withdrawal of the needle. When patients who are receiving heparin are to be placed on long-term anticoagulant therapy, the teaching plan discussed in the section on prothrombin time should be followed.

PLATELET COUNT

3

Description

Platelets, also called thrombocytes, are large, non-nucleated cells derived from the megakaryocytes produced in the bone marrow. Two-thirds are found in the blood and one-third in the spleen. One-tenth of the platelets found in the blood maintain endothelial integrity and the rest are available for hemostasis. The adhesive or sticky quality of platelets allows them to clump and adhere to injured surfaces. They form a platelet plug that occludes breaks in the integrity of small vessels. Along with fibrin, they form the network for a clot.

NORMAL RANGE	
Adults	150,000–400,000/mm³ or 150–400 10⁹/L
Children	200,000–473,000/mm³ or 200–473 10⁹/L
Newborns	140,000–300,000/mm³ or 140–300 10⁹/L

Specimen Required

A 5–10-ml sample of venous blood is collected in a tube containing disodium edetate (EDTA).

Preparation of the Patient

There are no food or fluid restrictions before venipuncture.

Causes of Deviation from Normal

It should be noted that an abnormal platelet count does not necessarily indicate that a pathological condition is present. Decreased platelet counts may be seen in newborns during the first few days of life or in women during the two weeks prior to the onset of menstruation. Increases may be seen in individuals living at high altitudes or following intense physical exercise. Platelet counts may also be higher in winter than in summer. Aspirin can alter platelet function for up to a week by interfering with the enzyme activity that gives platelets their "stickiness".

Disorders in the platelet count may result in a decrease or increase in the number of circulating platelets. A decrease in the number of platelets to below

100,000/cu mm is called thrombocytopenia, a disorder that may have several causes. These include idiopathic thrombocytopenic purpura, bone marrow injury or failure, lesions involving the bone marrow such as carcinoma, leukemia, and lymphoma, deficiencies of vitamin B_{12} or folic acid, infection, loss by hemorrhage and massive blood transfusion, and destruction caused by systemic lupus erythematosus, hemolytic anemias, and the toxic effects of drugs (see Table 2.6).

Platelets may be temporarily elevated, a condition called thrombocytosis. This may occur as a result of hemorrhage, surgery, splenectomy, iron deficiency, or chronic inflammatory disorders. Thrombocytosis may also be associated with carcinoma and Hodgkin's disease. A sustained elevation of the platelet count is called thrombocythemia. It may occur alone or be associated with polycythemia vera, chronic myelogenous leukemia, or myelosclerosis.

Nursing Implications of Abnormal Findings

Assessment and Interventions. The nursing care of a patient with an abnormal platelet count should focus on the possibility of spontaneous and prolonged bleeding, which can occur with either thrombocytopenia or thrombocytosis. (See the section on prothrombin time in this chapter for a detailed discussion of related nursing care.) In addition, patients with an increased platelet count may have venous or arterial thrombosis. Because a detailed discussion of these complications is not within the scope of this text, refer to a general medical-surgical textbook for this information.

PLATELET AGGREGATION

Description

Platelet aggregation tests measure the ability of platelets to adhere to each other when mixed with substances known to cause their aggregation. Adenosine Diphosphate (ADP) is added to a mixture of platelets, collagen, epinephrine, and thrombin after which the rate and percentage of aggregation is measured. If von Willebrand's disease or Bernard-Soulier syndrome is suspected, the antibiotic agent ristocetin is added.

NORMAL RANGE

Platelet aggregates should be visible in 3–5 minutes.

Specimen Required

A 5-ml sample of venous blood is collected in a tube containing sodium citrate. The sample must be kept at room temperature.

Preparation of Patient

Food and fluids except water are restricted overnight for eight hours before venipuncture. Aspirin or aspirin compounds should not be taken for 7–10 days prior to the test. Medications the patient is taking should be listed on the laboratory slip.

Causes of Deviation from Normal

A decrease in platelet aggregation may be caused by von Willebrand's disease, Bernard-Soulier syndrome, Glanzmann's thromboasthenia, acute leukemia, infectious mononucleosis, idiopathic thrombocytopenic purpura, cirrhosis of the liver, or uremia. Aspirin and aspirin compounds can also cause a decrease in platelet aggregation. An increase may be seen in diabetes mellitus and hyperlipidemia.

3

Nursing Implications of Abnormal Findings

Assessment and Interventions. The nursing care of a patient with decreased platelet aggregation should focus on the possibility of prolonged peripheral bleeding and excessive bruising. A medication history should be taken and patients advised not to take over-the-counter drugs containing aspirin or aspirin compounds. A medical-surgical textbook should be consulted for nursing care related to specific disorders which cause abnormal test results.

PROTHROMBIN CONSUMPTION TIME

Description

The *prothrombin consumption time* (PCT), or *serum prothrombin time*, is performed to measure the capacity of stage I to generate thromboplastin. When a clot forms, thromboplastin converts most of the available prothrombin to thrombin, leaving only about twenty-five percent or less prothrombin in the serum. When there is a defect in the factors in stage I of the clotting mechanisms that produce thromboplastin, a high concentration of prothrombin will be left in the serum.

NORMAL RANGE

Almost complete consumption occurs in fifteen to twenty seconds. More than eighty percent should be consumed in one hour.

Specimen Required

A 7-ml sample of venous blood is obtained in a syringe with no anticoagulant added. The specimen is then placed in a nonsiliconized glass tube. Care should be taken to prevent hemolysis or agitation of the blood, since both may accelerate prothrombin consumption.

Preparation of the Patient

There are no food or fluid restrictions before venipuncture.

Causes of Deviation from Normal

A deficiency in any of the factors involved in stage I of the coagulation process will cause a decrease in the prothrombin consumption time. A decrease in the number of platelets (thrombocytopenia) may also cause a shortened PCT, since normal platelet function is necessary for the generation of thromboplastin. DIC, liver disease, hemophilia, and heparin therapy may also decrease the PCT.

Nursing Implications of Abnormal Findings

The nursing care for patients with abnormal prothrombin consumption time is the same as that discussed in the sections on prothrombin time and partial thromboplastin time.

PROTHROMBIN TIME

Description

Prothrombin (factor II) is manufactured in the liver and synthesized by a process that requires vitamin K. Prothrombin is present in normal plasma and is an inactive precursor in the coagulation process, being enzymatically converted to thrombin during clot formation. The test of prothrombin time (pro. time, PT) determines defects in the extrinsic clotting mechanism by reflecting the activity of fibrinogen (factor I), prothrombin (factor II), and factors V, VII, and X.

N O R M A L R A N G E	
Adults	12–14 seconds
Children	11–14 seconds
Newborns	<17 seconds

The prothrombin time should be assessed by comparing the patient's PT to the control time that is also included in the laboratory report. When the prothrombin time is being used to determine the adequacy of anticoagulant therapy, the therapeutic range is 2–2.5 times the normal control. For example, if the normal control is 14 seconds, the patient's PT should be approximately 28–35 seconds.

3

The normal range (12–14 seconds) is considered to be 100% of normal activity. Because the curve relating the percent of normal activity to the prothrombin time in seconds is not a straight line, a strict percent is not an accurate reflection of the small changes that can occur in prothrombin activity.

Specimen Required

A 5-ml specimen of venous blood is collected in a tube that contains sodium citrate or a sodium oxalate solution. The tube should be filled to capacity.

Preparation of the Patient

Food and fluids are usually not restricted before venipuncture. Several medications may affect the prothrombin time (Table 3.4). If a patient is taking one of

TABLE 3.4. Drugs that Affect Prothrombin Time

Drugs Causing Increased Values	Drugs Causing Decreased Values
Alcohol	Barbiturates
Anabolic steroids	Chloral hydrate
Antibiotics	Corticosteroids
Anticoagulants (oral)	Digitalis
Cathartics	Ethchlorovynol (Placidyl)
Chlordiazepoxide (Librium)	Glutethimide (Doriden)
Chlorpromazine	Griseolfulvin
Cimetidine (Tagamet)	Metaproterenol (Alupent)
Clofibrate (Atromid-S)	Oral contraceptives
Methyldopa (Aldomet)	Rifampin
Morphine	Vitamin K
Phenylbutazone (Butazolidin)	
Phenytoin (Dilantin)	
Quinidine	
Quinine	
Reserpine	
Salicylates	
Sulfonamides	
Thyroid hormones	

these drugs, it should be noted on the laboratory slip. Digital pressure should be maintained over the puncture site for 2–3 minutes after the procedure. The venipuncture site should also be checked for further bleeding.

Causes of Deviation from Normal

When the prothrombin content of the blood is decreased, the prothrombin time is said to be prolonged and the clotting ability of the blood diminished. One of the most common causes of an increased prothrombin time is the presence of medically prescribed anticoagulants in the blood. The prothrombin time is used to monitor the effects of coumarin-type anticoagulants, and the dosage is adjusted depending on the test results. In general, the prothrombin time is kept within 2–2.5 times the normal, which is comparable to 20–30% of normal activity. The prothrombin time can also be prolonged if the plasma contains normal levels of most factors, lacking only a few specific factors.

Because vitamin K is essential for the synthesis of prothrombin, a deficiency in or malabsorption of this vitamin could cause a decrease in prothrombin activity and a prolonged prothrombin time. Hepatic disease may cause a prolonged prothrombin time, either by interference with the synthesis of prothrombin or the intestinal uptake of vitamin K. The hepatocellular necrosis that occurs in hepatitis and cirrhosis can interfere with prothrombin synthesis and result in a prolonged prothrombin time, which may give some indication of the severity of the damage. A severely prolonged prothrombin time is an indication that damage is extensive and the prognosis poor. On the other hand, in milder forms of hepatitis or cirrhosis the prothrombin time may be close to normal.

Obstructive jaundice also prolongs the prothrombin time because of interference with the bile salts necessary for the intestinal synthesis of vitamin K. When this interference occurs, the parenteral administration of vitamin K rapidly restores the prothrombin time to normal. This *vitamin K prothrombin time test* helps differentiate between obstructive and hepatocellular jaundice; however, it is not conclusive because patients with obstructive jaundice may have only a slightly prolonged prothrombin time that cannot be assessed with the administration of vitamin K.

The prothrombin time may also be affected by the ingestion of drugs (Table 3.4).

Nursing Implications of Abnormal Findings

Assessment. When the prothrombin time is prolonged, the patient should be assessed for any signs of bleeding, however subtle. The skin and mucous membranes should be examined for petechiae, ecchymoses, or hematomas. Stools should be checked for bright red bleeding or for the black tarry appearance that occurs with the passage of old blood. The urine should be examined for hematuria and the patient observed for any signs of nosebleeds. The nurse should also observe for signs of internal hemorrhage, such as tachycardia, hypotension, confusion, disorientation, air hunger, and faintness. When the prothrombin time is abnormal because of liver disease, the nurse should be aware of the poor prognosis that accompanies this sign and should observe the patient closely for evidence of deteriorating condition or sudden onset of a massive hemorrhage.

Interventions. When a patient's prothrombin time is prolonged, the physician should be informed if a drug that can interfere with the prothrombin level has been ordered. If the prothrombin time is being monitored for an anticoagulant therapy, the nurse must know what the therapeutic level for the patient is and must report any significant alterations in this as soon as the data are known. If the patient is receiving daily doses of an anticoagulant, the medication should be held and the physician consulted if the prothrombin time is far beyond the therapeutic range. The patient should also be protected from trauma, particularly when on bed rest. Any person with a prolonged prothrombin time should be advised to use a soft toothbrush to prevent trauma to the oral cavity, to use an electric razor to prevent cuts while shaving, and to avoid situations that may result in bruising of tissues. Parenteral injections should be given with caution. The nurse should use a small-gauge needle and apply pressure to the injection site for several minutes after administration. Rectal temperatures should not be taken because the irritation to the rectal mucosa may cause bleeding.

Patients who are receiving anticoagulants for a long period of time should be given an individualized teaching plan that includes information about the bleeding tendencies associated with a prolonged prothrombin time, as well as information about medications that can affect it. When a severe bump or bruise has occurred as a result of trauma, patients should be taught to apply ice packs to the area. They should also be told about the importance of informing any physician or dentist who cares for them that their prothrombin time is prolonged due to anticoagulant therapy.

Patients should call their physician if they cough up or vomit any bright red or dark brown blood. If gastrointestinal bleeding is or has been a problem, patients should be taught to test their stools periodically for occult blood (see Chapter 1).

THROMBIN TIME

Description

This test is done to measure the time required for a fibrin clot to form when thrombin is added to plasma. Because this test artificially bypasses stages I and II of the coagulation process, deficits due to fibrinogen abnormalities in stage

III (the last stage of coagulation) can be detected. Thrombin time can also be used to monitor a person's response to heparin therapy.

NORMAL RANGE

The normal range of thrombin time varies in different laboratories. In most places 10–15 seconds is considered normal. Test results are usually compared to a normal control value that is included in the laboratory report. In general, a thrombin time 1.3 times the normal control time is considered abnormal.

Specimen Required

A 7-ml sample of venous blood is collected in a collecting tube or syringe containing sodium citrate or sodium oxalate. Blood should be drawn 1 hour before heparin administration when the test is being used to monitor heparin therapy.

Preparation of the Patient

There are no food or fluid restrictions before venipuncture.

Causes of Deviation from Normal

The most common cause of an increased thrombin time is a defect or alteration in the structure of fibrinogen, which may include either afibrinogenemia or dysfibrinogenemia. Hypofibrinogenemia associated with acute leukemia, lymphoma, or poor nutrition may also be the cause. The thrombin time may also be prolonged in multiple myeloma and in cirrhosis of the liver. Heparin therapy also prolongs thrombin time.

Nursing Implications of Abnormal Findings

Assessment and Interventions. The nursing implications for a patient with a prolonged thrombin time are the same as those discussed for partial thromboplastin time, including the care of patients receiving heparin therapy.

TOURNIQUET TEST (RUMPEL-LEEDE POSITIVE PRESSURE TEST, CAPILLARY FRAGILITY TEST)

Description

The *tourniquet test* (Rumpel-Leede Positive Pressure Test, Capillary Fragility Test, or Negative Pressure Test) evaluates the ability of capillaries to remain intact under the stress of external pressure. When capillary fragility is increased, petechiae will appear if positive pressure is applied using a tourniquet. The ability of platelets to occlude small gaps between endothelial cells of the capillary walls also affects petechiae formation.

3

N O R M A L   R A N G E

Usually no petechiae form; however, formation of from 1–10 petechiae within an area the size of a quarter is considered normal. The presence of 5–10 petechiae after five minutes may be questionable, whereas the presence of more than twenty indicates abnormal hemostatic function. A grading of from 1+ to 4+ is used to describe positive results. The scale is as follows when an arm is used:

1+	a few petechiae over anterior forearm
2+	many petechiae over anterior forearm
3+	many petechiae over the whole arm and top of hand
4+	confluent petechiae in all areas of arm and top of hand

Some adults normally have a positive reaction depending on the texture, thickness, and temperature of their skin. In addition, capillary fragility may be increased in women over age 40 with decreasing estrogen levels, in patients with measles or influenza, or in women who are premenstrual.

Specimen Required

This test is performed by placing a blood-pressure cuff on the limb and inflating it to a point midway between systolic and diastolic pressure, with a maximum level of 100 mm Hg. The pressure is maintained for five minutes, following which the number of petechiae that have appeared on the forearm, wrist, hand, and fingers are counted. These areas should be inspected for the presence of any petechiae or eccyhmoses before the cuff is applied. Repeat tests should not be performed on the same arm for at least a week because the results will be unreliable.

Preparation of the Patient

The patient should be told about the way the test will be performed and that bruising may occur as a result of it.

Causes of Deviation from Normal

Minimally positive results may occur in several hematological conditions, such as polycythemia vera, vitamin K deficiency, von Willebrand's disease, and severe prothrombin, fibrinogen, and factor VII deficiencies. Strongly positive results accompany diseases in which capillary fragility and platelet formation are inadequate, such as idiopathic and secondary thrombocytopenic purpura and scurvy.

Nursing Implications of Abnormal Findings

Assessment and Interventions. Observation of the extent of petechiae and ecchymoses present and the ease with which bruising occurs are the most important areas of nursing assessment. Protection of the patient from trauma is the primary goal of nursing care. Specific interventions depend on the severity of the problem and the patient's daily activities. The precautions taken in the hospital can be discussed with the patient and used as a foundation for developing a teaching plan to use following discharge. If the patient must make a change in life-style or job, the nurse will have to provide guidance and support.

BIBLIOGRAPHY

Byrne, C.J., D.F. Saxton, P.K. Pelikan, and P.M. Nugent. *Laboratory Tests: Implications for Nursing Care*. Menlo Park: Addison-Wesley, 1986.

Gaedeke-Norris, M.K. "Lab Test Tips—How To Evaluate Platelet Values." *Nursing 91*, 21:20 (February 1991).

Henry, J.B. *Clinical Diagnosis and Management by Laboratory Methods*. Philadelphia: W.B. Saunders Co., 1991.

Ignatavicius, D.D., and M.V. Bayne. *Medical-Surgical Nursing: A Nursing Process Approach*. Philadelphia: W.B. Saunders, 1991.

Lucas, F. "Lab Tests Plus Diagnostic Clues Equals Diagnosis of Bleeding Disorders." *Diagnostic Medicine*, 6:65–66, 68, 70 (November–December, 1983).

Lewis, S.M., and I.C. Collier. *Medical-Surgical Nursing: Assessment and Management of Clinical Problems*. St. Louis: Mosby Yearbook, 1992.

Luckman, J., and K.C. Sorensen. *Medical-Surgical Nursing: A Psychophysiological Approach*. Philadelphia: Saunders, 1987.

Phipps, W.S., B.C. Long, N.F. Woods, and V. Cossmeyer. *Medical-Surgical Nursing*. St. Louis: Mosby Yearbook, 1991.

Ravel, R. *Clinical Laboratory Medicine*. Chicago: Year Book Medical Publishers, 1989.

Rifkind, R.A. *Fundamentals of Hematology*. Chicago: Year Book Medical Publishers, 1986.

Sacher, R.A., and R.A. McPherson. *Widmann's Clinical Interpretation of Laboratory Tests*. Philadelphia: F.A. Davis, 1991.

Sacher, R.A. "Laboratory Tests for Cost-Effective Evaluation." *Consultant*, 26:60–66 (November, 1986).

Smetzer, S.C., and B.G. Ball. *Brunner and Sudarth's Medical-Surgical Nursing.* New York: J.B. Lippincott, 1992.

Vander, A.S., S.H. Sherman, and D.S. Luciano. *Human Physiology: The Mechanisms of Body Function.* New York: McGraw-Hill, 1990.

Williams, W.J., E. Beutler, and A.J. Erslen. *Hematology.* New York: McGraw-Hill, 1990.

Wilson, J., et al. *Harrison's Principles of Internal Medicine.* New York: McGraw-Hill Inc., 1991.

3

4

Laboratory Tests of Cardiovascular Function

Creatine Phosphokinase
(Creatine Kinase, CPK Isoenzymes)

Aspartate Aminotransferase
(Glutamic Oxaloacetic
Transaminase)

Lactic Dehydrogenase

Alpha-Hydroxybutyrate
Dehydrogenase

Plasma Lipids
Cholesterol
Triglycerides
Lipoproteins

CREATINE PHOSPHOKINASE
(CREATINE KINASE, CPK ISOENZYMES)

Description

Creatine phosphokinase (CPK), also called *creatine kinase* (CK) is an enzyme. Its storage contributes to energy in the cell. Specifically, CPK is a catalyst in the reversible reaction of creatine phosphate and adenosine diphosphate (ADP) to creatine and adenosine triphosphate (ATP). It is normally found in high concentrations in skeletal muscle, brain tissue, and myocardium, with small amounts being present in a few other organs. There are three CPK isoenzymes of differing molecular structure labeled CPK_1 (BB), CPK_2 (MB), and CPK_3 (MM). CPK_1 (BB) is found in the brain, lungs, bladder, and bowel; CPK_2 (MB) is found almost exclusively in the myocardium; CPK_3 (MM) is found in skeletal and heart muscle.

N O R M A L R A N G E		
Adults		
Men	55–170 U/l at 37°C	5–35 µg/ml
Women	30–135 U/l at 37°C	5–35 µg/ml
Children		
Male	0–70 IU/l at 30°C	
Female	0–50 IU/l at 30°C	
Newborns	10–300 IU/l at 30°C	
Isoenzymes		
CPK_1 (MM)	94–100%	5–70 IU/l
CPK_2 (MB)	0–6%	0–7 IU/l
CPK_3 (BB)	0%	0 IU/l

4

Specimen Required

A 5-ml sample of venous blood is obtained in a plain collecting tube or syringe. When completed enzyme studies or isoenzyme analyses are to be done, a 15–30-ml sample of blood may be needed. Because the value of enzyme studies for diagnosis depends on serial analysis of enzymes, each specimen must be labeled with the time the blood was drawn.

Preparation of the Patient

Food and drink are not usually restricted before venipuncture. Because intramuscular injections may cause an elevation of CPK, a note should be made on the laboratory slip if the patient has received an intramuscular injection during the previous 24–48 hours.

Causes of Deviation from Normal

An elevation of serum CPK is most often associated with myocardial damage, specifically myocardial infarction (MI). CPK also rises during diseases of the striated muscle fibers, after muscular trauma such as vigorous exercise, in alcoholic myopathy, after major surgery, and after intramuscular injections. Other less frequent causes of an elevated CPK are electrical cardioversion, cardiac catheterization, and stroke.

The value of CPK as a diagnostic aid is increased when the isoenzymes are separated by electrophoresis. Since CPK_2 (MB) is found only in myocardial tissue, it is present in the serum for forty-eight hours after an acute MI. It may also be present in patients with severe myocardial ischemia. The rise and fall of this enzyme in association with acute MI are shown in Figure 4.1.

Elevation of the isoenzyme CPK_1 (BB) occurs after a cerebrovascular accident (CVA). When isoenzyme levels are reported, percentage levels of each are given. Table 4.1 compares isoenzyme levels after an MI or a CVA with the normal levels.

Nursing Implications of Abnormal Findings

Assessment. When a patient has an elevated CPK, it is important to remember that an increase in the serum level of this enzyme alone is not an absolute indicator that a specific disease is present. Some people with diseases that destroy muscle fiber have an increase in serum CPK; however, a common cause of an elevated CPK is damage to the myocardium. When the nursing assessment shows strong evidence that an MI has occurred, the nurse must determine if any intramuscular injections have been given to the patient. This step is particularly important when a person has received an injection for chest pain that may not be of cardiac origin. The resulting elevation in CPK, along with the symptom of pain, can lead to a false assumption that an MI has occurred. It is also important to note the number of intramuscular injections that have been given. When a series of enzyme studies have been done to determine the extent of damage, intramuscular injections can cause a higher level of CPK than that resulting from an MI. If given repeatedly, injections can also result in a prolonged elevation of this enzyme. When serial enzyme levels are ordered, results should be evaluated to determine the extent of the patient's infarction or if reinfarction has occurred. CPK normally appears in the blood serum within six hours after an MI has occurred and returns to normal in 48–72 hours if there has been no further damage.

All clinical manifestations exhibited by the patient must also be followed. If

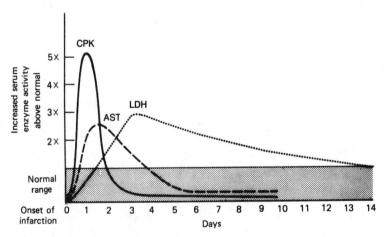

FIGURE 4.1. Serum enzyme level changes after myocardial infarction (CPK—creatinine phosphokinase; AST—aspartate aminotransferase; LDH—lactic dehydrogenase)

TABLE 4.1. CPK Isoenzyme Levels during Myocardial Infarction and Cardiovascular Accident

	CPK$_1$ (BB)	CPK$_2$ (MB)	CPK$_3$ (MM)
MI	0	60%	40%
CVA	80%	0	20%
Normal	0	0	100%

4

it is known that the patient has a disease affecting muscle fibers, the nursing assessment and related interventions should focus on problems related to that specific disease. When myocardial damage is the suspected cause of an elevated CPK, the patient should be evaluated for the presence of the heavy, crushing, squeezing substernal chest pain associated with the presence of an MI. In addition, the presence of pallor, cyanosis, and moisture of the skin, fatigue, the apical and radial pulse rate and rhythm, blood pressure, temperature, respirations, the presence of abnormal heart sounds, and the presence of peripheral edema should be noted. The patient's fluid balance should also be assessed daily. When an acute MI has occurred, an attempt should be made to determine the patient's life-style before the infarction, as well as the patient's psychological response to the diagnosis.

Interventions. Nursing interventions depend on the problems identified and the severity of the myocardial damage. The extensive nursing care that must be planned for a patient who has had an MI is described in medical-surgical nursing texts. The following is a brief discussion of some of the nursing interventions planned for a patient who has had an MI.

When pain is present, its extent and location must be evaluated and vital signs (blood pressure, pulse, respirations) taken before and after morphine sulfate (the analgesic usually ordered) is administered, since this drug can depress respirations and lower the blood pressure. A patient who is dyspneic may be placed in a modified Fowler's position to lower the diaphragm and increase lung expansion. A footboard and pillows may be used to help the patient maintain a comfortable position. When oxygen has been ordered, the patient's need for, and response to, oxygen therapy must be evaluated.

The nurse can provide the supplies needed to perform simple tasks so that an anxious patient may be allowed to participate in morning care. The change in activity caused by an MI should be explained and attempts made to establish a trusting relationship. If a mild sedative has been ordered, the patient should be observed for any side effects of the drug. Nursing care should also focus on reducing or eliminating the potential sources of stress and anxiety that are present in a coronary-care unit.

When a patient is exhibiting signs of denial, nursing interventions must be planned to assist the patient through the stages of grief and grieving. Consultation with a psychiatric nurse specialist may be helpful in this situation.

The amount of time the patient remains on bed rest depends on the extent of myocardial damage and the physician's plan of care. Whatever the medical plan, the nurse should provide for adequate rest periods during the day, place call light and supplies within easy reach, and omit baths when excessive fatigue is observed.

When changes in vital signs occur, the nurse should determine if there is an apparent cause for the change, such as increased anxiety or the administration of an analgesic, such as morphine. A report of the change should be noted. When arrhythmias are observed, medication should be administered as ordered and the patient's response reported. Life-threatening arrhythmias should be treated according to the protocols established by the medical and nursing staff in each hospital.

ASPARTATE AMINOTRANSFERASE (GLUTAMIC OXALOACETIC TRANSAMINASE)

Description

Aspartate aminotransferase (AST) is an enzyme that contributes to protein metabolism. Specifically, it is important in the biosynthesis of amino acids because it catalyzes the reversible transfer of an amino group between glutamic and aspartic acid. The old term for this enzyme was glutamic oxaloacetic transaminase (GOT). This enzyme is found in cardiac tissue; lesser amounts are found in hepatic tissue, skeletal muscle, and renal and cerebral tissue. When cell damage occurs, AST is released into the bloodstream.

N O R M A L R A N G E	
*Adults and children	0–40 Frankel U/ml
	4–36 IU/l
	16–60 Karmen U/ml
Newborns	Higher values—up to four times the adult level.
	Consult each laboratory for normal ranges.
*Women may have slightly lower values than men.	

Specimen Required

A 5-ml sample of venous blood is obtained in a plain collecting tube or syringe. When complete enzyme studies or isoenzyme analyses are to be done, a 15–30-ml sample of blood may be needed. Because the value of enzyme studies for diagnosis depends on serial analysis of enzymes, each specimen must be labeled with the time the blood was drawn.

Preparation of the Patient

Food and drink are usually not restricted before venipuncture. However medications should be withheld until after blood is drawn as some medications increase levels of this enzyme (Table 4.2). If medications cannot be withheld, note them on the laboratory slip. If the specimen cannot be taken to the laboratory immediately, refrigerate it and note the time it was drawn.

Causes of Deviation from Normal

4

A patient who has had an acute MI will have elevated concentrations of AST in the serum. Levels begin to rise 8–12 hours after the chest pain has occurred, peak in 36–48 hours, and return to normal in 3–5 days. Because of the high level of AST present in cardiac tissue, the destruction of less than 1g of myocardium is sufficient to produce an elevation in AST. Furthermore, 96–98% of patients with EKG changes consistent with the diagnosis of acute MI have a significant elevation in AST activity. High serum levels of AST are also present in people with acute hepatic necrosis (see Chapter 8).

Nursing Implications of Abnormal Findings

Assessment. Although an elevated AST level occurs most often with myocardial damage, the presence of AST in so many other body tissues reduces its specificity for the presence of MI. Thus, all aspects of the patient's illness must be assessed when there is an increase in this enzyme. Knowledge of the level in a patient who has had a diagnosed MI helps the nurse to establish the length of time that has elapsed after the infarct (Fig. 4.1). For example, by following the rise and subsequent peaking of the AST level, the nurse can check for early complications, such as cardiac arrhythmias. In addition, the amount of damage that has taken place can be estimated because the peak AST levels are

TABLE 4.2. Drugs that May Cause an Increase in AST

Antibiotics	Narcotics
Cortisone	Oral contraceptives
Digitalis preparations	Pyridoxine
Flurazepam	Rifampin
Guanethidine	Salicylates
Indomethacin (Indocin)	Theophylline
Isoniazid	Vitamin A
Mithramycin	

a semiquantitative index of the amount of myocardial damage that has occurred unless there are rises attributable to accompanying liver damage or shock.

Interventions. The nursing care for a patient who has had an MI is discussed in the section on creatine phosphokinase. The interventions chosen depend upon the severity of the MI and the number of days that have elapsed since the initial attack.

LACTIC DEHYDROGENASE

Definition

Lactic dehydrogenase (LDH) is a cellular enzyme that contributes to carbohydrate metabolism. Specifically, it catalyzes the reversible oxidation of lactate to pyruvate. LDH is present in almost all metabolizing cells, present especially in the liver, heart, kidneys, skeletal muscles, brain, and erythrocytes and is released during tissue injury. LDH is composed of five different components (isoenzymes) that can be separated and identified by several methods; heat and electrophoresis are the most common. Different quantities of each isoenzyme are found in various organs and tissues. LDH_1 and LDH_2, also known as the cardiac fraction, are present in heart, kidneys, and erythrocytes, and in small amounts in other body tissues. LDH_3 is found in the lungs, spleen, pancreas, thyroid, adrenal glands, and lymph nodes. LDH_4 and LDH_5 are the hepatic fractions found mainly in the liver and in skeletal muscle. Serum levels of each isoenzyme are different. LDH_2 level is the highest, then LDH_1, LDH_3, LDH_4, and LDH_5. LDH_1 is the only isoenzyme of the five that remains stable when heated at sixty-five degrees centigrade for thirty minutes. This quality is used to identify what proportion of total LDH is LDH_1, and provides information useful in diagnosing cardiac disease.

N O R M A L   R A N G E

LDH

Adult	165–400 Wroblewski units/ml
	80–120 Wacher units/ml
	71–200 IU/l
Children	50–150 IU/l
Newborns	300–2000 IU/l

Normal values may vary with each laboratory and the test used.

LDH Isoenzyme Electrophoresis

	Range of % of Total LDH
LDH$_1$	17–33
LDH$_2$	27–37
LDH$_3$	18–25
LDH$_4$	3–8
LDH$_5$	0–5

Normal values may vary with each laboratory.

4

Specimen Required

A 5-ml sample of venous blood is obtained in a plain collecting tube or syringe. When complete enzyme studies or isoenzyme analyses are to be done, a 15–30-ml sample of blood may be needed. Since the value of enzyme studies for diagnosis depends on serial analysis of enzymes, each specimen must be labeled with the time the blood was drawn. Note on the laboratory slip if the patient has received any of the following drugs:

Clofibrate

Codeine

Meperidine (Demoral)

Mithramycin

Morphine

Procainamide

Preparation of the Patient

Food and drink are usually not restricted before venipuncture. Freezing, heating, or shaking the sample should be avoided because hemolysis of red blood cells releases their LDH and can cause falsely elevated levels.

Causes of Deviation from Normal

Serum elevations of LDH occur with damage to the organs or tissues that contain this enzyme. See Chapter 8 for discussion of elevations in hepatic disease. The measurement of LDH and its isoenzymes has a predictive value from 90–95% when used to determine if myocardial damage has occurred. Increased serum LDH activity generally appears within twenty-four hours after an MI, peaks on the third day, and may remain elevated for as long as fourteen days (Fig. 4.1). This prolonged course is very helpful in confirming the diagnosis of an MI, since elevations in other cardiac enzymes released during myocardial damage may return to normal before blood samples are obtained.

When an MI has occurred, a rise in LDH_1 often takes place before there is an increase in total LDH. Therefore, a rise in heat-stable LDH with a normal total LDH is usually a sign of myocardial damage. When all the LDH isoenzymes are measured by electrophoresis, myocardial necrosis must be considered if the amount of LDH_1 exceeds that of LDH_2. This reversal in the normal ratio of these two isoenzymes is often referred to as a "flipped pattern".

Nursing Implications of Abnormal Findings

Assessment. LDH must be evaluated in relation to the person's clinical manifestations and any other laboratory data that have been obtained, since evaluating levels of this enzyme alone is not helpful. If the elevation appears to be an isolated finding unrelated to other laboratory data or to the clinical assessment, the test may have to be repeated, as it may be a false-positive reading due to hemolysis of red cells. When the patient being assessed is thought to have myocardial damage, the serum LDH must be looked at in relationship to (1) the time the rise began after the occurrence of signs and symptoms, (2) the course of that rise over time, and (3) its relationship to CPK and AST levels (Fig. 4.1). If the rise and fall of the serum LDH is compared to the rise associated with a typical MI, the amount of time that has elapsed since the initial attack can be estimated and progressive nursing interventions planned. For example, when LDH levels are still rising, patient activity should be minimized.

Interventions. The nursing care for a patient who has had an MI is discussed in the section on creatine phosphokinase. The interventions chosen as appropriate will depend upon the severity of the MI and the number of days that have elapsed since the initial attack.

ALPHA-HYDROXYBUTYRATE DEHYDROGENASE

The measurement of *serum alpha-hydroxybutyrate dehydrogenase* (HBD) has been used as a substitute for measurement of the isoenzymes of LDH when isoenzyme assay is unavailable. HBD is actually the total LDH forced to act on alpha-ketobutyric acid rather than lactic or pyruvic acid. Recently, measurement of HBD has been less widely used than that of LDH and its isoenzymes. Discussion is therefore referred to the section on lactic dehydrogenase. Once the diagnosis of myocardial infarction has been established, HBD measurements may be used to indicate the duration of tissue injury, since HBD elevation may last up to 2 weeks.

> **N O R M A L   R A N G E**
>
> Adults   110–290 IU/l
> Normal values may vary with each laboratory.

Specimen Required
See the section on lactic dehydrogenase.

4

PLASMA LIPIDS

Description
Plasma lipids (cholesterol, triglycerides, and phospholipids) are used by the body in the formation of various enzymes, hormones, and body structures. Because they are not soluble in water, they require vehicles for circulation, which are called *lipoproteins*. There are four major categories of lipoproteins, each containing differing amounts of cholesterol, triglycerides, phospholipids, and protein. These categories are *chylomicrons, very low density lipoproteins* (VLDL, or pre-beta), *low-density lipoproteins* (LDL, or beta), and *high-density lipoproteins* (HDL, or alpha).

CHOLESTEROL

Cholesterol is a steroid alcohol endogenously derived from fat metabolism. It is of great importance in the synthesis of steroid hormones, the formation of bile salts for fat digestion, and the composition of cell membranes. The cholesterol synthesized within the body is transported in the plasma as LDL or HDL. The LDL transports cholesterol to the cells and the HDL removes it. Nearly three-fourths of the total serum cholesterol is esterified by the liver and transported with LDL of blood for delivery to tissues.

TRIGLYCERIDES

Triglycerides are naturally occurring fats (neutral fats) that are formed by esterification. When glycerides are ingested in food, they are hydrolyzed and absorbed in the intestinal lumen and reformed into triglycerides in the intestinal mucosa. Triglycerides are transported in the bloodstream as chylomicrons. They are stored as lipids in adipose tissue or used for energy.

LIPOPROTEINS

Lipoproteins are macromolecular complexes that transport insoluble lipids in the plasma. Lipoproteins, while closely related metabolically, can be divided into broad classifications based on their density, flotation characteristics, and electrophoretic mobility. These classifications are *chylomicrons; pre-beta lipoproteins* (VLDL); *beta lipoproteins* (LDL); and *alpha lipoproteins* (HDL). These types of lipoproteins can be separated by the process of electrophoresis.

N O R M A L R A N G E	
Adults	
HDL	
Men	44 mg/dl
Women	55 mg/dl
LDL	62–185 mg/100 ml
VLDL	25–50%
Cholesterol	less than 200 mg/dl
Triglycerides	less than 100 mg/dl
Children	
Cholesterol	130–175 mg/dl
Triglycerides	10–135 mg/dl
Infants	
Cholesterol	70–170 mg/dl
Triglycerides	5–40 mg/dl

Note. The normal levels for cholesterol and triglycerides are difficult to establish because conditions such as coronary atherosclerosis, dietary hypercholesterolemia, and obesity, which are common in the United States, cause frequent elevations that may be considered normal.

Specimen Required

A 5-ml sample of blood is obtained in a plain collecting tube or syringe for any of the plasma lipid tests.

Preparation of the Patient
CHOLESTEROL

Food and beverage restrictions before obtaining the blood sample vary among laboratories. Because the ingestion of large amounts of cholesterol during the twelve hours preceding the test may affect the results, fasting is often required. If no restrictions exist, the patient should be told to avoid a fatty meal for at least twelve hours before the test. A repeat test may be ordered to confirm elevated levels.

TRIGLYCERIDES

There appear to be many drugs that affect serum triglycerides. Because all the specific drugs that have this effect are not known, all drugs should be discontinued for 24 hours before the blood sample is taken, if possible. The patient should be told to eat a normal diet for two weeks before the test but not to eat or drink anything except water for twelve hours before the test.

LIPOPROTEIN ANALYSIS

The patient should be told to eat a normal diet for three weeks before the test but not to eat anything or drink anything but water for twelve hours before the blood specimen is taken.

Causes of Deviation from Normal

The causes of elevated plasma lipids may be either genetic (hereditary), induced, or both.

4

Low levels of HDL have been associated with an increased incidence of coronary vascular disease. Regular physical activity can raise the level of HDL in some people. High levels of LDL are also closely associated with an increase in coronary heart disease and atherosclerosis.

Nursing Implications of Abnormal Findings

Assessment. Once hyperlipidemia has been identified, the cornerstone of treatment is dietary alteration. The goal is to attain and maintain an ideal weight. The nursing assessment for patients with hyperlipidemia should begin with a comparison of each patient's weight with the ideal body weight of other people of the same age, sex, and height. A nutrition history should be taken over several weeks, beginning in the hospital, clinic, or doctor's office and continuing in the patient's home. It should include the types of food the patient normally eats, the effect food has on daily habits, and the social meaning food has for the patient. Demographic data should also be obtained.

Interventions. After the nursing assessment has been done, education of the patient and family should begin. Problems such as limited financial resources, the need to cook one meal acceptable to all family members, and the frequent consumption of ethnic foods with high fat content must be considered when a teaching plan is developed. The patient should be helped to incorporate the diet that has been prescribed into daily activities. Emphasis should be placed on the importance of adhering to the diet and the benefit of the diet to family members who do not have hyperlipidemia, especially children. This point is particularly important. Some forms of hyperlipidemia tend to run in families, with atherosclerosis originating in childhood and progressing throughout life. Occasionally, people who are accustomed to ethnic foods with a high lipid content find it difficult to avoid these foods. When this situation occurs, the patient may not cooperate completely with the dietary modifications recommended. Continual support and assistance should be given to these people so that they will not feel rejected for not having completely given up their former life-styles. Referral to home care for reinforcement of dietary alterations after discharge from the hospital is recommended.

BIBLIOGRAPHY

Byrne, C.J., D.F. Saxton, P.K. Pelikan, and P.M. Nugent. *Laboratory Tests: Implications for Nursing Care*. Menlo Park: Addison-Wesley, 1986.

Cohen, J.A., N. Pantaleo, and W. Shell. "A Message From the Heart: What Isoenzymes Can Tell You About Your Cardiac Patient." *Nursing 82*, 12:46–49, (April 1982).

Fisher, M.L., et al. "Serum Creatine Kinase in the Diagnosis of Acute Myocardial Infarction." *Journal of the American Medical Association*, 249:393–394 (January 1983).

Guzetta, C.E., and B.M. Dossey. *Cardiovascular Nursing: Holistic Practice*. Philadelphia: Mosby Yearbook, 1992.

Grundy, I.M. "The Place of HDL in Cholesterol Management." *Archives of Internal Medicine*, 149:505–510 (March 1989).

Henry, J.B. *Clinical Diagnosis and Management by Laboratory Methods*. Philadelphia: W.B. Saunders Co., 1991.

Hurst, J.W., et al. *The Heart*. New York: McGraw-Hill Information Services Company, 1990.

Ignatavicius, D.D., and M.V. Bayne. *Medical-Surgical Nursing: A Nursing Process Approach*. Philadelphia: W.B. Saunders, 1991.

Lewis, S.M., and I.C. Collier. *Medical-Surgical Nursing: Assessment and Management of Clinical Problems*. St. Louis: Mosby Yearbook, 1992.

Luckman, J., and K.C. Sorensen. *Medical-Surgical Nursing: A Psychophysiological Approach*. Philadelphia: Saunders, 1987.

Nowakowski, J.F. "Use of Cardiac Enzymes in the Evaluation of Acute Chest Pain." *Annals of Emergency Medicine*, 15:354–360 (March 1986).

Phipps, W.S., B.C. Long, N.F. Woods, and V. Cossmeyer. *Medical-Surgical Nursing*. St. Louis: Mosby Yearbook, 1991.

Ravel, R. *Clinical Laboratory Medicine*. Chicago: Year Book Medical Publishers, 1989.

Roberts, R. "Diagnostic Assessment of Myocardial Infarction Based on Lactate Dehydrogenase and Creatine Kinase Isoenzymes." *Heart and Lung*, 10:486–506 (May–June 1981).

Ryan, M.A. "What Cardiac Enzymes Tell You About Acute M.I." *RN*, 47:46–49 (March 1984).

Sacher, R.A., and R.A. McPherson. *Widmann's Clinical Interpretation of Laboratory Tests*. Philadelphia: F.A. Davis, 1991.

Smetzer, S.C., and B.G. Ball. *Brunner and Sudarth's Medical-Surgical Nursing*. New York: J.B. Lippincott, 1992.

Underhill, S.C., S.L. Woods, E.S. Froelicher, and C.J. Halpenny. *Cardiac Nursing,* Philadelphia: J.B. Lippincott Co. 1989.

Vander, A.J., J.H. Sherman, and D.S. Luciano. *Human Physiology: The Mechanisms of Body Function.* New York: McGraw-Hill Publishing Co., 1990.

Wilson, J., et al. *Harrison's Principles of Internal Medicine.* New York: McGraw-Hill Co., Inc., 1991.

4

5

Laboratory Tests of Fluid and Electrolyte Balance

Serum Sodium	**Serum Copper**
Serum Potassium	**Serum Osmolality**
Serum Chloride	**Urine Osmolality**
Serum Calcium	**Urine Sodium**
Serum Magnesium	**Urine Potassium**
Serum Phosphorus	**Urine Calcium (Sulkowitch Test)**
Serum Zinc	

SERUM SODIUM

Description

Sodium is the principle cation of the extracellular fluid and is the most important electrolyte in the maintenance of fluid balance in the body. Sodium accounts for more than 90% of the total body cations. Therefore, changes in the serum sodium level occur during any change in body cations. Sodium is found predominantly in the extracellular fluid and does not easily move into the cell. The sodium pump moves sodium out of the cells. Because of the intricate relationship between sodium and water, sodium has a primary role in the distribution of body water.

Sodium balance is maintained by the daily ingestion of sodium in food and the excretion of excess sodium by the kidneys. Daily replacement is necessary because of obligatory losses in urine, feces, and perspiration. The normal diet contains at least 100 mEq of sodium daily, which exceeds the minimum of 12–15 mEq needed for daily replacement. Normal serum sodium levels are maintained by two hormones, *aldosterone* and the *antidiuretic hormone* (ADH). Aldosterone is secreted by the adrenal cortex in response to (1) a decrease in sodium concentration in the extracellular fluid, (2) an increase in intracellular potassium, (3) decreases in blood volume and cardiac output, or (4) either physical or emotional stress. Aldosterone moves to the renal tubules and increases the reabsorption of sodium from them. An exchange is made with potassium, which is then diffused into the urine. Along with sodium reabsorption, water is retained.

ADH regulates sodium balance more indirectly by means of the regulation of body water. A number of factors have been related to ADH secretion by the posterior pituitary gland. The most common stimulants are increases in body tonicity and osmolality, and decreases in blood volume and pressure. Additional factors that stimulate ADH secretion include surgery, trauma, fear, pain, infection, and vigorous exercise. ADH functions in the distal and collecting tubules of the kidney and regulates the size of the pores in the epithelial lining of the tubules. As ADH increases, the pores become larger and water is reabsorbed into the epithelial lining and retained by the body. As ADH decreases, the pores become smaller and water can no longer be reabsorbed but is lost in dilute urine. Water reabsorption then has an effect on the concentration of extracellular sodium.

5

N O R M A L R A N G E	
Adults	135–148 mEq/L
Children	138–144 mEq/L
Newborns	133–144 mEq/L

Specimen Required
A 5-ml sample of venous blood is obtained in a plain collecting tube or syringe.

Preparation of the Patient
Food and fluids are not usually restricted before collection of the specimen.

Causes of Deviation from Normal
Because sodium is the predominant cation in extracellular fluid, changes in serum sodium levels generally reflect changes in water balance as well. Thus, the deviations discussed here relate to changes in serum sodium or body water, or both. These deviations can be classified as *isotonic* if the resulting body fluid concentration is equal to the normal concentration of body fluids. Deviations that result in a concentrated body fluid state are referred to as *hypertonic*, whereas deviations that result in a diluted body fluid state are referred to as *hypotonic* (Table 5.1).

Isotonic fluid imbalances can result from an *isotonic depletion* or an *isotonic excess*. In isotonic depletion, both sodium and water are lost, and the imbalance may be referred to as *fluid volume deficit*. Clinically, this may be referred to as

TABLE 5.1. Sodium and Water Imbalances

| Imbalances | Clinical Diagnosis | Serum Sodium Value | Body Levels | | Example |
			Sodium	Water	
Isotonic depletion	Fluid volume deficit	Normal	Decreased	Decreased	"Dehydration" Diabetic ketoacidosis
Isotonic excess	Fluid volume excess	Normal	Increased	Increased	Renal failure Congestive heart failure
Hypertonic fluid imbalances	Hypernatremia	Increased	Increased	Normal	Congestive heart failure, cirrhosis with ascites
		Increased	Normal	Decreased	Diabetes insipidus Tube feeding syndrome
Hypotonic fluid imbalances	Hyponatremia	Decreased	Normal	Increased	Dilutional hyponatremia: e.g., SIADH, water intoxication
		Decreased	Decreased	Normal	Chronic low sodium intake, renal salt wasting

dehydration, a term that is erroneous, since it means only lack of water. In isotonic depletion the serum sodium level is within normal limits. The most common cause of this abnormality is loss of gastrointestinal fluids, as when prolonged vomiting and diarrhea occur. Other causes include excessive enemas, diabetic ketoacidosis, and hemorrhage.

In isotonic excess, both sodium and water excesses are present in the body, and this imbalance is referred to as *fluid volume excess*. The serum sodium level is within normal limits. One cause of this imbalance is excessive and rapid intake of intravenous fluids associated with normal renal functioning or occurring in the postoperative patient with decreased renal function. It is common during renal shutdown or renal failure. Additional causes of this imbalance are situations in which inefficient excretion of body fluids occurs, as with patients in renal failure, with congestive heart failure, with cerebral damage, or on prolonged cortisone therapy.

Hypertonic fluid imbalance is caused by either a sodium excess or a water deficit and is mainifested as a hypernatremia with serum sodium levels above 150 mEq/l. The excess sodium can be caused by ingestion of salt without water, near drowning in salt water, high solute tube feedings without adequate water, extensive burns, or primary aldosteronism.

Hypotonic fluid imbalance is caused by either an excess of body water or a decrease in sodium intake and is reflected as hyponatremia with serum sodium levels below 120 mEq/l. Excessive body water can result from excessive tap water enemas, excessive water intake, which may occur in schizophrenia, inability to excrete body water, as seen in kidney disease, and continued fluid intake by patients with syndrome of inappropriate secretion of ADH (SIADH). Decreases in sodium intake are associated with a low-sodium diet, chronic or massive diuretic therapy, generally poor nutrition, and renal salt wasting.

Nursing Implications of Abnormal Findings

Assessment. The nurse is in a key position to detect and prevent sodium and water imbalances. To detect isotonic imbalances, the nurse should assess patients whose serum sodium levels are normal but whose intake and output records and clinical pictures indicate either an excess or a deficit of body fluids. Isotonic depletion can occur gradually, over a period of days, or be an acute episode that arises over a period of hours. *Slow-onset isotonic depletion* can occur in patients who are suffering from increased gastrointestinal fluid losses along with decreased intake of either oral or intravenous fluids. *Rapid-onset isotonic depletion* is seen in patients with acute losses, such as those due to hemorrhage. Daily weights, vital signs with specific attention to the pulse and blood pressure, and examination of intake and output records provide quantitative data for the nurse to examine. When checking the condition of the patient, the nurse should note the condition of the mucous membranes and skin turgor. If mucous membranes are dry and skin turgor is decreased, a deficit may be occurring and should be reported to the physician. In isotonic excess or fluid volume excess the nurse should assess patients for an increase in body weight, pitting edema, pulmonary edema, puffy eyelids, and ascites. These observations are especially important in patients with heart or renal disease or those in the early stages of total parenteral nutrition therapy. Once the diagnosis of isotonic depletion is made, the nurse is responsible for accurate monitoring of replacement fluids. If the patient's condition is acute, rapid treatment may be necessary, and assessment of the patient every 5–10 minutes may be needed to prevent fluid volume overload.

In preventing and detecting early hypernatremia or hypertonic fluid imbalance, the nurse should be aware of the patient's clinical condition, laboratory results, excessive fluid losses, and decreased water intake. For example, patients receiving high solute feedings, patients with extensive burns, patients with primary aldosteronism, elderly patients with decreased renal concentrating ability, and patients with diabetes insipidus should be followed carefully. The nurse should monitor the laboratory test results for serum sodium levels, which may gradually move toward the upper limits of normal. Other related abnormal laboratory results include elevated hemoglobin, hematocrit, blood urea nitrogen (BUN), and serum protein. These elevations reflect concentrated serum and not actual increases in red cells or protein. Signs and symptoms are related to dehydration and include thirst, decreased blood pressure, poor skin turgor, dry mucous membranes, soft eyeballs, loss of body weight, increased temperature, and apprehension leading to restlessness and coma. The urinary output is decreased, urine has high specific gravity, and renal shutdown may occur. For patients with hypernatremia the nurse should keep accurate intake and output records and should record temperature, pulse, respirations, and daily body weight. The urine specific gravity should be checked and if it is high, should be monitored with each urination.

Hyponatremia or hypotonic fluid imbalance is seen more frequently than hypernatremia by the clinical nurse. The older patient undergoing diagnostic X-ray preparation is particularly prone to this disorder and should be watched carefully for initial signs of fatigue and cerebral confusion. These signs should be reported to the physician and followed up by the nurse with continued monitoring of signs and symptoms and implementation of safety measures to prevent patient injury.

Interventions. When patients with fluid volume overload (isotonic excess) are receiving intravenous fluids, fluids should not be administered too rapidly or too slowly. Trying to catch up on fluid administration when it gets behind schedule is contraindicated, since this may overload the kidneys and cause fluid imbalance. When the diagnosis of fluid volume overload has been made, the nurse is involved in the careful administration of diuretics and measurement of output. The nurse should teach the patient to expect an increased urinary output and should make arrangements for ready access to the bedpan or urinal or assistance in getting up to the bathroom. Making sure a device for measuring urine is in the patient's bathroom will help the nurse obtain the necessary information on urinary output. The nurse should pay attention to signs of sodium or potassium depletion that may occur with diuretic therapy. These signs and symptoms are discussed later in the sections on Hypotonic Fluid Imbalances and Potassium Imbalances. Patients with isotonic excess are prone to skin breakdown, especially in edematous areas. Meticulous skin care and frequent changes in position are essential. If dyspnea occurs, the patient should be placed in Fowler's position and the physician notified.

The major goal of nursing care of patients with hypernatremia is the accurate administration of intravenous fluids. Fluids should be infused carefully so that rapid correction of the problem does not send the patient into fluid overload.

The nurse can prevent hyponatremia by means of cautious administration of intravenous fluids for patients who may have compromised renal function and the use of normal saline, rather than water, for nasogastric tube irrigation. The careful use of tap water enemas for patients having a bowel preparation will also help prevent this imbalance from occurring. Patients prone to hyponatremia include those whose inability to excrete water excesses is caused by the syndrome of inappropriate antidiuretic hormone secretion (Table 5.2). This group of patients should be watched for signs of mental confusion and decreasing fluid output as compared with fluid intake. Edema is generally not seen in patients with SIADH.

SERUM POTASSIUM

Description

Potassium is one of the major electrolytes in body fluid. It is the predominant cation in intracellular fluid, with only 2% found in the extracellular space. *Serum potassium* has a narrow range of normal and is responsible for maintaining life-sustaining neuromuscular functioning. Potassium functions in initiating and sustaining muscular contraction in both cardiac and skeletal muscles. In addition, it functions in maintaining normal acid-base balance by serving as an exchange electrolyte for the hydrogen ion, and by moving out of the cell during acidosis and into the cell during alkalosis. In healthy people, potassium intake is maintained by diet. Normal levels of potassium are maintained by kidney elimination of the potassium ingested in excess of the amount needed to maintain normal serum levels. Aldosterone increases the elimination of potassium by causing retention of sodium and excretion of potassium in the renal tubules. There is no known mechanism by which the body stores potassium.

NORMAL RANGE	
Adults	3.5–5.0 mEq/L
Children	3.4–4.7 mEq/L
Newborns	3.7–5.9 mEq/L

TABLE 5.2.   Causes of SIADH

Drugs
  Vincristine
  Oxytocin
  Vasopressin
  Sulfonylurea hypoglycemic agents
  Diuretics
Intrathoracic pressure increases
  Infection
  Positive pressure breathing
  Postcommissurotomy syndrome
Central nervous system disorders
  Tumors
  Head trauma
  Meningitis
  Cerebral infarction
  Encephalitis
ADH-secreting tissues
  Bronchogenic carcinoma
  Tumors of the pancreas, duodenum, prostate, thymus, and ureters
  Lymphosarcoma
  Tuberculosis tissue
Excessive fluid administration during periods of normal ADH depression
  Postoperative states
  Trauma
  Hemorrhage
  Stress

Specimen Required

A 5-ml sample of venous blood is obtained in a plain collecting tube or syringe. Care should be taken to draw the sample with as little trauma as possible to decrease the occurrence of false elevations of potassium from hemolysis. This can be done by (1) applying the tourniquet loosely enough to prevent venous stasis, (2) avoiding excessive traction on the collection device, and, (3) using a 20-gauge needle, which allows the blood to flow into the container rather than be withdrawn from the vein under suction.

Preparation of the Patient

Food and drink are usually not restricted before collection of the specimen.

Causes of Deviation from Normal

Changes in potassium levels can occur in both directions. An excess is called *hyperkalemia* and a deficit is called *hypokalemia*. Hyperkalemia occurs when the serum level of accumulated potassium rises above 5.5 mEq/l. The most common cause for this rise is kidney disease, such as renal shutdown, in which there is interference with the elimination of potassium through the kidney tubules. Hyperkalemia also results from administering intravenous fluids containing potassium at too rapid a rate, especially in patients who have decreased renal function. An unusually high serum potassium can result from the release of cellular potassium from injured body tissues. This occurs in such instances as burns, crushing injuries, and myocardial infarction, and is related to an inability of the kidney to eliminate potassium rapidly enough to keep the serum levels normal. Hyperkalemia may be compounded in these instances by decreased kidney functioning due to accompanying shock. Hyperkalemia also occurs in Addison's disease, when inadequate amounts of glucocorticoids and mineral corticoids are secreted; the decrease in hormones causes excessive loss of sodium and a resulting retention of potassium. Metabolic acidosis and administration of medications known to cause accumulation of potassium, such as spironolactone or high doses of aldactone, can also lead to hyperkalemia.

5

Hypokalemia also has several causes. The administration of thiazide diuretics without potassium replacements, the long-term administration of potassium-free intravenous fluids to a patient who is not eating, and cirrhosis from chronic alcoholism are the most frequent causes of hypokalemia. Excessive elimination of potassium through the bowel can occur with diarrhea, prolonged gastrointestinal suction, and Crohn's disease. In these instances, potassium-rich gastrointestinal secretions, generally reabsorbed in healthy people, are lost from the gastrointestinal tract. Hypokalemia can also be caused by increases in aldosterone, which occur with Cushing's syndrome and during episodes of congestive heart failure. In these conditions, sodium is retained in large quantities by the renal exchange of potassium.

There is a relationship between decreased serum levels of potassium and alkalosis. Hypokalemia can be produced during alkalosis as the kidney exchanges potassium and hydrogen ions in an attempt to retain hydrogen ions and decrease the degree of alkalosis. Hypokalemia can also lead to alkalosis, since a decrease in cellular potassium causes a shift of hydrogen ions into the cell to maintain a more normal cellular chemical environment.

Nursing Implications of Abnormal Findings

Assessment. In assessing patients for the onset and occurrence of either hypokalemia or hyperkalemia, the nurse should consider the patient's total clinical picture, since symptoms of potassium decrease are very similar to those of potassium increase. Overlapping symptoms include muscle weakness, nausea, anorexia, and mental changes, such as lethargy and drowsiness. When these symptoms occur, the nurse should include the patient's history and current therapy in the assessment. A serum potassium determination will be needed for final confirmation.

In assessing the possible presence of hyperkalemia, the nurse should evaluate patients who have either increased potassium intake or decreased potassium output. In patients with burns or multiple trauma, beginning hyperkalemia can be detected by means of careful assessment of symptom changes combined with monitoring of the EKG. Peaked T-waves may be seen in patients with hyperkalemia. The nurse should look for weakness, fatigue, paresthesias, and lethargy. Deep tendon reflexes may become decreased.

The nurse should frequently assess patients who have an increased potential for developing hypokalemia, such as (1) patients who are receiving aggressive diuretic therapy in which rapid excretion of fluids can quickly deplete normal serum potassium levels, and (2) patients being treated for diabetic acidosis, in which the rapid movement of potassium into the cell can cause a drop in serum potassium levels. In these acute situations patients should be evaluated as frequently as every 10–15 minutes. Mental status, neuromuscular changes, vital signs, and EKG monitoring should be included in the evaluation. Depressed T-waves may be seen in patients with hypokalemia. Accurate intake and output records will provide essential information to the physician prescribing replacement therapy.

Interventions. One of the ways nurses can clinically prevent hyperkalemia is to administer potassium-containing intravenous solutions cautiously. Patients should not receive more than 40 mEq in 8 hours. The amount administered should be lower in patients with reduced renal functioning. If hyperkalemia is present, the nurse may need to prepare the patient for dialysis or the administration of cation-exchange resins such as sodium polystyrene sulfonate (Kayexalate), either orally, rectally, or both. This drug promotes removal of the excessive potassium by way of the gastrointestinal tract. Management of the patient with hyperkalemia should include prevention of infection, decubitus ulcers, and injury, as these will add to the imbalance by releasing additional potassium.

For patients with hypokalemia who are receiving intravenous potassium replacement, the potassium should be carefully diluted to prevent vein irritation and cardiac arrest. Patients receiving potassium intravenously should be checked for adequate urinary output to prevent unexpected hyperkalemia.

Hypokalemia associated with prolonged diuretic therapy has a slower onset and is harder to distinguish from other fluid and electrolyte imbalances. The nurse should be especially alert to this imbalance in patients who are receiving a digitalis product. Digitalis toxicity can occur with low-normal potassium levels of 3.5–4.0 mEq/l and can cause cardiac irregularities and gastrointestinal symptoms. The patient on diuretic therapy for fluid retention or hypertension should receive either a daily potassium replacement or a potassium-rich food in the daily diet (see Table 5.3). Potassium replacements should be diluted in at

| TABLE 5.3. | Foods High in Potassium |

Apricots	Nuts
Bananas	Orange juice
Cola drinks	Oranges
Dates	Peaches
Figs	Prunes
Instant coffee	Raisins
Meat base	Tomato juice

least four ounces of water to prevent irritation to the mouth, esophagus, and stomach mucosa. The nurse should formulate a teaching plan for these patients that emphasizes sources of dietary potassium and identification of symptoms to be reported to the physician. Intravenous potassium replacement is done slowly to prevent cardiac toxicity. The intravenous site should be monitored regularly for possible infiltration since tissue necrosis can result.

5

SERUM CHLORIDE

Description

Chloride is the primary anion found in the extracellular fluid. It functions primarily with sodium in the maintenance of osmotic pressure of the blood and arterial pressure. It is regulated indirectly by aldosterone, which causes reabsorption of sodium by the kidney. As each sodium ion is reabsorbed, a chloride or a bicarbonate ion is reabsorbed as well. Chloride also has a part in maintaining acid–base balance in that it functions along with bicarbonate in providing the total number of anions necessary to equal the total number of cations. If bicarbonate is lost from the body, chloride is retained to make up the loss. Conversely, when chloride is lost, bicarbonate is retained. A relatively large amount of chloride is found in gastrointestinal secretions, primarily as hydrochloric acid in the stomach. It provides the acid medium necessary for digestion in the stomach and activates enzymes, such as pepsinogen to pepsin.

N O R M A L R A N G E	
Adults	95–105 mEq/L
Children	98–105 mEq/L
Newborns	94–112 mEq/L

Specimen Required

A 5-ml sample of venous blood is obtained in a plain collecting tube or syringe. Fresh serum is required for precise measurement; therefore, the specimen should be analyzed within 24 hours after it is drawn from the patient.

Preparation of the Patient

Food and fluids are not usually restricted before venipuncture.

Causes of Deviation from Normal

Chloride abnormalities are less common than other electrolyte abnormalities and are often associated with other abnormal electrolyte levels. Both increases and decreases in serum chloride occur. *Hypochloremia* can occur following continued vomiting, diarrhea, or prolonged gastric suction. This decrease is caused by the loss of gastrointestinal secretions, which contain the body's largest reservoir of chloride. Hypochloremia leads to metabolic alkalosis as bicarbonate increases to maintain the essential amount of anions in the serum. Administration of potent diuretics, such as ethacrynic acid and furosemide, causes hypochloremia by direct loss through the kidneys. In addition, hypochloremia may occur following several days of administering intravenous electrolyte-free solutions to patients who are not eating.

Hyperchloremia, which is less common than hypochloremia, is also associated with other electrolyte abnormalities. In dehydration, chloride ions are concentrated because of a decrease in body fluid. In *hyperparathyroidism*, the kidneys waste phosphate, and chloride levels rise to compensate for this anion loss. Two acid-base disorders are associated with chloride increases: *metabolic acidosis*, during which the bicarbonate ions are replaced by chloride ions; and *respiratory alkalosis*. Drugs associated with chloride increases include ammonium chloride, ion exchange resins, phenylbutazone, and excessive sodium chloride administration.

Nursing Implications of Abnormal Findings

Assessment. When the development of hypochloremia is anticipated, the nurse should maintain accurate intake and output records for patients who have sustained losses of gastrointestinal secretions such as diarrhea, vomiting, or are on continuous nasogastric suction. The nurse should continually assess the development in these patients of symptoms of increased nervous system irritability, such as hypertonicity of muscles, tetany, and depressed respirations. In anticipating the development of hyperchloremia, the nurse must watch those patients prone to the development of metabolic acidosis, such as those with renal tubular acidosis and hyperparathyroidism. These patients should be observed for the development of stupor, deep, rapid breathing, weakness, and unconsciousness. Laboratory values reflecting developing metabolic acidosis should be watched (Chapter 6).

Interventions. During replacement therapy following the diagnosis of hypochloremia, the nurse should continue keeping accurate intake and output records, recording the time and amounts of chloride replacements, so that accurate calculations of the total replacement needed can be made. Although the medical treatment of metabolic acidosis is very complex, the following measures can be taken: If intravenous injections of bicarbonate are given, patients should be assessed every few minutes for decreasing signs and symptoms of acidosis. Intravenous fluid administration must be monitored carefully and accurate intake and output records kept.

SERUM CALCIUM

Description

Calcium is an important cation found, predominantly in bones and teeth, combined with phosphate and carbonate. This combination, deposited in bony tissue, provides the mineralization and resulting strength of the skeleton. The remaining 10% of the body calcium is found in the blood serum and is essential for normal functioning of neuromuscular tissue, cardiac activity, and the coagulation of blood. Approximately one-half of the serum calcium is free (oxidized), and the other half is bound to protein. When serum calcium levels fall below normal, rapid replacement is available from the bones. This replacement is regulated by a negative feedback mechanism involving the parathyroid glands and serum calcium levels. As calcium levels drop below normal, parathyroid hormone is secreted, thus causing increased gastrointestinal calcium absorption and resorption of calcium in the renal tubules, as well as release of calcium from the bones. When normal serum calcium levels are reestablished, parathormone secretion decreases. Normal calcium levels are maintained by daily calcium ingestion. Calcium is excreted daily in both urine and stool. Calcium and phosphorus have a reciprocal relationship in the serum: As one is elevated, the other is decreased.

NORMAL RANGE	
Adults	4.5–5.5 mEq/L
Children	5.0–6.0 mEq/L
Newborns	3.7–7.0 mEq/L

Specimen Required

A 5-ml sample of venous blood is obtained in a plain collecting tube or syringe.

Preparation of the Patient

Food and drink are not usually restricted before collection of the specimen.

Causes of Deviation from Normal

Both *hypercalcemia* and *hypocalcemia* can occur. When serum calcium levels rise above 5.6 mEq/l, hypercalcemia occurs. The most common cause of serum calcium excess is immobilization, during which calcium moves from the bones and teeth into the bloodstream. Hypercalcemia also occurs from hyperparathyroidism, multiple myeloma, and other diseases involving bone catabolism, such as bone tumors and leukemia. In these diseases there is decreased mineralization of body tissue. *Hypervitaminosis D* is associated with hypercalcemia via different mechanisms. As vitamin D is absorbed from the gastrointestinal tract, calcium accompanies it and can reach excessive serum levels with toxic vitamin D ingestion. Hypercalcemia can occur during renal disease when renal shutdown prevents loss of excess serum calcium.

A variety of conditions can lead to hypocalcemia. In diseases of the small intestine in which decreased absorption occurs, inadequate serum calcium results. These diseases include sprue, pancreatitis, and Crohn's disease. Excessive protein intake causes calcium to move out of the bone and be excreted, resulting in osteoporosis. The administration of excessive amounts of citrated blood can also cause hypocalcemia, since the citrate binds with calcium, lowering blood levels. Primary hypoparathyroidism causes hypocalcemia by decreased formation of parathyroid hormone. With improved methods of thyroid surgery, the inadvertent removal of parathyroid tissue during thyroidectomy occurs less freqently. However, it may still occur after the removal of large or malignant thyroid tumors that disrupt the normal anatomical demarcation of tissues.

Nursing Implications of Abnormal Findings

Assessment. The nurse should observe the patient with an elevated serum calcium for decreased muscular tone, deep bone and flank pain, bony cavitation, and a variety of gastrointestinal problems including nausea, anorexia, vomiting, thirst, and constipation. A pathological fracture may occur due to demineralization of the bones. As calcium levels increase, nervous system depression may produce lethargy and coma. Vital signs should be checked frequently, since cardiac arrest may occur from the inability of the cardiac muscle to contract.

The nurse should observe the patient with decreased serum calcium for increased neuromuscular irritability, signified by abdominal cramps, leg muscle cramps, tingling of the fingertips, tetany, and convulsions. An acute deficit of serum calcium can be identified by a bedside assessment of the patient. Significantly, a positive Trousseau's sign, defined as the occurrence of carpopedal spasm while the arm is constricted with a blood-pressure cuff, along with

Chvostek's sign, indicate a lowered serum calcium level. Chvostek's sign is checked by tapping the patient's face over the facial nerve in the front of the temple. Calcium deficit causes the face to twitch on the same side of the face. Respiratory symptoms may include stridor and dyspnea. EKG changes involve lengthening of the QT interval and prolongation of the ST segment. If hypocalcemia occurs with a hypoproteinemia, the patient may be asymptomatic. Symptoms of hypocalcemia may occur in a patient with a normal serum calcium when alkalosis is present. This occurs because the alkalotic state decreases the amount of physiologically active calcium.

Interventions. The nurse is in a key position to decrease the occurrence of hypercalcemia by promoting early ambulation of all eligible patients and establishing a daily passive exercise program for patients confined to bed. The use of a tilt table for some patients should be explored. If immobility is inevitable or beginning hypercalcemia is present, the nurse should take steps to prevent renal calculi formation. This is accomplished by increasing the patient's fluid intake to 3,000–4,000 ml/day, increasing the acidity of urine by ingesting 250 ml of cranberry or prune juice daily, and preventing urinary tract infections. The increased fluid intake dilutes the excreted calcium and thus decreases the likelihood of calcium precipitation. Likewise, precipitation is less likely in an acid environment. Urinary tract infections are associated with renal calculi in two ways—urea-splitting organisms produce ammonia, resulting in alkaline urine, and the organisms act as foreign objects around which calcium precipitation can occur. Prevention of urinary tract infections includes a careful assessment of the patient's voiding pattern, checking for urinary retention, and using means other than catheterization to promote bladder emptying. If a catheter is required, it should be inserted under strict medical aseptic technique, perineal care should be carried out at least once daily, and the urinary drainage system should be kept sterile.

Because excess serum calcium can cause cardiac arrhythmias and cardiac arrest, the nurse should monitor the patient's vital signs. If acute increases in serum calcium are anticipated, EKG monitoring should be carried out as well. Careful handling of the patient's extremities during positioning is essential in controlling bone pain and preventing pathological fractures due to osteoporosis.

The prevention and early detection of hypocalcemia also has implications for nurses. The gradual onset of hypocalcemia begins shortly after menopause. Nutritional education of menopausal women should include the need for a daily intake of foods high in calcium such as milk and milk products, and in protein. Intestinal absorption of calcium is enhanced by protein. Patients with diagnosed hypocalcemia should be observed for changes in neuromuscular activity, and seizure precautions should be used to maintain the patient's safety. Because low serum calcium levels increase sensitivity to digitalis, patients receiving digitalis products should be followed carefully. For acute episodes of hypocalcemia, the nurse should be prepared to administer calcium chloride or calcium gluconate intravenously. Chronic hypocalcemia is generally controlled with oral replacement of calcium salts.

SERUM MAGNESIUM

Description

Magnesium is an important cation in the body fluids. It is second only to potassium in predominance in intracellular fluids. Only 1% of magnesium is located in the serum, and of this about one-third is bound to protein. About 50–60% of the body magnesium is located in an insoluble state in bones; the rest is located in muscle and soft tissues. Magnesium is active in cellular metabolism as a coenzyme in phosphate transfer reactions. It affects neuromuscular functioning by acting on the myoneural junction and by depressing acetylcholine release at the synaptic junction. It may participate in the enzyme functions that affect the sliding filament mechanism for muscle contraction and relaxation.

Magnesium is required for chemical reactions involving adenosine triphosphate (ADP), and thus is needed for carbohydrate metabolism as well as protein and nucleic acid synthesis. It also plays an important role in the clotting mechanism. Magnesium has a sedative effect on the body that is opposed by calcium. Magnesium balance is maintained by means of daily ingestion of foods containing magnesium. Magnesium is found in most foods and is abundant in chlorophyll-containing fruits and vegetables. Absorption of magnesium from the intestinal tract is stimulated by parathyroid hormone and inhibited by the presence of excess fat, phosphates, and calcium, and by alkalosis. Magnesium is excreted in both the feces and urine.

NORMAL RANGE	
Adults	1.5–2.5 mEq/L
Children	1.6–2.6 mEq/L
Newborns	1.4–2.9 mEq/L

Specimen Required

A 5-ml sample of venous blood is obtained in a plain collecting tube or syringe.

Preparation of the Patient

Food and drink are not usually restricted before venipuncture.

Causes of Deviation from Normal

Both *hypermagnesemia* and *hypomagnesemia* can occur. Both of these imbalances are fairly rare compared with other fluid and electrolyte problems.

Measurement of serum magnesium levels is somewhat difficult, and atomic absorption spectroscopy is the method of choice. However, current hospital treatment can produce magnesium imbalances. Hypomagnesemia occurs more frequently than hypermagnesemia and is associated with a decrease in the intake of magnesium or an increased loss of the ion through the kidney or bowel. Decreases in intake may be associated with intestinal malabsorption problems, such as chronic diarrhea, nontropical sprue, or steatorrhea, and may occur following bowel resection or in an inherited defect in magnesium absorption. Administration of long-term intravenous therapy or total parenteral nutrition without magnesium can lead to hypomagnesemia. Increased losses of magnesium accompany chronic alcoholism, diuretic therapy, starvation, hypoparathyroidism, and prolonged gastrointestinal suction.

Hypermagnesemia occurs less commonly and is associated primarily with a decreased ability to eliminate magnesium. This condition can occur during chronic renal failure when renal shutdown is present. The high serum level of magnesium may signal the need for a chronic dialysis program for the patient. Increased serum magnesium levels can also accompany overdoses of magnesium sulfate or sedative treatment. The administration of too many magnesium-containing enemas or the use of large doses of magnesium-containing antacids, especially for patients with compromised renal functioning, can also lead to increased serum magnesium levels.

Nursing Implications of Abnormal Findings

Assessment. Magnesium imbalances are found infrequently in clinical practice. However, the nurse should keep the possibility of these imbalances in mind when assessing patients with altered intake, particularly those whose intake does not include normal table foods and who have decreased renal functioning. Prevention and early detection of magnesium deficits may be accomplished by means of careful assessment of patients on non-magnesium-containing intravenous fluids over a period of time and of patients with chronic alcoholism or decreased intestinal absorption. Susceptible patients may demonstrate increased neuromuscular and central nervous system irritability. Clinical signs include tetany, hyperactive reflexes, a positive Chvostek's sign, facial twitching, convulsions, and plucking at the bed sheets. Behavior changes may include hallucinations, delusions, wild combative behavior, and extreme confusion. It can be difficult to distinguish these symptoms from those of calcium deficit. However, a possible calcium deficit that remains unimproved with treatment may in reality be a magnesium deficit and may respond to magnesium replacement therapy dramatically.

Hypermagnesemia should be anticipated in patients with chronic renal failure and in patients who have had multiple rectal enemas with magnesium-containing solutions. The nurse should assess these patients for muscle weakness, hypotension, EKG changes, sedation, and confusion.

Interventions. When hypomagnesemia is present, the nurse must administer magnesium replacement carefully to prevent toxic increases in serum magnesium. The patient's cardiac rhythm should be watched and the patient's reflexes observed for indications of sedation. As long as deep tendon reflexes are present, it is unlikely that the patient will go into respiratory depression from magnesium toxicity. As a safety precaution, emergency respiratory equipment should be available at the bedside. Calcium gluconate injection should be readily available to counteract the effects of magnesium toxicity. Tetany may occur but can be decreased or minimized by means of provision of a quiet, stress-free environment. The patient should be watched for seizures and protected from injury should seizures occur. Rapid correction of the underlying cause of the deficiency is crucial. When treatment involves long-term supplements of magnesium for patients with chronic problems, the nurse should implement a teaching program to ensure accurate patient self-medication. The program should include information about the importance of taking accurate doses, taking medication on time, and watching for signs of increased or decreased serum magnesium levels. Follow-up medical care should be emphasized.

When hypermagnesemia is present, the nurse should check the patient's deep tendon reflexes. If the magnesium rises to toxic levels, respiratory depression and paralysis can result in respiratory arrest, and cardiac depression can result in heart block. Respiratory support equipment should be available, and the patient's vital signs should be monitored every 2–3 minutes until the danger of respiratory arrest has passed. Calcium salts should be available for administration for quick antagonism of toxic magnesium levels. Once the immediate danger has passed and correction of the underlying cause of the increased magnesium levels has been undertaken, nursing care may involve teaching the patient about the dangerous practices of having multiple magnesium-containing enemas and of taking excessive amounts of magnesium-containing antacids and cathartics.

SERUM PHOSPHORUS

Description

Phosphorus is found in the body in the form of phosphate and is the major anion within the cells. Over 80% of the phosphate is found in the bones and teeth along with calcium.

In addition to its importance in the formation and maintenance of the skeleton, phosphorus is an important constituent of nucleic acids, phospholipids, and nucleotides. Every calcium ion in the circulation is accompanied by a phosphate radical, and the phosphate buffering system is essential in maintaining acid–base balance. Parathyroid hormone affects the serum phosphate levels differently than it does the calcium levels. As serum calcium levels drop, parathyroid hormone is released, causing release of calcium and phosphate from bone. The calcium is retained in the bloodstream and the phosphorus is lost in the urine. Parathyroid hormone increases calcium absorption from the intestine and decreases the rate of calcium reabsorption from the renal tubules. Therefore, with excess parathyroid hormone, phosphate loss occurs by means of renal excretion. Phosphorus is present in nearly all foods, and dietary needs are easily met with phosphorus found in milk or other foods.

N O R M A L R A N G E	
Adults	2.5–4.5 mg/dL
	1.7–2.6 mEq/L
Children	4.5–5.5 mg/dL
Newborns	4.5–6.7 mg/dL

Specimen Required

A 5-ml sample of venous blood is obtained in a plain collecting tube or a syringe. The specimen required must be free of hemolysis. The blood must therefore be separated as quickly as possible after collection.

Preparation of the Patient

The patient should fast before the morning blood collection to eliminate the effects of circadian rhythm and carbohydrate metabolism on the serum phosphate level.

Causes of Deviation from Normal

Deficits in serum phosphate are more common than are increased levels. Until recently, the most common cause associated with *hypophosphatemia* was an excess of parathyroid hormone from hyperparathyroidism. However, a report of a 21.6% incidence of hypophosphatemia in hospitalized patients led to examination of this high incidence. The causes identified include the intravenous administration of carbohydrate, increased use of diuretics, hyperalimentation, and alcoholism, all of which occurred far more commonly than hyperparathyroidism. Decreases in serum phosphate occur in conjunction with carbohydrate administration due to insulin release, which leads to the movement of both glucose and phosphate into skeletal muscle, liver, and other tissues. This rapid movement of phosphate into cells can occur in patients with diabetic acidosis. Additional causes of hypophosphatemia include dialysis, vomiting, ingestion of phosphate-binding antacids, and Gram-negative sepsis.

Hyperphosphatemia is found primarily in patients with chronic glomerular disease and elevated blood urea nitrogen and creatinine levels. Hypoparathyroidism also causes hyperphosphatemia, and the elevated serum phosphorus levels may be the key diagnostic tool in identifying this disorder. Hyperphosphatemia is associated with certain bone diseases, such as multiple myeloma, Paget's disease, and osteolytic metastatic tumor. It also occurs during fracture healing.

Nursing Implications of Abnormal Findings

Assessment. Nursing care for patients with deficits in serum phosphate includes careful monitoring of blood levels and observation of nervous system manifestations. When phosphate depletion has occurred, multiple clinical manifestations are seen, affecting the nervous system, musculoskeletal system, renal and hepatic tissue, and hematological tissue. Patients may differ in the extent of symptoms experienced. Nervous system manifestations include changes in consciousness status, weakness, slurred speech, and anorexia. Musculoskeletal disorders include weakness, stiffness of joints, and bone pain. Renal problems include hypercalciuria, and hepatic problems involve impaired response of the liver to glucagon. Most patients in hepatic coma are hypophosphatemic. Hematological disturbances involve changes in red cell metabolism, which results in increased hemolysis. White cells also have abnormalities, such as impaired chemotaxis, impaired phagocytosis, and impaired bactericidal activity. Increases in serum phosphate levels should be anticipated in patients with glomerulonephritis. As treatment for renal failure occurs, patients should be evaluated for changes in phosphate levels.

Interventions. When lowered serum phosphate levels occur, safety measures should be implemented to prevent patient injury. If bone pain is present, care must be taken when moving the patient and support given to the long bones during position changes. If hematological changes are present, the patient should be protected from secondary infections, and care should be given during intravenous and intramuscular injections to prevent tissue bruising and injury.

For patients with hyperphosphatemia associated with glomerulonephritis, accurate intake and output records are needed. Additional care should focus on the nursing problems the patient presents. For example, if the patient is retaining fluids, protective skin care should be implemented.

SERUM ZINC

Description

Zinc is one of the trace elements found in the body (Table 5.4). Zinc is a coenzyme for more than 80 enzymes in the body and is active in many catabolic processes. It is necessary for synthesis of cell division.

N O R M A L R A N G E	
Adults	50–150 Ug/dL
Children	Consult laboratory for reference values.
Newborns	Consult laboratory for reference values.

Specimen Required

A 5–10-ml sample of venous blood is obtained. Serum is used for the analysis.

TABLE 5.4. Trace Elements

Arsenic	Manganese
Cadmium	Molybdenum
Chromium	Nickel
Cobalt	Selenium
Copper	Silicone
Fluorine	Tin
Iodine	Vanadium
Iron	Zinc

5

Preparation of the Patient

Food and drink are not usually restricted before venipuncture.

Causes of Deviation from Normal

Decreased levels of serum zinc are found in patients on long-term alternate feeding regimens that are deficient in zinc. Critically ill patients are also susceptible to large losses of all trace elements, including zinc. Deficiencies in zinc have been related to a number of pathological problems, including anorexia, cachexia, alopecia, difficult wound healing, and lowered immune responses to infection. Decreases in serum zinc have been demonstrated in various malignant tissues, such as carcinoma of the prostate and cancer of the head and neck. Although it is known that zinc is essential for all cellular growth, including growth of cancerous cells, the metabolic mechanisms involved in its activity have not been demonstrated.

Nursing Implications of Abnormal Findings

Assessment and Interventions. When caring for patients on long-term alternate nutrition, the nurse should observe the patients for zinc deficiencies as well as for copper deficiencies. Because cancer patients may be particularly prone to this problem, the nurse should assess these patients for cachexia, anorexia, difficulties with wound healing, and infections. Nursing interventions should include protecting the patient from infection, planning nutritional intake using the patient's food preferences, and providing for emotional support. Food sources of zinc include shellfish, meat, milk and milk products, legumes, nuts, and whole grains.

SERUM COPPER

Description

Copper is one of the trace elements found in the body (Table 5.4). It is found in small amounts in the serum. It is required for hemoglobin synthesis and is a constituent of various enzymes, including cytochrome oxidase, which is important in cellular respiration.

NORMAL RANGE	
Adults, male	70–140 Ug/dL
Adults, female	80–155 Ug/dL
Pregnant females	140–300 Ug/dL
Children	30–190 Ug/dL
Newborns	20–70 Ug/dL

Specimen Required
A 5-ml sample of venous blood is obtained. Serum is used for the analysis.

Preparation of the Patient
Food and drink are not usually restricted before venipuncture.

Causes of Deviation from Normal
Decreases in serum copper are found in patients whose long-term feeding regimens are deficient in copper-containing nutrients. Patients with kwashiorkor, or those on long-term parenteral and enteral nutrition programs, are potentially vulnerable. Some childhood anemias are manifested by decreases in copper and iron and require replacement of both elements. Serum copper is decreased in Wilson's disease, a rare disease in which copper accumulates in neurological tissues, causing degenerative changes. Increases in serum copper are found in other adult anemias such as pernicious, aplastic, and iron deficiency anemias. Increases in serum copper levels occur in both acute and chronic leukemia and in thyroid and collagen diseases.

Nursing Implications of Abnormal Findings
Assessment and Interventions. When caring for patients on long-term parenteral and enteral nutrition programs, serum copper determination is important in identifying deficiencies. If decreased copper is found in childhood anemia, replacement therapy should include both iron and copper supplements. Education of the parents regarding accurate dosage administration is an important nursing responsibility. For patients with Wilson's disease, nursing management varies according to the amount of neurological degeneration present. Protection of the patient from injury is a prime responsibility. When a high serum copper level is associated with a malignant disease, nursing interventions vary according to specific patient needs.

SERUM OSMOLALITY

Description

Serum osmolality is a measurement of the total concentration of dissolved particles per unit of water in serum. These particles include electrolytes, such as sodium and potassium, as well as electrically inactive substances dissolved in serum, such as urea and glucose. Serum sodium is responsible for 85–90% of the serum osmolality. The measurement of serum osmolality reflects the osmolality in all body compartments because the cell membranes do not permit an osmolar gradient. Serum osmolality is regulated by two mechanisms that affect body water. First, the thirst mechanism is activated by *osmoreceptors* that are sensitive to increases in osmotic pressure and that thus stimulate a person with an increased osmotic pressure to drink water. Second, *antidiuretic hormone* (ADH) is secreted by the posterior pituitary gland in response to increases in serum osmolality; in the collecting ducts in the kidney, ADH allows for progressive diffusion of water into the medulla and results in excretion of concentrated urine into the renal pelvis. The term *osmolarity* is sometimes used interchangeably with *osmolality* in discussing fluids and electrolytes. *Osmolality* refers to particles per unit of water expressed as milliosmoles per kilogram of water, and *osmolarity* refers to particles per unit of solution expressed as milliosmoles per liter of solution.

5

N O R M A L R A N G E	
Adults	280–300 mOsm/kg water
Children	270–290 mOsm/kg water
Newborns	as low as 266 mOsm/kg water

Specimen Required

Serum is used for the examination. It may be obtained by means of venipuncture and collected in a plain or heparinized collecting tube or syringe. Oxalated plasma is not satisfactory. If urine osmolality is also being tested, the specimens should be collected at approximately the same time.

Preparation of the Patient

No special preparation of the patient is required. If both urine and serum osmolality tests are ordered, the patient should be informed of the need for simultaneous collection of the specimens.

Causes of Deviation from Normal

Serum osmolality can increase with dehydration and loss of body water and decrease with water excess. *Hyperosmolar* states may occur in (1) elderly patients who cannot take fluids well, (2) infants with mild diarrhea who are losing more water than solutes, (3) patients on high protein feedings with inadequate water intake, (4) patients with acute brain trauma and brain surgery in which ADH secretion is depressed, (5) patients in chronic renal failure caused by increased blood urea nitrogen and increased serum sodium, (6) patients in hyperglycemic hyperosmolar nonketotic coma, and (7) patients with diabetes insipidus in which the secretion of ADH is impaired. During hyperosmolar states, cellular water decreases and cells shrink.

Hypoosmolar states occur when the kidneys are unable to excrete the free water derived from ingestion, intravenous fluids, and metabolism. Hypoosmolar states occur when water is used to replace sodium and water losses from excessive perspiration, gastric suction and irrigation, during compulsive water drinking, from excessive tap-water enemas, and during inappropriate ADH secretion or production (see Table 5.2). Hypoosmolar states also occur after cerebral injury and trauma and in postoperative patients treated with excessive water replacement. Patients with congestive heart failure and cirrhosis are also frequently hypoosmolar. During a hypoosmolar state, the excess in water causes an increase in cell water and cell size, resulting in cellular edema.

Nursing Implications of Abnormal Findings

Assessment. Careful observation may prevent shock and renal shutdown in patients with elevated serum osmolality. The nurse should carefully monitor weight, urinary output, vital signs, neurological status, and changes in skin and mucous membranes.

Nursing observations are needed to detect deterioration in the neurological status of patients with decreased serum osmolality. The nurse should carefully note the patient's vital signs and neurological status and keep accurate and complete intake and output records. A change in neurological status should be reported promptly.

Interventions. When the nurse is caring for a patient in a hyperosmolar state, prevention of additional fluid losses from elevations in body temperature is necessary. If the patient is lethargic or becoming stuporous, safety precautions should be instituted to prevent accidents.

When a patient has a decrease in serum osmolality, the nurse should avoid additional dilution of body fluids by (1) replacement of lost fluids with electrolyte solutions, (2) careful use of tap-water enemas, (3) irrigation of nasogastric tubes with saline rather than water, and (4) not forcing fluids on postoperative or post-trauma patients without a careful evaluation of the fluid-balance state. Medical management of a patient in a hypoosmolar state generally involves fluid restriction. The nurse should plan a 24-hour distribution of allowed fluids so that some fluids are available at all times. If oral medications are ordered, adequate fluid must be allowed so that the patient has sufficient fluid for swallowing the medications. For patients on diuretics and low-sodium diets, patient education should include the appropriate use of medications, signs of a decrease in osmolality, and the need for regular medical evaluation.

URINE OSMOLALITY

Description

Urine osmolality is a measurement of the total concentration of dissolved particles per unit of water in the urine. The substance contributing most to urine osmolality is urea. The osmolality of urine varies greatly with diet and with fluid intake. It reflects the ability of the kidney to vary the concentration of urine in order to maintain fluid balance.

N O R M A L   R A N G E

5

The osmolality of urine can range from 50–1400 mOsm/kg. When both urine and serum osmolality determinations are performed, the usual ratio of urine to serum osmolality is 4:1. This ratio may fall to 1:1 when excess water is being excreted, but is abnormal if it is less than 1:1. Values for children are the same as those for adults.

Specimen Required

Urine is collected in a plain tube. If both serum and urine osmolality tests are ordered, both specimens should be collected at the same time.

Preparation of the Patient

The urine osmolality may be tested along with a simultaneously collected serum sample. If this occurs, the patient should be told to expect to have both specimens collected as close together in time as possible. A more complex preparation is sometimes ordered. This involves (1) eating a high-protein diet for three days before the test, (2) eating a dry supper and no liquids the evening before the test, (3) emptying the bladder and discarding the urine at six AM on the morning of the test, and (4) collecting the urine specimen at eight AM in a clear tube. With this latter method, careful patient instruction regarding diet restriction is needed.

Causes of Deviation from Normal

Abnormalities of urine osmolality reflect abnormalities in renal function. Diabetes insipidus causes low serum osmolality levels, due to the impaired secretion of ADH. In chronic renal disease, a fixed urine osmolality reflects the inability of the kidney to concentrate and dilute the urine to maintain fluid balance. This is evident when simultaneous serial serum and urine osmolalities are taken at different times during the day but remain at a ratio of 1:1. In the syndrome of inappropriate secretion of ADH (SIADH), the high serum osmolality present is related to additional body water retention from excess ADH activity (see Table 5.2). A dehydrated patient with normal kidney function will have a urine osmolality of greater than 1,000 mOsm/l, while patients with shock, hyperglycemia, hemoconcentration, and acidosis will have elevations in both urine and serum osmolality.

Nursing Implications of Abnormal Findings

Assessment and Interventions. When caring for patients with diabetes insipidus, the nurse should plan for adequate availability of fluids for the patient. Careful intake and output records are needed for all patients with abnormalities in urine osmolality. For patients with chronic renal failure, nursing interventions vary depending on the stage of illness and the medical treatment plan. When caring for a patient with SIADH, the nurse should plan distribution of the restricted fluid intake over a 24-hour period so that the patient is as comfortable as possible and there is liquid available on all shifts for administering oral medications. The nurse should monitor bowel functioning daily to prevent fecal impaction, a complication of SIADH. In critically ill patients with dehydration, shock, or acidosis, the nurse should expect to see urine osmolalities of greater than 100 mOsm/l. If the level drops, the nurse should be alert to the potential occurrence of renal failure and should notify the physician of the patient's status. The nurse should expect dilution of the urine in patients on diuretic therapy. With potent diuretics such as mannitol, the urine may become isoosmolar with serum.

URINE SODIUM

Description

Sodium is the principal cation in the extracellular fluid. Urine contains sodium as a result of the normal excretion of excess sodium through the kidneys. Control of sodium excretion is regulated by the hormone *aldosterone*, which is secreted by the adrenal cortex. Aldosterone causes reabsorption of sodium from the renal tubules in response to (1) a decrease in sodium concentration in the extracellular fluid, (2) an increase in intracellular potassium, (3) decreases in blood volume and cardiac output, and (4) both physical and emotional stress.

NORMAL RANGE	
Adults	130–200 mEq/24 h
Children	130–200 mEq/24 h

Specimen Required

A 24-hour urine specimen is obtained in a plain collecting bottle. Refrigerate the specimen or place it on ice during the collection period.

Preparation of the Patient

There are no food or fluid restrictions before or during the specimen collection period.

Causes of Deviation from Normal

To distinguish specific causes, abnormal values of urine sodium should be considered in relation to other signs and symptoms. A variety of conditions may lead to increased urine sodium levels (Table 5.5).

Conditions associated with decreased urine sodium levels include acute renal failure, congestive heart failure, decreased salt intake, and primary aldosteronism.

Nursing Implications of Abnormal Findings

Assessment and Interventions. Because of the variety of conditions that can cause increases in urine sodium levels, the nursing assessment and interventions depend on the specific condition. The nurse may expect to collect additional urine specimens.

URINE POTASSIUM

Description

Potassium is one of the major electrolytes in the body. It is primarily involved in life-sustaining neuromuscular functioning of cardiac and skeletal muscles.

TABLE 5.5. Conditions Associated With Increased Urine Sodium Levels

Acute renal failure	Diaphoresis
Adrenal cortical deficiency	Diarrhea
Aldosteronism	Diuretic therapy
Chronic renal failure	Malabsorption syndrome
Congestive heart failure	Pulmonary emphysema
Cushing's disease	Pyloric obstruction
Dehydration	Salicylate toxicity
Diabetic acidosis	Starvation

Normal serum potassium levels are maintained by means of renal elimination of the excess amounts remaining from protein metabolism and dietary ingestion. Aldosterone increases the rate of elimination of potassium through the retention of sodium and excretion of potassium in the renal tubules.

N O R M A L R A N G E	
Adults	25–125 mEq/24 hr
Children	Consult laboratory for reference values.
Newborns	Consult laboratory for reference values.

Specimen Required

A 24-hour urine specimen is collected. The laboratory should be consulted about the correct container.

Preparation of the Patient

There are no food or fluid restrictions before or during the specimen-collection period.

Causes of Deviation from Normal

Urine potassium levels are increased in a variety of conditions, including chronic renal failure, diabetic renal disease, acute tubular necrosis, dehydration, starvation, primary aldosteronism, Cushing's disease, salicylate toxicity, and diuretic therapy. Urine potassium levels are decreased in malabsorption syndrome, diarrhea, acute renal failure, adrenal cortical insufficiency, and excessive mineralocorticosteroid activity. As urinary potassium increases, the urine pH decreases, since hydrogen ions are secreted along with potassium.

Nursing Implications of Abnormal Findings

Assessment and Interventions. The assessment and interventions planned by the nurse depend on the underlying cause of the urinary potassium abnormality. Fluid and electrolyte problems are likely to be present, and the nurse should prepare the patient for additional diagnostic testing. If the patient is hypokalemic, assessment should include checking for diminished reflexes, rapid, weak, or irregular pulse; confusion; hypotension; anorexia; weakness; and paresthesia. ECG changes also occur with signs of ventricular fibrillation, respiratory paralysis, and cardiac arrest.

URINE CALCIUM (SULKOWITCH TEST)

Description

Calcium is a cation found primarily in bones and teeth combined with phosphate and carbonate. Most excess body calcium is excreted daily in the stool. However, serum calcium levels are regulated by parathyroid hormone. When serum calcium levels drop, parathyroid hormone is secreted, causing increased intestinal absorption of ingested calcium and resorption of calcium in the renal tubules.

N O R M A L   R A N G E

For qualitative analysis, the Sulkowitch test is done, with normal ranges running from 1+ to 2+. For quantitative analysis, a 24-hour urine specimen is analyzed. The normal range is 100–250 mg/24 h on an average diet and 150 mg/24 h on a low-calcium diet. Values for children are similar to those for adults.

5

Specimen Required

A random urine specimen is needed for the Sulkowitch test. For the quantitative urine calcium measurement, a 24-hour urine specimen is required.

Preparation of the Patient

Although food and fluid restrictions are not usually required before or during specimen collection, false-positive results may be caused by diets high in calcium (high milk and milk-product intake), elevated sodium and magnesium intake, which binds calcium, and administration of androgens, vitamin D, parathyroid hormone, and cholestyramine. False-negative results may be caused by increased intake of phosphates and administration of thiazides, viomycin, and sodium phytate. If the urine is alkaline, false-negative results may occur.

If a metabolic disorder is suspected, the patient may be asked to eat a low-calcium diet and to restrict calcium medications for one to three days before the collection of the specimen.

Causes of Deviation from Normal

Increases in urine calcium level occur in conjunction with hyperparathyroidism, breast and lung cancers, metastatic cancer involving the bone, Wilson's disease, renal tubular acidosis, and glucocorticoid excess. These increases in urine calcium may be accompanied by the formation of calcium stones in the urinary tract.

Decreases in urine calcium level occur in conjunction with hypoparathyroidism, vitamin D deficiency, and malabsorption syndrome.

Nursing Implications of Abnormal Findings

Assessment. When a patient's urine calcium level is elevated, the nurse should assess the patient for decreased muscle tone, deep bone and flank pain, and gastrointestinal symptoms, including nausea, vomiting, thirst, anorexia, and constipation. Pathological fractures may occur from bony cavitation. At toxic levels of increase, nervous-system depression may occur and cardiac arrest may result from the inability of the cardiac muscle to contract.

When a patient's urine calcium level is decreased, the nurse should watch for increased neuromuscular irritability, which is indicated by abdominal cramps, leg cramps, tingling of the fingertips and the area around the mouth, tetany, and convulsions.

Interventions. When a patient's urine calcium level is increased, there is likely to be an elevated serum calcium as well. The nurse should provide for adequate fluid intake to prevent the formation of calculi. The acidity of the urine can be increased by the ingestion of cranberry or prune juice daily. This also may prevent formation of calcium calculi. The patient's extremities should be handled with care to prevent pathological fractures and to control bone pain.

Patients whose urine calcium level is decreased will likely be taking oral replacement of calcium. A teaching plan should be carried out to assist these patients with accurate long-term administration of this calcium replacement.

BIBLIOGRAPHY

Brady, S. "Urodynamics: an overview." *Urological Nursing*, 9(1):837–841 (January/March 1990).

Corbett, J.V. *Laboratory Tests and Diagnostic Procedures with Nursing Diagnoses*. Norwalk, Connecticut: Appleton and Lange, 1992.

Fischbach, F.T. A *Manual of Laboratory and Diagnostic Tests*. Philadelphia: J.B. Lippincott Company, 1992.

Ignatavicius, D.D., and M.V. Bayne. *Medical-Surgical Nursing: A Nursing Process Approach*. Philadelphia: W.B. Saunders, 1991.

Lewis, S.M., and I.C. Collier. *Medical-Surgical Nursing: Assessment and Management of Clinical Problems*. St. Louis: Mosby Yearbook, 1992.

Phipps, W.S., B.C. Long, N.F. Woods, and V. Cossmeyer. *Medical-Surgical Nursing*. St. Louis: Mosby Yearbook, 1991

Ravel, R. *Clinical Laboratory Medicine*. Chicago: Year Book Medical Publishers, Inc., 1989.

Smetzer, S.C., and B.G. Ball. *Brunner and Sudarth's Medical-Surgical Nursing*. New York: J.B. Lippincott, 1992.

Wallach, J. *Interpretation of Diagnostic Tests*. Boston: Little, Brown and Company, 1992.

Wilson, J.D., et al. *Harrison's Principles of Internal Medicine*. New York: McGraw-Hill, 1991.

5

Laboratory Tests of Acid–Base Balance

Arterial Blood Gas Analysis
pH
Pa$_{O_2}$
Oxygen Saturation (S$_a$O$_2$)
Pa$_{CO_2}$
Bicarbonate
Base Excess

Anion Gap

Lactic Acid

ARTERIAL BLOOD GAS ANALYSIS

Description

Blood gas analysis (analysis of pH, Pa$_{O_2}$, oxygen saturation (SaO$_2$), Pa$_{CO_2}$, HCO$_3$, base excess, and CO$_2$ combining power) is the measurement of pH, Pa$_{O_2}$, and Pa$_{CO_2}$ in arterial blood. It is done to determine the respiratory status (adequacy of oxygenation and ventilation) and the acid–base status of the patient.

pH

pH is the term used to express the hydrogen ion (H$^+$) concentration of a solution. pH is a measurement of the overall acid–base status of the blood. It is defined as the negative logarithm of hydrogen ions in solution. When hydrogen ions are added to a solution, the *increased* H$^+$ concentration is reflected in a *lower* pH, and the solution becomes more acidic. When hydrogen ions are

136

removed from a solution, the concentration of H^+ is *decreased*, the pH becomes *higher*, and the solution becomes more alkaline.

Pa_{O_2}

Pa_{O_2} is a measurement of the partial pressure of oxygen in the arterial blood. Oxygen is carried in the blood in two forms: physically dissolved and chemically bound to hemoglobin. Since oxygen is relatively insoluble in plasma, the amount of oxygen carried in physically dissolved form is only slightly more than 1%. This amount is not sufficient to meet even the lowest tissue needs at rest. The greatest portion of oxygen (over 98%) is transported by the red cells as oxyhemoglobin. Each hemoglobin molecule has four sites that can carry oxygen. When all sites carry oxygen, the hemoglobin is 100% saturated. Each gram of hemoglobin can carry 1.36 ml of oxygen; therefore, when hemoglobin in a concentration of 15 g% is completely saturated, it carries 20.4 ml of oxygen.

The extent to which oxygen can combine with hemoglobin is primarily determined by the Pa_{O_2} of the blood. The oxyhemoglobin dissociation curve (Fig. 6.1) illustrates the relationship between Pa_{O_2} and percent saturation. The shape of the curve, which has a steep slope between 10 and 60 mm Hg and a plateau between 70 and 100 mm Hg, illustrates the body's physiological adaptation to its environment. When situations arise that cause the arterial Pa_{O_2} to fall from 100 to 60 mm Hg, the total amount of O_2 carried by hemoglobin decreases by only 10%. The steeper portion of the curve allows large amounts of oxygen to dissociate from the hemoglobin in response to small changes in the Pa_{O_2} of systemic capillaries.

6

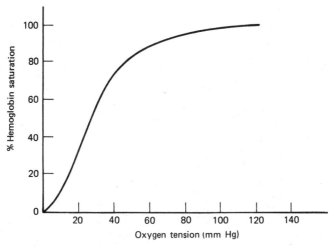

FIGURE 6.1. Oxyhemoglobin Dissociation Curve.

The ability of O_2 to combine with hemoglobin is also affected by the body temperature and blood pH. When the temperature is elevated or acidosis is present, the curve shifts downward and to the right (Fig. 6.2). When this change occurs, the affinity of hemoglobin for O_2 is less than normal; however, O_2 is more readily released to the cells. For example, it takes a Pa_{O_2} of 40 mm Hg to achieve 50% saturation (normal = 27 mm Hg for 50% saturation). The opposite effect occurs when the body temperature is below normal or when alkalosis is present; that is, the curve shifts upward and to the left (Fig. 6.3). When this change occurs, it takes a Pa_{O_2} of only 20 mm Hg to achieve 50% saturation and oxygen is not as readily released to the tissues.

OXYGEN SATURATION (SaO₂)

The *oxygen saturation* is a report of the quantity of oxygen in the blood. It is a ratio of the amount of oxygen in the blood that is combined with hemoglobin compared to the total amount of oxygen that can combine with hemoglobin. The relationship of oxygen saturation to the Pa_{O_2} can be seen on the oxyhemoglobin dissociation curve (Fig. 6.1). This value does not reflect the quantity of oxygen that is delivered to the tissues.

Pa_CO2

Pa_{CO_2} is a measurement of the partial pressure of CO_2 in the arterial blood. Most of the body's CO_2 comes from food that is metabolized to form energy. H_2O and CO_2 are by-products of this metabolism. The body produces two hundred ml of CO_2 every minute, most of which is transported by the blood from the tissues to the lungs, where it is eliminated. Carbon dioxide is carried in the blood in three forms: physically dissolved, chemically bound to hemoglo-

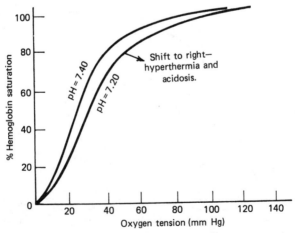

FIGURE 6.2. Effect of decreased pH on oxyhemoglobin dissociation curve.

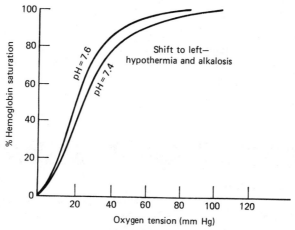

FIGURE 6.3. Effect of increase in pH on oxyhemoglobin dissociation curve.

6

bin, and converted to bicarbonate. Conversion to bicarbonate occurs when carbon dioxide in the blood is hydrated to form carbonic acid and then dissociated to bicarbonate and hydrogen ions. The following equation illustrates this process:

$$CO_2 + H_2O \leftrightharpoons H_2CO_3 \rightleftharpoons HCO_3 + H^+$$

The amount of carbon dioxide in arterial blood is in equilibrium with the amount of carbon dioxide in the alveoli. Therefore, as ventilation of the alveoli is increased, carbon dioxide tension in the blood decreases.

BICARBONATE

Bicarbonate (HCO_3) is a part of the carbonic acid–bicarbonate buffer system. It helps to stabilize pH by combining reversibly with H^+. Most of the body's bicarbonate is produced in the red cells, where the enzyme carbonic anhydrase accelerates the conversion of CO_2 to carbonic acid. The following reversible equation illustrates the production of bicarbonate:

$$CO_2 + H_2O \overset{\text{carbonic}}{\underset{\text{anhydrase}}{\leftrightharpoons}} H_2CO_3 \rightleftharpoons HCO_3 + H^+$$

When there is an increased concentration of hydrogen ion in the extracellular space, the reaction of this equation shifts toward the left. A decreased concentration of hydrogen ion drives the reaction to the right.

BASE EXCESS

The *base excess* of whole blood is a commonly used measurement of acid–base status. This value represents the amount of acid or base that must be added to each liter of blood to return it to a normal pH when the Pa_{CO_2} is equilibrated at 40 mm hg. This value gives information about the amount of excess acid or base per unit volume of blood.

N O R M A L R A N G E		
Adults and children		
	Range	*Mean*
Arterial pH	7.36–7.44	7.4
Arterial Po_2	85–100 mm Hg	
Arterial Pco_2	38–42 mm Hg	40 mm Hg
Arterial HCO_3^-	22–26 mEq/l	24 mEq/l
Base excess	−3 to +3 mEq/l	
Oxygen saturation	95% of Po_2	

Note. Arterial Po_2 varies with age. Older people have values near the lower part of the normal range and younger people in the upper portion. Some of the normal values for arterial blood gases are influenced by altitude. At an altitude of one mile above sea level, the arterial Po_2 and Pco_2 are:

Arterial Po_2	65–75 mm Hg
Arterial Pco_2	34–38 mm Hg

Specimen Required

Arterial blood is obtained from the femoral, radial, or brachial artery. A 2.5–10-ml sample is obtained in a glass syringe whose interior has been coated with heparin. After the blood has been drawn, any air that has been aspirated accidentally must be expelled. After the needle is removed, an airtight cap should be placed over the tip of the syringe, which should then immediately be placed in ice and sent to the laboratory. (See Chapter 1 for a more detailed description of the method for arterial puncture.)

Total CO_2 may be obtained from venous blood during a routine test for serum electrolytes. The total CO_2 value in venous blood is 23–30 mM/l. When the venous CO_2 is being used to assess acid–base parameters, the following measures should be taken when the blood is drawn:

The skin and arm of the hand must be warm.

The tourniquet must not be applied too tightly or for too long.

The fist must not be clenched repeatedly before and during the drawing of the blood sample.

Preparation of the Patient

The nurse should explain the need for obtaining an arterial blood sample and describe how it differs from a venipuncture. If the patient is receiving oxygen therapy, there must be a minimum of ten minutes of uninterrupted oxygen flow. The Pa_{O_2} will not be accurate if suctioning, intermittent positive pressure breathing (IPPB), or a change in FI_{O_2} has taken place during the ten minutes prior to the arterial puncture.

Causes of Deviation from Normal

pH, Pa_{CO_2}, HCO_3

Since the pH, Pa_{CO_2}, and HCO_3, readings are obtained to determine the acid–base status of the patient, they will be discussed together. Disturbances in acid–base balance are caused by either respiratory or non-respiratory (metabolic) abnormalities. The carbonic acid–bicarbonate buffering system can be used to identify the source of acid–base disturbances. The following equation illustrates this.

$$\underset{\substack{\uparrow \\ \text{metabolism}}}{\overset{\overset{\text{lung}}{\uparrow}}{CO_2}} + H_2O \leftrightharpoons H_2CO_3 \rightleftharpoons \underset{\substack{\uparrow \\ \text{metabolism} \\ NH_4Cl, \text{ etc.}}}{\overset{\overset{\text{kidney}}{\overset{\text{stomach, etc.}}{\uparrow}}}{H^+}} + \underset{\substack{\uparrow \\ \text{oral} \\ \text{intake, etc.}}}{\overset{\overset{\text{GI tract,}}{\overset{\text{kidney, etc.}}{\uparrow}}}{HCO_3}}$$

RESPIRATORY ABNORMALITIES

If the lungs do not ventilate fast enough to eliminate CO_2 in proportion to the rate at which it is being formed, the equation will shift to the right. This change occurs because the CO_2 that is being produced cannot be eliminated. As a result, hydrogen ions accumulate and acidemia occurs. Conversely, if more CO_2 is eliminated by the lungs than is being produced by the body's metabolism, alkalemia results from overventilation. These disturbances are called *respiratory acidosis* and *respiratory alkalosis*, respectively, because they are caused by a change in lung status. Since the Pa_{CO_2} is directly proportional to the concentration of CO_2 in the blood, the extent of deviation from normal Pa_{CO_2} will indicate the severity of the acid–base disturbance present. When the Pa_{CO_2} is greater than 42 mm Hg, respiratory acidosis is present. When it is below 38 mm Hg, respiratory alkalosis is the acid–base abnormality.

METABOLIC ABNORMALITIES

If hydrogen ions accumulate on the right side of the reversible equation as a result of an increase in their rate of formation or a decrease in their rate of

TABLE 6.1.　Causes of Respiratory Acidosis

Obstructive lung diseases
Oversedation with analgesics, hypnotics, etc.
Head injuries that depress respiratory centers
Primary alveolar hypoventilation
Cardiopulmonary arrest
Poliomyelitis
Congestive heart failure
Burns of the respiratory tract
Mechanical obstruction of the respiratory tract

excretion by the kidney, acidemia results. Acidemia also occurs when bicarbonate is lost at a rapid rate from the gastrointestinal tract because of severe diarrhea. Alkalosis may be caused by severe vomiting or gastric suctioning resulting in an excessive loss of hydrogen ions from the stomach. It can also occur in persons who have a high oral intake of bicarbonate. Diuretic therapy and hyperadrenocorticism also produce it when bicarbonate retention occurs as a result of potassium and chloride excretion. Tables 6.1 to 6.4 provide lists of causes of respiratory and metabolic acid–base disturbances.

When the blood pH is abnormal and the Pa_{CO_2} is normal, a metabolic acid–base disturbance must be present. The plasma bicarbonate level is the most useful criterion to use in detecting metabolic acid–base disturbances. If this value is not included in the blood gas analysis reported by the laboratory, it can be determined by means of a nomogram (Fig. 6.4). When the bicarbonate level is greater than 26 mEq/l, metabolic alkalosis is present, and when it is below 22 mEq/l, metabolic acidosis is the acid–base abnormality.

TABLE 6.2.　Causes of Respiratory Alkalosis

Acute or chronic hypoxemia
Hyperventilation attributable to anxiety, fever, exercise, etc.
Pulmonary embolus
Hyperventilation of pregnancy
Mechanical ventilation
Salicylate intoxication

TABLE 6.3. Causes of Metabolic Acidosis

Diabetic ketoacidosis
Starvation ketosis
Poisonings—salicylate, ethylene glycol, methyl alcohol, paraldehyde
Lactic acidosis
Renal failure
Diarrhea
Ureteroenterostomy
Treatment with Diamox. NH_4Cl
Renal disease—chronic renal failure, renal tubular acidosis, renal failure

COMPENSATORY STATES

In addition to the initial buffering that occurs in response to acid–base distur-bances, physiological compensatory responses also take place. These are very important in minimizing the changes in pH that result when any of the four types of acid–base disturbances occurs. When a respiratory acid–base imbal-ance is present, it is compensated for by a physiologically induced metabolic disturbance. Metabolic acid–base imbalances are compensated for by respira-tory mechanisms (Table 6.5).

Respiratory Acidosis. When respiratory acidosis occurs, the kidneys begin to increase the production and retention of bicarbonate. This renal compensa-tion begins immediately but takes several days to reach its peak effectiveness. When compensation is occurring, the pH returns toward normal. Renal disease or diuretic therapy may impair the ability of the kidneys to compensate.

TABLE 6.4. Causes of Metabolic Alkalosis

Diuretic therapy
Treatment with corticosteroids
Cushing's disease
Hyperaldosteronism
Fluid losses from upper gastrointestinal tract due to vomiting
    or nasogastric suctioning
Excessive intake of alkalis, such as sodium bicarbonate

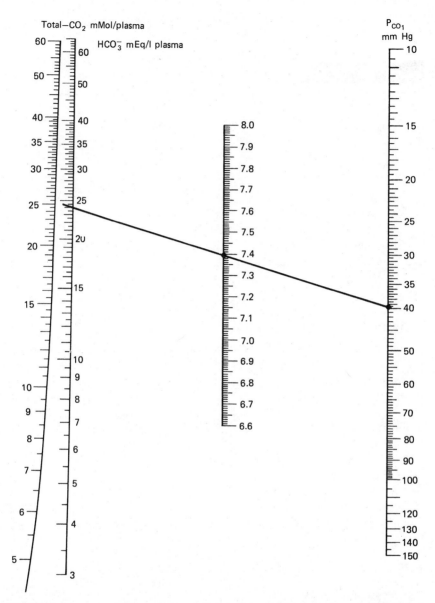

FIGURE 6.4. A nomogram used to determine the [HCO$_3^-$] from measured pH and Pa$_{CO_2}$. If arterial pH is 7.39 and P$_{CO_2}$ is 40 torr, the [HCO$_3^-$] in that sample is 24 mEq. To determine [HCO$_3^-$], mark the values of Pa$_{CO_2}$ and pH obtained from blood gas analysis in the appropriate columns. Draw a straight line through the two points marked and extend the line through the column labeled HCO$_3^-$ mEq/l of plasma. The [HCO$_3^-$] is read directly in mEq/l from the intersection of the extended line and the HCO$_3^-$ column. (Adapted from the alignment nomogram by O. Siggard-Andersen. Reprinted by permission of Jack L. Keyes, "Blood Gas Analysis and the Assessment of Aud–Base Status." *Heart and Lung,* 5:248 (March–April 1976.)

144

TABLE 6.5. Blood Parameters of Acid–Base Balance during Uncompensated and Compensated States

Respiratory Acidosis

	Uncompensated	Compensated
pH	↓	Low normal
Pa_{CO_2}	↑	↑
HCO_3	Normal	↑

Respiratory Alkalosis

	Uncompensated	Compensated
pH	↑	High normal
Pa_{CO_2}	↓	↓
HCO_3	Normal	↓

Metabolic Acidosis

	Uncompensated	Compensated
pH	↓	Low normal
Pa_{CO_2}	Normal	↓
HCO_3	↓	↓

Metabolic Alkalosis

	Uncompensated	Compensated
pH	↑	High normal
Pa_{CO_2}	Normal	↑
HCO_3	↑	↑

6

Respiratory Alkalosis. In primary respiratory alkalosis, compensation occurs by metabolic means. Bicarbonate reabsorption by the kidneys is reduced and bicarbonate is excreted through the urine. Occasionally the hyperventilation that causes respiratory alkalosis is followed by an increase in lactate and pyruvate in the blood, which aids in compensation by producing a base deficit.

Metabolic Acidosis. In primary metabolic acidosis, the major compensatory mechanism is hyperventilation, which induces a respiratory alkalosis by means of stimulation of chemoreceptors in the aortic-carotid area and in an area near the floor of the fourth ventricle. This compensation is not complete. The process stops when stimulation of respirations stops as the initially high pH approaches normal. If the kidneys are not diseased, they may participate in the compensation for metabolic acidosis by increasing their rate of synthesis of HCO_3.

Metabolic Alkalosis. When metabolic alkalosis occurs, the increased pH depresses respiration and reduces ventilation, causing a rise in the Pa_{CO_2}. Respiratory compensation does not return the pH to normal, because depression of respiration caused by a low pH ceases as the pH approaches normal. Kidneys that are not diseased may also help the compensatory response by excreting HCO_3 through the urine.

MIXED ACID–BASE DISTURBANCES

In clinical situations, more than one primary acid–base disturbance may be present simultaneously. Most commonly, a respiratory acidosis or alkalosis occurs at the same time as its metabolic counterpart. Mixed acidosis often occurs when a person has developed hypoventilation so extreme that lactic acidosis occurs due to the anaerobic metabolism that accompanies hypoxemia. Mixed alkalosis may occur in patients with adult respiratory distress syndrome (shock lung).

Pa$_{O_2}$

A decrease in the total arterial oxygen content of the blood may be related to hypoventilation (Fig. 6.5), physiological capillary shunting, ventilation/perfusion abnormalities (Fig. 6.6), anatomical right-to-left shunts (Fig. 6.7), or the decreased inspired oxygen tension that occurs at high altitudes. Hypoventilation may be caused by:

1. Airway obstruction due to vomitus, foreign objects, large mucous plugs, or cramped neck position.

2. Central nervous system injury.

3. Thoracic injury.

4. Ingestion of drugs that inhibit breathing centers.

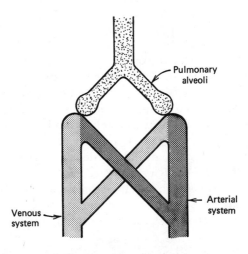

HYPOVENTILATION

FIGURE 6.5. Hypoventilation—cardiac output perfusing poorly ventilated alveoli.

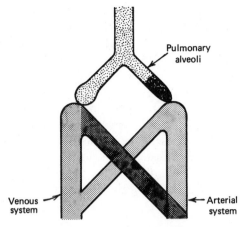

PHYSIOLOGIC–CAPILLARY SHUNT

FIGURE 6.6. Physiological capillary shunt—portion of cardiac output perfusing non-ventilating alveoli.

6

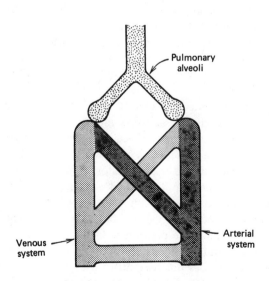

ANATOMIC RIGHT–TO–LEFT SHUNT

FIGURE 6.7. Anatomical right-to-left shunt—portion of cardiac output by passing pulmonary capillaries.

In these situations, the P_{CO_2} rises in the alveolar gas, limiting the amount of oxygen present and resulting in a fall in the arterial oxygen content. Physiological shunting occurs when blood flows through the pulmonary capillaries but the alveoli are not well ventilated because of a pulmonary problem such as pneumonia, pulmonary edema, or atelectasis. When anatomical right-to-left shunts occur, blood is shunted from the venous to the arterial system without passing through the pulmonary capillaries. Pulmonary arteriovenous (A-V) fistulas and congenital heart anomalies cause this shunting to occur.

An increase in the Pa_{O_2} is caused by the inspiration of high oxygen concentrations. It has been reported that patients may show symptoms of pulmonary irritation after exposure to 70–100% O_2 for more than 24 hours. Damage to lung tissue will result if exposure to these high concentrations of oxygen is prolonged.

Nursing Implications of Abnormal Findings

The nursing care of patients with abnormal blood gas analyses will be discussed first in relation to alterations in acid–base balance and then in relation to abnormalities in the oxygen content of the arterial blood.

RESPIRATORY ACIDOSIS

Assessment. The nursing care of patients with respiratory acidosis should focus on the presence of signs and symptoms related to this abnormality and whether the disease causing the problem is chronic or acute. The typical signs and symptoms are somnolence, decreased attention span, restlessness, hypoventilation, hypoxia, low blood pressure, and tachycardia and other arrhythmias. The physical assessment may also reveal rales, rhonchi, wheezes, and grunting expirations. If the patient has a chronic disease, a barrel chest, distended neck veins when the patient is upright, and the use of accessory muscles to breathe may be observed. Cyanosis, a late sign of respiratory failure, may also be present.

Interventions. For patients with chronic obstructive pulmonary disease, oxygen should be given judiciously, at a flow rate not greater than 3–4 liters per minute. This restriction is essential, because hypoxia is the only stimulus to breathe for most of these patients. When sedatives have been ordered they should be given cautiously and the respiratory rate monitored closely. When the condition causing the respiratory acidosis is acute, emergency measures should be started to improve ventilation. The airway should be cleared of secretions or foreign bodies and oxygen should be administered. The patient should also be placed in a comfortable position to facilitate lung expansion. Nursing actions should be continually evaluated and blood drawn for further blood gas analysis. If the patient does not respond to the nursing measures, the nurse should be prepared for endotracheal intubation or surgical tracheostomy.

A patient who has a chronic respiratory condition with mild respiratory acidosis should be taught how to live with the condition. Such patients should be told to avoid chemical irritants such as cigarette smoke, hot dusty rooms, air pollution, and toxic gases. The patient should be taught to observe sputum and to report any changes in color and consistency to the physician or nurse. Unless contraindicated, large amounts of fluid should be given to the patient to keep secretions loose and easy to expectorate. Humidified air can also help to keep secretions thin and mobile. The patient and family should be taught techniques to aid in expectorating secretions, such as postural drainage, vibration, and percussion. Exercises to promote abdominal breathing should also be included in a teaching plan.

RESPIRATORY ALKALOSIS

Assessment. The presence and severity of the clinical manifestations of respiratory alkalosis must be assessed. In mild cases, the patient may complain of light-headedness and numbness and tingling of the fingers and toes. In more severe cases, tetany may result from the shift of free ionized calcium. Since refractory cardiac arrhythmias may also occur in patients who have chronic respiratory alkalosis, frequent assessment of the heart beat should be made. If a patient in respiratory alkalosis is receiving assisted ventilation, the rate and depth of respirations delivered to the patient must be evaluated. The patient's emotional status should also be part of the assessment, since fear and anxiety often causes the hyperventilation that leads to respiratory alkalosis.

When this abnormality is caused by a pathophysiological alteration, such as pulmonary embolism, atelectasis, fever, pain, or salicylate intoxication, the nursing assessment and care are related to the primary disease process. Because an arterial puncture may cause severe pain, anxiety, and apprehension, the nurse must always consider the procedure itself as the cause of respiratory alkalosis.

Interventions. An anxious patient who has self-induced hyperventilation should be taught to breathe into a closed paper bag. This will help the patient focus on controlling respirations as well as improve arterial P_{CO_2} by forcing the patient to rebreathe carbon dioxide. The patient should be reassured that the uncomfortable symptoms, such as dizziness, light-headedness, and numbness and tingling of the extremities, will be relieved by this activity. When the mechanical ventilation is thought to be the cause, the number of breaths given to the patient per minute may be decreased or the volume of air delivered to the patient with each breath reduced. Patients who frequently hyperventilate when anxious can be taught relaxation techniques and guided imagery which may prevent continuous episodes of hyperventilation.

METABOLIC ACIDOSIS

Assessment. The nursing assessment for patients with metabolic acidosis should be related to the disease process that caused the abnormality and to the clinical manifestations that are present. Perception and coordination may be altered in metabolic acidosis, resulting in headaches, lethargy, mental dullness,

6

drowsiness, and stupor. Respirations should be assessed, because when patients in metabolic acidosis attempt to compensate for the abnormality an increase in the rate and depth of respirations (Kussmaul respirations) results.

Interventions. Nursing interventions are related to the clinical manifestations of the disorder as well as to the underlying cause. Patients who exhibit signs and symptoms of neurological dysfunction should be protected from injury and should be observed continuously if disorientation and delirium are severe. These patients should also be given good pulmonary care to facilitate respiratory compensation by allowing the lungs to excrete carbon dioxide. When lactic acidosis is present, nursing care should include plans to improve oxygenation and circulation. The nurse should also be aware of the possible development of hyperkalemia and should take the nursing actions necessary to prevent cardiac arrest (see Chapter 5).

METABOLIC ALKALOSIS

Assessment. The nurse should collect data about the underlying cause of metabolic alkalosis, including the signs and symptoms manifested by the patient. A low potassium level in a patient who is taking diuretics should alert the nurse to the possibility of metabolic alkalosis.

Interventions. If the alkalosis was caused by vomiting or gastric suctioning, the nurse must be sure that any replacement fluids given to the patient are isotonic. The nasogastric tube should also be irrigated with an isotonic solution rather than with sterile water. If the metabolic alkalosis was caused by the ingestion of too many alkaline substances at home, a teaching plan should be developed to focus on the prevention of recurrence. Patients must be instructed about the excessive use of baking soda to relieve indigestion. If the problem was caused by prescribed alkaline substances, the patient should be told to discontinue medications and call the physician if a dry mouth, anorexia, weakness, or a distaste for milk occurs.

ABNORMAL Pa_{O_2}

Assessment. The nursing assessment of a patient with a low Pa_{O_2} should include the following:

The normal oxygen value, if it is known.

The concentration of inspired oxygen.

The method of administering oxygen.

The length of time of uninterrupted oxygen flow.

The patient's temperature and pH and their effect on the oxyhemoglobin dissociation curve (Fig. 6.2).

In addition, the nurse should remember that the signs and symptoms exhibited by a patient with a low Pa_{O_2} result from the effects of tissue hypoxia on the various organ systems. Responses to hypoxemia differ because of individual variations in the amount of circulation and metabolic uptake of oxygen for each type of tissue. The organs most commonly affected are the brain and the myocardium. Confusion, anxiety, irritability, and disorientation indicate the presence of cerebral anoxia, whereas tachycardia and hypertension indicate a cardiovascular response. Cyanosis may also be present, but is a late sign. It does not appear until arterial oxyhemoglobin saturation falls to 83% and the arterial P_{O_2} to 48 mm Hg. At least 5 g of deoxygenated hemoglobin per 100 ml of blood must be present in the systemic capillary circulation to produce the typical color of cyanosis.

The mouth and upper airway should also be inspected for obstruction. The lungs should be auscultated to assess breath sounds. The presence of adventitious sounds, such as rales, wheezes, and friction rubs, may indicate that a serious respiratory disorder is present. When the effort to breathe is so strenuous that accessory respiratory muscles are being used, the patient's status may be critical and immediate attention needed.

Interventions. Nursing interventions for a patient who has a low Pa_{O_2} must be planned to restore ventilation. If the patient is comatose, the first nursing action is to pull the patient's tongue forward and position the head to provide maximum ventilation. The administration of oxygen has a high priority in the care of patients with respiratory insufficiency; however, oxygen must be used judiciously. Giving no oxygen to a person with a Pa_{O_2} of below 50 mm Hg might lower the Pa_{O_2} further and possibly cause tissue damage. Giving a continuous high flow of oxygen might block the hypoxic drive to breathe in patients with underlying chronic pulmonary disease. For this reason, the nurse should be aware of the patient's normal blood gas levels before administering oxygen. It is unnecessary and often harmful to attempt to raise the oxygen content to normal levels in a patient with a normally low Pa_{O_2}.

In patients who are confused or unconscious due to hypoxemia, high concentrations of oxygen may be needed until danger has passed. When the Pa_{O_2} reaches about 60 mm Hg, the amount of oxygen administered should be adjusted to prevent a rapid rise in the Pa_{O_2}. The administration of 2–4 liters of oxygen at between 30% and 40% concentrations is usually safe for less critically ill patients. Many patients can be maintained at this flow rate. Because clinical observations provide only a rough assessment of patient progress, frequent blood gas analyses should be the primary guide for therapy. In many critical-care situations it is the nurse's responsibility to draw blood gases as needed, based on assessment of the patient.

Additional nursing interventions include frequently changing the patient's position to increase Pa_{O_2} by increasing ventilation to all areas of the lungs and preventing a physiological shunt. Removal of secretions by means of good bronchial hygiene is another important nursing intervention. Effective coughing, deep breathing, and chest physiotherapy (percussion, vibration, and postural drainage) promote clearing of the airway. Suctioning may also be used if the patient is unable to raise secretions.

6

The nursing care plan for patients with chronic respiratory problems should include a teaching program planned to improve ventilatory function and prevent frequent infections. Patients should be taught pursed-lipped and abdominal diaphragmatic breathing in order to increase tidal volume, decrease respiratory rate, and provide some subjective improvement. The methods of bronchial hygiene used during hospitalization should be adapted to the home setting. Daily graded exercises may also be taught but must be individualized according to the degree of respiratory impairment. If a low Pa_{O_2} level is caused by respiratory acidosis, the teaching plan discussed previously should also be included.

ANION GAP

Definition

The *anion gap* is a mathematical estimation of the difference between the number of measured cations (sodium and potassium) and measured anions (chloride and bicarbonate) in the serum. It is calculated by subtracting the sum of chloride and bicarbonate anion concentrations from the concentration of sodium and potassium cations.

$$[\text{anion gap} = (\text{sodium} + \text{potassium}) - (\text{chloride} + \text{bicarbonate})]$$

The gap is made up of unmeasured anions such as phosphate and sulfate, organic ions, and anionic groups of plasma proteins. When the anion gap exceeds the normal range, there is an increase in one or more of the unmeasured anions that preserve the electrical neutrality of the serum.

NORMAL RANGE

The range of the normal anion gap is 12–18 mmol/L.

Note: When newer instruments are used to measure sodium, chloride, and bicarbonate, the normal range is 7+ or −4 mmol/L. This is due to an upward shift of chloride values as measured by a new chloride electrode.

Specimen Required

A 5–10-ml specimen of venous blood is required.

Preparation of the Patient

The anion gap is a mathematical approximation that uses serum sodium, potassium, chloride, and bicarbonate values previously obtained. Patient preparation is not necessary.

Causes of Deviation from Normal

An increased anion gap occurs when hydrogen ions have been added to body fluids containing an anion other than chloride. This most commonly occurs in metabolic acidosis caused by diabetic ketoacidosis, lactic acidosis, azotemic renal failure, and drug toxicity from salicylates, ethylene glycol, methyl alcohol, and paraldehyde. Hyperchloremic metabolic acidosis may occur without an increase in the anion gap. This occurs with diarrhea, renal tubular acidosis with hyperchloremia, ureterosigmoidostomy, and the therapeutic use of ammonium chloride or carbonic anhydrase inhibitors.

Nursing Implications of Abnormal Findings

The nursing assessment and interventions for metabolic acidosis are covered in the section on blood gas analysis. Calculation of the anion gap may be helpful to the nurse in caring for a patient with metabolic acidosis of unknown etiology. It is the first step in identifying the cause of metabolic acidosis.

6

LACTIC ACID

Description

Lactic acid is a product of massive anaerobic metabolism when cells are unable to receive an adequate amount of oxygen. Lactic acidosis results when the body is unable to remove excess amounts of lactic acid.

N O R M A L R A N G E	
Adults	0.5–2.2 mEq/L venous blood
	0.5–1.6 mEq/L arterial blood
Children	Consult laboratory for reference values.

Specimen Required

A 5-ml sample of venous or arterial blood is obtained in a tube containing heparin.

Note: The tourniquet must not be applied too tightly or for too long. The fist must not be clenched repeatedly before and during the drawing of the blood sample. The specimen must be placed on ice and delivered to the laboratory immediately.

Preparation of the Patient

Food and fluids are not restricted before collection of the specimen. If an arterial sample is drawn, the nurse should explain how it differs from venipuncture. Increased levels of lactic acid may result from tissue hypoxia due to circulatory collapse, systemic hypoxemia, shock, hemorrhage, renal or liver disease, severe infection, or the presence of drugs or toxins. Strenuous exercise may cause a temporary increase in lactic acid levels which will return to normal following exercise.

Nursing Implications of Abnormal Findings

Assessment and Interventions. Nursing implications are included in the section on metabolic acidosis.

BIBLIOGRAPHY

Brenner, M., and J. Welliver. "Pulmonary and Acid–Base Management." *Nursing Clinics of North America,* 25:761–770 (December 1990).

Buckingham, A.K. "Arterial Blood Gases." *Nursing Life,* 5:48–51 (November–December 1985).

Davenport, H.W. *The ABCs of Acid–Base Chemistry.* Chicago: University of Chicago Press, 1974.

Handerhan, B. "Computing the Anion Gap." *RN,* 54:30–31 (July 1990).

Henry, J.B. *Clinical Diagnosis and Management by Laboratory Methods.* Philadelphia: W.B. Saunders Co., 1991.

Hricik, D.E., and J.P. Kassirer. "Understanding and Using the Anion Gap." *Consultant,* 23:130–134, 143 (July 1983).

Keyes, J.L. "Blood Gases and Blood Gas Transport." *Heart and Lung,* 3:945–954 (November–December 1974).

Keyes, J.L. "Basic Mechanisms Involved in Acid–Base Homeostasis." *Heart and Lung,* 5:239–246 (March–April 1976).

Keyes, J.L. "Blood Gas Analysis and the Assessment of Acid–Base Status." *Heart and Lung,* 5:247–255 (March–April 1976).

Laschinger, H.K. "Demystifying Arterial Blood Gases." *The Canadian Nurse,* 80:45–47 (November 1984).

Lewis, S.M., and I.C. Collier. *Medical-Surgical Nursing: Assessment and Management of Clinical Problems.* St. Louis: Mosby Yearbook, 1992.

Luckman, J., and K.C. Sorensen. *Medical-Surgical Nursing: A Psychological Approach.* Philadelphia: Saunders, 1987.

Mims, B.C. "Interpreting ABGs." *RN*, 54:42–47 (March 1991).

"New Anion Gap Reference Values." *Emergency Medicine*, 22:48–50 (May 15, 1990).

Pfister, S.M. "Arterial Blood-Gas Evaluation: Metabolic Acidemia." *Critical Care Nurse*, 8:14–15, 19 (November–December 1988).

Phipps, W.S., B.C. Long, N.F. Woods, and V. Cossmeyer. *Medical-Surgical Nursing.* St. Louis: Mosby Yearbook, 1991.

Ravel, R. *Clinical Laboratory Medicine.* Chicago: Year Book Medical Publishers, 1989.

Stein, J.M "Interpreting Blood Gases." *Emergency Medicine*, 18:61–68 (January 15, 1986).

Sacher, R.A., and R.A. McPherson. *Widmann's Clinical Interpretation of Laboratory Tests.* Philadelphia: F.A. Davis, 1991.

Smetzer, S.C., and B.G. Ball. *Brunner and Sudarth's Medical-Surgical Nursing.* New York: J.B. Lippincott, 1992.

Vander, A.J., J.H. Sherman, & D.S. Luciano. *Human Physiology: The Mechanisms of Body Function.* New York: McGraw-Hill Publishing Co., Inc., 1990.

Wilson, J., et al. *Harrison's Principles of Internal Medicine.* New York: McGraw-Hill Publishing Co., Inc., 1991.

York, K., and Moddeman, G. "Arterial Blood Gases." *AORN*, 49:1308–1329 (May 1989).

6

7

Laboratory Tests of Genitourinary Disorders

Urinalysis
Urine Specific Gravity
Urine pH
Urine Blood or Hemoglobin
Urine Protein
Urine Glucose
Urine Ketones
Urine Cells and Casts

Blood Urea Nitrogen

Creatinine

Creatinine Clearance

Uric Acid

Phenolsulfonphthalein Excretion Test

Myoglobin, Urine

Myoglobin, Blood

Acid Phosphatase

Carcinoembryonic Antigen (CEA)

Prostate Specific Antigen (PSA)

Urine Uric Acid

URINALYSIS

Description

Urinalysis is done as a general screening test for a variety of diseases. Following an evaluation for color and clarity, a urinalysis includes measurements of specific gravity, pH, protein, glucose, and ketones, plus microscopic examination for casts, red cells, white cells, and epithelial cells. Each of the determinations is discussed separately in this section.

Definition

URINE SPECIFIC GRAVITY

Specific gravity is a measurement of the concentration of urine. The specific gravity of water is 1.0. As the concentration of minerals, salts, and compounds in urine increases, the specific gravity increases. Substances contributing primarily to the specific gravity of normal urine are urea and uric acid.

The normal range of urine specific gravity is between 1.010 and 1.025; however, it may range from 1.001 when dilute to 1.030 when concentrated.

Specimen Required

A freshly voided specimen is needed to determine urine specific gravity. The amount of specimen needed depends on the method used to test for specific gravity. The most common and most accurate method involves use of a hydrometer or urinometer. A specimen of 30 ml is required when using the urinometer, since it has to float in a sufficient amount of fluid. Other methods, such as a reagent stick are less accurate, but require only a few drops of urine, and can be very useful in serial determinations. If tested at the bedside or on the nursing unit, the specimen is put into a clean cylinder. If the patient has a urinary catheter the specimen should be obtained using a sterile syringe and needle from the porthole in the catheter. It should not be obtained from the collecting bag.

Preparation of the Patient

Food and fluid restrictions are not necessary before collection of the specimen.

7

Causes of Deviation from Normal

Increases in urine specific gravity are caused by increased concentrations of the various substances contributing to the concentration of urine. In diabetes mellitus, when glucose is present, the specific gravity of the urine increases, as does the volume of the urine. Concentration of urine results from increased water loss in the body, thus increasing the specific gravity of the urine. These water losses occur in association with fear, gastrointestinal fluid losses, and third-space accumulation of fluid.

Decreases in urine specific gravity occur in association with renal diseases that interfere with the kidney's ability to concentrate urine. Such diseases include glomerulonephritis, acute tubular necrosis, and pyelonephritis. As the renal damage increases, urine volume decreases, but the specific gravity remains fixed, indicating inability of the kidney to concentrate the urine.

When decreased urine specific gravity occurs in association with a large daily urine output, there is absence of antidiuretic hormone (ADH), a hormone that triggers reabsorption of water from the renal tubules. The most common cause of decreased ADH production is diabetes insipidus, a disorder of the posterior pituitary gland characterized by diminished ADH production.

Nursing Implications of Abnormal Findings

Assessment. When specific gravity of urine is increased, determination of the components in urine contributing to this increase is needed. Urine glucose testing will determine whether hyperglycemia is also present. If it is, assessment of the patient should be directed toward identifying additional signs of hyperglycemia. If urea is the principle factor causing the increase in specific gravity, the patient should be assessed for additional signs and symptoms of fluid loss, for example, draining wounds, nausea, vomiting, diarrhea, increased pulse and respirations, increased temperature, and decreased blood pressure. If the patient is acutely ill, the physician should be notified so that fluid replacement can start immediately.

If a decreased amount of urine with a low specific gravity is present and the patient has renal disease, the nurse should assess the patient for changes in daily urine output, skin integrity, and neurological status. When the patient is on dialysis, assessment should include observations for fluid and electrolyte imbalances and complications of the dialysis procedure. Additional assessment should depend on the kind of dialysis the patient is receiving and the stage of illness.

For patients with abnormal urine specific gravity, it may be necessary for the nurse to institute bedside monitoring of the specific gravity each time the patient voids.

Interventions. If a patient has an increased specific gravity and hyperglycemia from diabetes mellitus, nursing interventions may include administration of hypoglycemic agents, such as insulin or oral hypoglycemics. If fluid losses have occurred, the nurse should carefully administer the fluids needed to restore the patient's blood volume. Continual teaching about the various self-care aspects of diabetes should also be included in the nursing care plan.

If decreased specific gravity and low urine volume occur in a patient with kidney disease, the nurse should check with the physician about long-range patient treatment so that education of the patient for potential dialysis and kidney transplant can be initiated. The patient with chronic renal failure needs emotional support from both the professional staff and the family. For a patient with decreased urine specific gravity and high urine output due to diabetes insipidus, fluids need to be given in larger-than-normal amounts to prevent dehydration.

Description
URINE pH

The pH of the urine is defined as the hydrogen ion concentration of the urine. It is a measurement of the acid or alkaline status of urine. The secretion by the kidney of acidic or alkaline urine is one of the mechanisms by which the normal acid–base balance of the body is maintained.

N O R M A L R A N G E	
Adults	4.5–8.0
Children	4.5–8.0
Newborns	5.0–7.0

Specimen Required

A small amount of fresh urine is required, enough to moisten a small strip of pH paper.

Preparation of the Patient

There are no food or fluid restrictions before collection of the specimen. If a urinary catheter is in place, the specimen should be obtained from the catheter junction or port using a sterile syringe and needle.

Causes of Deviation from Normal

Acid urine is found in patients with acidosis associated with diabetes mellitus, emphysema, starvation, diarrhea, and dehydration. Alkaline urine is found in patients with urinary tract infection, salicylate poisoning, renal tubular acidosis, and chronic renal failure.

7

Nursing Implications of Abnormal Findings

Assessment and Interventions. A patient with an abnormal urine pH needs additional testing to determine the underlying cause of the abnormality. Nursing assessments and interventions vary depending upon the disease present.

Description

URINE BLOOD OR HEMOGLOBIN

Hemoglobin is a component of red cells and is found in the bone marrow and within red cells. It transports oxygen from the lungs to the body cells. When red cells break down, hemoglobin is collected by the liver and eliminated through the gastrointestinal tract.

N O R M A L   R A N G E
Normally there are no hemoglobin or red cells in the urine.

Specimen Required

A small amount of fresh urine is required for the measurement of hemoglobin using a reagent strip. At least 30 ml of urine is required for the measurement of red cells, which is done after centrifuge.

Preparation of the Patient

There are no food or fluid restrictions before collection of the specimen.

Causes of Deviation from Normal

Red cells appear in the urine in the presence of renal disease, when red cells leak into the glomerular filtrate. Hemoglobin appears in the urine in association with conditions in which red cells are destroyed at a rate higher than the liver can metabolize the end products of their destruction. These conditions include extensive tissue trauma, burns, transfusion reactions, malaria, prostatic irrigation during surgery, and hemolytic anemia.

Nursing Implications of Abnormal Findings

Assessment and Interventions. Urine that has a dark color or a reddish-brown color may contain red cells or hemoglobin. These color changes should be reported so that further urine examination can be ordered by the physician. Note whether the patient is taking any of the following medications that can discolor the urine: Azo-Gantrisin, cascara, Elavil, phenolphthalein (Ex-Lax), Pyridium, sulfonamides, or phenothiazine tranquilizers. Because protein is found along with hemoglobin and red cells, the nurse can test the specimens at the patient's bedside with protein reagent strips. Additional nursing care needs depend upon the cause of the abnormal findings and should include specific nursing assessment of related problem areas.

Description

URINE PROTEIN

Protein found in the urine is *albumin*, a serum protein that normally does not leak into the glomerular filtrate.

NORMAL RANGE

Normally no protein is found during qualitative analysis of the urine. In quantitative analysis, 10–100 mg/24 h is normal.

Specimen Required

For quantitative analysis a small amount of freshly voided urine is required, since reagent strips are used for measurement. A 24-hour specimen is required for quantitative measurement.

Preparation of the Patient

Procedures may vary from laboratory to laboratory. The patient may be asked to empty the bladder upon rising in the morning and then collect a second specimen after standing or walking. No food or fluid restrictions are required before collection of the specimen.

Causes of Deviation from Normal

The most common causes of protein in the urine is glomerular damage from renal disease, including glomerulonephritis, nephrosis, polycystic kidney, kidney stones, and cancer of the kidney. Renal distress resulting in proteinuria also occurs in association with fear, trauma, burns, anemias, leukemia, cardiac disease, and various poisonings.

Nursing Implications of Abnormal Findings

Assessment and Interventions. Because the causes of proteinuria vary, nursing assessment and care planning depend on the underlying cause of the abnormality.

Description

URINE GLUCOSE

Urine normally contains no glucose. When the blood glucose level exceeds the renal threshold for the reabsorption of glucose, some glucose spills into the urine. Renal threshold levels vary among individuals, but an average of 180 mg/dl of blood glucose is associated with glucose in the urine. In diabetics this can rise to much higher levels.

7

N O R M A L   R A N G E

Normally, urine tests for glucose are negative. However, normal individuals who have eaten a meal very high in concentrated carbohydrates can have transient glucosuria. Pregnancy may also cause temporary glucosuria. Urine glucose test results are reported in percentage of glucose or in number of pluses; that is, one plus (+), two plus (++), and so forth. A variety of products are available to test urine glucose levels. Differences in percentages and pluses for different products illustrated in Table 7.1 indicate the need to report urine glucose levels as percentages as well as product-specific results. *TesTape* and *Diastix* are specific for glucose, whereas the reducing-agent products measure all reducing substances. If the specimen is rated using a color chart, evaluate results in a good light and make sure the chart is specific to the product being used.

TABLE 7.1. Urine Glucose Testing Products

Product	0%	1/10%	1/4%	1/2%	3/4%	1%	2%	>2%
Benedict's	neg	trace	+	++	++	+++	+++	++++
Clinitest	neg		trace	+	++	+++	++++	
Clinistix		light	medium	medium		dark		
Diastix	neg	trace	+	++		+++	++++	
TesTape	neg	+	++	+++			++++	

Specimen Required

A freshly voided urine specimen of at least 15 ml is required. A sequence of timed specimens during the day is frequently ordered; for example, a fasting morning specimen, specimens taken from 30–60 minutes before lunch and dinner, and a bedtime specimen. If the tests on the urine specimen are not done immediately, the specimen should be stored in the refrigerator or kept cool until transported to the laboratory.

Because a urinary glucose determination represents a lag time of at least 20 minutes from the serum glucose level, the collection of a second-voided specimen has been recommended as the most accurate reflection of serum glucose levels. That is, the bladder is emptied 30–60 minutes before the specimen is due, and a second-voided specimen is collected 30 minutes later. Some physicians prefer to have both specimens analyzed; however, the second specimen is believed to be more reflective of current blood glucose status. Present studies of first- and second-voided specimens have not revealed significant differences. However, study samples may not have included adequate numbers of unstable diabetics or may have included diabetics with neurogenic bladders, who cannot completely empty the bladder.

Preparation of the Patient

Food and fluids are restricted overnight for eight hours before collection of a fasting urine specimen. If a double-voided specimen is collected, the bladder should be emptied 30–60 minutes before the time the specimen is ordered. The patient may have a glass of water after the first specimen is taken to ensure adequate urine formation for the collection of the second-voided specimen.

Causes of Deviation from Normal

The most common cause of the presence of glucose in the urine is diabetes mellitus. As blood glucose levels rise above the renal threshold level, the urine glucose level rises as well. The higher the urine glucose level, the higher the blood glucose level. Urine glucose can also be present in patients who receive intravenous hyperalimentation with a high glucose concentration.

Nursing Implications of Abnormal Findings

Assessment. When a diabetic patient has glycosuria, the same urine specimen used for glucose testing should be assessed for ketone bodies. In carrying out the glucose test, the nurse must make sure that the directions are followed exactly and the products used have not deteriorated. If urine glucose levels are high, the patient should be assessed for other indications of hyperglycemia including peripheral blood glucose levels, if allowed, acetone breath, drowsiness, abdominal cramps, Kussmaul respirations, and decreased muscle tone and reflexes. These symptoms should be reported to the physician so that treatment can be ordered. The patient's history should include recent unusual emotional distress, since such episodes can increase release of glucocorticoids, adding additional glucose to the serum. The patient should also be assessed for infection and fever, which can also trigger release of serum glucose from epinephrine and cortisol secretion. If the patient is a diabetic receiving treatment, the nurse should determine whether the patient has been taking the prescribed insulin or oral hypoglycemic and whether the prescribed diet has been followed.

If urine glucose is present in a patient who is not a diagnosed diabetic, the nurse should determine whether the patient has received high-carbohydrate intravenous hyperalimentation or has had an unusually highly concentrated carbohydrate meal.

Interventions. If the patient with urinary glucose is a diabetic, the nurse should implement a teaching program for the patient that includes urine testing and other pertinent self-care information. Since diabetes mellitus requires lifelong adaptations and changes in daily routine, emotional support should be provided by the nursing staff as well as by the family. For patients who are on hyperalimentation and who have urinary glucose, the nurse may be responsible for adding insulin to the hyperalimentation solution. For all patients with urinary glucose, perineal hygiene after urination should be carried out, since residual glucose on the perineal tissues may lead to inflammations, vaginitis, and urinary-tract infections.

7

Description

URINE KETONES

Ketones are composed of acetone, keto hydroxybutyric acid, and acetoacetic acid. These products result from fatty acid metabolism and are normally completely metabolized by the liver.

NORMAL RANGE

Normally there are no ketone bodies in the urine.

Specimen Required

A small amount of freshly voided urine is required, since reagent strips are used for measurement. A note should be made on the laboratory slip if the patient is taking any of the drugs that may interfere with urine ketones (Table 7.2).

Preparation of the Patient

Food and fluids are restricted for eight hours before collection of fasting urine specimens. If double-voided specimens are being used for glucose and ketone determinations, the patient's bladder should be emptied 30–60 minutes before the time the specimen is ordered, and a second specimen should be collected at the specified time. The patient may have a glass of water after the first specimen is collected to ensure adequate urine formation for the second specimen.

Causes of Deviation from Normal

Ketones collect in the body and are eliminated via the urinary tract during abnormal fat and protein metabolism. *Ketonuria* is most common in unregulated diabetes mellitus with ketoacidosis, but can also occur in patients with cachexia, febrile diseases, excess exposure to cold, starvation, and strenuous exercise. As ketoacidosis increases, ketone levels in the urine increase.

Nursing Implications of Abnormal Findings

Assessment. The patient with ketonuria should be assessed for other evidence of ketoacidosis, such as acetone breath, elevated temperature, poor skin turgor, dry mucous membranes, electrolyte imbalances, nausea, vomiting, and Kussmaul respirations. The presence of infection should be noted, and the nurse should anticipate follow-up blood ketone analysis. Intravenous fluids and insulin should be administered carefully and the patient's responses should be observed.

Interventions. The diabetic patient with ketoacidosis is generally a type I insulin-dependent diabetic who needs to adjust to lifelong adaptations of diet and exercise. Nursing interventions should include teaching the various aspects

TABLE 7.2.	Drugs that May Cause a False-Positive for Urine Ketone Bodies	
Levodopa	Phthalein compound (BSP or PSP)
Pyridium	Ether
Isopropyl alcohol	Insulin
Metformin	Paraldehyde

of diabetes care and should be geared to the individual patient's needs and resources.

Description

URINE CELLS AND CASTS

Casts are formed within the kidney tubules from agglutination of protein cells, of red and white cells, or of epithelial cells.

NORMAL RANGE

Normally there are two or fewer red cells or casts, four or fewer white cells or casts, and an occasional epithelial cell or cast in the urine sample.

Specimen Required

A freshly voided urine specimen is required. At least 30 ml of urine is needed, as the specimen is centrifuged and the sediment examined under the microscope. Care should be taken to prevent any menstrual contamination of the urinary specimen.

7

Preparation of the Patient

Food and fluid restrictions are not required before collection of the specimen.

Causes of Deviation from Normal

The size of the cast is an important determinant of the source of origin. It may indicate the amount of renal damage that is present. If the cast is broad, for example, the collecting tubule is probably the site of origin, indicating severe renal damage.

Accumulation of red cells indicates bleeding within the glomeruli or tubules, hemorrhagic cystitis, or the presence of calculi in the renal pelvis. Tumors or tuberculosis of the kidney can also cause bleeding into the tubules. Accumulation of red cell casts indicates glomerulonephritis.

Accumulation of white cells indicates an infection of the urinary tract, whereas accumulation of white cell casts occurs in glomerulonephritis, pyelonephritis, nephrotic syndrome, and inflammation of the kidney.

Epithelial cells accumulate from cast-off tubular cells damaged by nephrosis, eclampsia, and poisoning from heavy metals and toxins.

Nursing Implications of Abnormal Findings

Assessment and Interventions. Abnormal cells and casts in the urine may indicate a variety of diseases and problems. Patients need careful assessment of developing problems and support during further follow-up diagnostic testing.

BLOOD UREA NITROGEN

Description
Blood urea nitrogen (BUN) is the major nitrogenous waste resulting from protein metabolism. It is produced by the liver and eliminated from the body primarily by the kidneys.

N O R M A L R A N G E	
Adults	4–22 mg/dl
Children	5–20 mg/dl
Newborns/infants	5–15 mg/dl

Specimen Required
A 3–5-ml sample of venous blood is collected in an oxalated tube.

Preparation of the Patient
There are no food or fluid restrictions before venipuncture. Since many drugs affect the test results, any medications that the patient is receiving should be noted on the patient's laboratory slip.

Causes of Deviation from Normal
Elevations in BUN (azotemia) are caused primarily by diseases of the kidney and obstructions of the urinary tract. The most common obstructive disease is prostatic enlargement. Kidney diseases associated with elevated BUN include glomerulonephritis, nephrosis, tumor, calculi, and congenital anomalies. Elevations occur because of an inability of the body to excrete urine or because of increases in protein metabolism. These increases are seen in catabolic diseases such as starvation, infection, trauma, surgery, bleeding into the gut, and during therapy with corticosteroids and tetracyclines.

Decreases in BUN are rare, and occur during liver failure, when protein metabolism is inhibited, and in a negative nitrogen balance when protein breakdown exceeds protein intake. Negative nitrogen balance may occur during anorexia, malnutrition, or intravenous therapy in patients receiving inadequate oral nutrition.

Nursing Implications of Abnormal Findings
Assessment. When an elevated BUN is caused by a kidney disease, the nurse should determine whether the patient has (1) had a decrease in urinary output,

(2) had a change in urine concentration, (3) been on medications that cause kidney damage, or (4) been exposed to nephrotoxic substances in the work environment. Bedside urine examination should include analysis for protein, glucose, pH, and occult blood. The patient should be observed for fluid over-load, evidenced by weight increases, distended neck veins, edema, and puffy eyelids. The skin may reveal a yellow tinge and bruises may be noticeable. Vital signs should also be monitored for fluid overload. The patient should be observed for changes in mental status, metabolic acidosis, and fluid and elec-trolyte imbalances. When an elevated BUN occurs without renal disease, the nursing assessment is specific to the cause and includes monitoring of vital signs and careful intake and output recording.

Nursing assessment of patients with decreased BUN levels is specific to the precipitating cause. If malnutrition or negative nitrogen balance is present, the nurse should monitor intake and output and carefully observe, promote, and record the patient's dietary intake.

Interventions. When an elevation in BUN is caused by renal disease and fluid overload is present, the patient should be positioned to provide for ade-quate respiratory exchange and protection of edematous body parts. Fluid restriction may be ordered and should be planned with the patient to allow for distribution of the allotted fluid over a 24-hour period. If changes in mental status occur, safety precautions should be instituted to prevent accidental injury. Daily hygiene is essential to prevent pruritus and skin breakdown. Psychosocial support is essential for patients with chronic kidney diseases and should include involvement of the family or significant others in order to foster supportive care after hospital discharge. If dialysis is ordered, specialized nursing care, as described in comprehensive nursing texts, is needed. When the eleva-tion in BUN is caused by obstructive kidney disease, a surgical treatment approach is likely and nursing interventions should focus on preoperative preparation and appropriate postoperative care.

If decreases in BUN are associated with negative nitrogen balance and a malnourished state, the patient's oral intake should be increased. This may include consideration of food preferences, dividing the intake into five or six small meals daily, and providing an environment conducive to eating.

CREATININE

Description

Creatinine is a nitrogenous waste product produced during protein metabolism in muscle tissue. The amount produced each day, which is related to the muscle mass, seldom changes rapidly. Creatinine is eliminated from the body by the kidneys.

```
N O R M A L   R A N G E
```

Adults	0.6–1.2 mg/dl
Children	0.3–0.7 mg/dl
Newborns	0.8–1.4 mg/dl

Since serum creatinine and the BUN both measure kidney function in slightly different ways, the ratio of one to the other is important diagnostically. The normal ratio of BUN to creatinine is 20:1.

Specimen Required

A 3–5-ml sample of venous blood is collected in a collecting tube or syringe.

Preparation of the Patient

There are no food or fluid restrictions before venipuncture. However, phenolsulfonphthalein (PSP) and bromsulphalein (BSP) dyes can give false positives and thus should not be administered before the test. Drugs that influence normal creatinine levels include diuretics, chloral hydrate, sulfonamides, chloramphenicol, ascorbic acid, and marijuana. A diet high in red meat can cause abnormally high levels.

Causes of Deviation from Normal

Increases in creatinine levels are associated primarily with renal disease and obstructive urinary tract disease. Decreased levels occur with muscular dystrophy.

BUN–creatinine ratio changes are used to differentiate the patient's pathology. If kidney disease is present, both the BUN and the creatinine are elevated. If conditions causing protein catabolism are present, such as trauma, infection, or bleeding, the BUN is elevated and the creatinine is normal or only slightly elevated. If conditions causing volume depletion are present, the BUN is elevated and the creatinine is normal or slightly elevated.

Nursing Implications of Abnormal Findings

Assessment and Interventions. Elevations in serum creatinine and the related nursing assessment and interventions are discussed in the section on blood urea nitrogen. Since elevated serum creatinine indicates potential kidney disease, the nurse should clarify administration of nephrotoxic chemotherapy when creatinine levels are elevated. Examples of the medications that may need to be held include methrotrexate, cisplatin, cytoxan, mithramycin, and semustine.

CREATININE CLEARANCE

Description

Clearance measurements are used to evaluate the glomerular filtration rate of the kidney. They involve identification of the rate at which specific substances are filtered by the glomeruli and eliminated in the urine. When *creatinine clearance* is conducted, the body's own sustained production of creatinine is used as the test agent. Both serum and urine are required.

<table>
<tr><th colspan="2">N O R M A L   R A N G E</th></tr>
<tr><td>Urine Creatinine</td><td></td></tr>
<tr><td>   Men</td><td>107–141 ml/min</td></tr>
<tr><td>   Women</td><td>87–132 ml/min</td></tr>
<tr><td>Serum Creatinine</td><td></td></tr>
<tr><td>   Men</td><td>0.6–1.5 mg/dl</td></tr>
<tr><td>   Women</td><td>0.5–1.0 mg/dl</td></tr>
<tr><td>   Infants</td><td><0.6 mg/dl</td></tr>
</table>

7

Specimen Required

A 24-hour urine specimen is required and a 5–10-ml venous blood specimen is collected in a plain tube or syringe.

Preparation of the Patient

Food and fluids are not restricted before venipuncture. The patient should be instructed on collection of the 24-hour urine sample. A collection specimen bottle should be readily available to the patient. Check whether any medications that the patient is receiving can affect creatinine clearance. These medications need to be restricted before conducting the test.

Causes of Deviation from Normal

Decreases in creatinine clearance result from any renal disease that affects glomerular filtration rate. Creatinine clearance may also be decreased in congestive heart failure, shock, cirrhosis, and dehydration. As the patient with renal disease improves, increases in creatinine clearance occur. Up to 50% of the nephrons can be damaged before changes in glomerular filtration rate are demonstrated.

Nursing Implications of Abnormal Findings

Assessment and Interventions. Patients with decreases in creatinine clearance should be assessed for other indications of renal or cardiovascular disease.

If patients with chronic renal disease are being evaluated for dialysis with a clearance test, the nurse should be prepared to provide education for the patient about dialysis. The nurse may carry this out individually or may consult with another nurse more skilled in the nursing care of patients with acute renal failure. Nursing interventions should relate to the specific nursing problems identified after the establishment of a definitive medical diagnosis.

URIC ACID

Description

Uric acid is one of the nitrogenous waste products formed when nucleonic acids are split. These acids are formed during amino acid metabolism and are the end product of purine metabolism. The metabolism of amino acids may occur within the liver or, to a lesser extent, in the intestinal mucosa. The primary excretion mechanism for uric acid is through the kidneys.

NORMAL RANGE	
Men	3.9–9.0 mg/dl
Women	2.2–7.7 mg/dl
Children	2.5–5.5 mg/dl
Infants	1.5–7.5 mg/dl

Specimen Required

A 5-ml sample of serum is used for the test. The serum should be separated from the cells at once and refrigerated. The specimen should be delivered to the laboratory promptly.

Preparation of the Patient

No food or fluid restrictions are needed before venipuncture.

Causes of Deviation from Normal

Increased uric acid in the serum is called *hyperuricemia*. It is associated with either an inability to excrete uric acid, an increased release of uric acid, or both. Increased production of uric acid occurs in metabolic disorders. In gout, purine metabolism is abnormal and a large amount of uric acid is formed; the increase may be slight in the early stages of the disease. Uric acid crystals accumulate in joints, causing an acute inflammatory response and forming deposits called *tophi*. Accumulations may also occur within the renal endothelium, leading to the formation of renal calculi.

During renal failure, uric acid levels rise, as do levels of other nitrogenous products, such as urea and creatinine. These rises are associated with the decreased ability of the kidney to excrete wastes. Other diseases associated with increases in uric acid include leukemia, lymphomas, metastatic cancer, severe eclampsia, and metabolic acidosis.

Decreased uric acid may occur in response to acute hepatic failure and in defective tubular absorption, as seen in Fanconi's syndrome and Wilson's disease. When patients with metastatic neoplastic disease or gout are being treated with uricosuric drugs such as allopurinol, probenecid, or sulfinpyrazone, a falling uric acid level is an expected response to the medication.

Nursing Implications of Abnormal Findings

Assessment. When caring for a patient with hyperuricemia, the nurse should note whether a specific diagnosis has been made. If the patient is known to have gout, uric acid levels will be tested at regular intervals and used to evaluate the patient's response to the prescribed medications. Assessment should include identification of any bony joints that appear to be involved. For patients with renal failure, uric acid levels will be monitored regularly, as will blood urea nitrogen and creatinine, to determine the progression of the disease and the need for specific therapies. The nurse should monitor bedside symptoms as well, including consciousness status, level of irritability, edema, and intake–output ratios. The physician may use these factors to determine the need for dialysis.

Interventions. The care plan for patients with gout should include the location of any involved joints so caution may be used in positioning, moving, and touching the patient. The nurse should plan patient teaching sessions for the long-term diet and medication approaches ordered. The sessions should also include the person in the family primarily responsible for cooking, if other than the patient. Medication instruction should include what toxic effects may occur and specific approaches to take if they occur. For example, when colchicine is being administered, the dosage increases until pain is relieved or diarrhea begins, whichever occurs first. For diarrhea, the patient is taught to stop the medication and call the physician to determine what dose level should be continued. Teach the patient not to take aspirin, as it increases the acidity and nullifies the action of uricosuric medications. Acetaminophen (Tylenol) may be used instead of aspirin.

For patients with renal failure, dietary and medication instructions are important aspects of the care plan. In addition, the nurse should look for and support psychological responses to the chronic and debilitating condition. If changes in consciousness status occur, safety measures should be implemented to prevent injury. Increasing serum levels of uric acid and other nitrogenous waste products may signal the need for dialysis, at which time nursing care should involve preparation of the patient for this procedure and observation of the patient for complications and reactions.

7

PHENOLSULFONPHTHALEIN EXCRETION TEST

Description
Phenolsulfonphthalein (PSP) is a dye administered to measure tubular secretion and renal blood flow in the kidney. It is a frequently used test of kidney function involving the injection of a specific amount of dye, after which urine specimens are collected at regular intervals to test the rate of dye excretion. The more severe the renal involvement, the less PSP is excreted.

N O R M A L R A N G E	
Adults	
15 minutes	25–35%
30 minutes	40–60%
60 minutes	50–75%
120 minutes	75–80%
Children	
5–10% higher than adults at each time interval	

Specimen Required
Specimens of total urine output are collected 15, 30, 60, and 120 minutes after injection of the dye.

Preparation of the Patient
While no food or fluid restrictions are needed, medications are omitted 24 hours before the test as they may interfere with results. The test is begun by having the patient drink several glasses of water; once the patient feels able to void, the PSP (1 ml or 6 mg) is administered intravenously. Timed specimens of total urinary output are collected 15, 30, 60, and 120 minutes after dye injection. The timing should be precisely recorded on the specimen.

Note: Bromsulphalein (BSP) can interfere with the results of this test.

Causes of Deviation from Normal
The most common cause of a decrease in the total percentage of PSP excreted is renal disease or decrease in renal circulation. As renal damage increases, the percentage of PSP excretion decreases.

Nursing Implications of Abnormal Findings
Assessment and Interventions. If a patient has decreased PSP excretion, a number of other tests will be ordered to determine the specific cause of the

decreased renal function. The nurse should prepare the patient for further diagnostic testing. Nursing assessment and interventions vary with individual patients, depending on the degree of illness and the problems presented.

MYOGLOBIN, URINE

Description

Myoglobin is a protein similar to hemoglobin that is found in highly oxidative muscle fibers. It binds oxygen and increases the rate of oxygen diffusion into the muscle cell. It also stores small amounts of oxygen within the muscle that can be called upon during sudden changes in activity.

N O R M A L   R A N G E

Adults
      Qualitative (random sample)   Negative
      Quantitative (24-hour sample)   <4 mg/l
Children   Consult laboratory for
                                 reference values.

7

Specimen Required

A fresh morning urine specimen is obtained and sent to the laboratory when a qualitative sample is requested. A 24-hour specimen is required for a quantitative analysis.

Preparation of the Patient

There are no food or fluid restrictions before collection of the specimen. Specific instructions for the collection of urine specimens are given in Chapter 1.

Causes of Deviation from Normal

Myoglobin appears in the urine when there is severe destruction of muscle fibers. This can be caused by (1) infarction of large skeletal or cardiac muscles, (2) trauma from crush injuries, excessive exertion, bullet wounds, convulsions, or beatings, (3) familial myoglobinuria, and (4) miscellaneous events, including hyperthermia, infections such as polymyositis, and ingestion of fish that has been poisoned by factory wastes. When muscle damage has occurred, myoglobin is released from the cells, rapidly cleared from the blood, and excreted in the urine. In some instances large amounts of myoglobin precipitate in the renal tubules, causing kidney damage.

Nursing Implications of Abnormal Findings

Assessment and Interventions. The dark red or brown urine associated with hemoglobinuria may be an indication of myoglobinuria. When a patient has severe muscle damage from either trauma or myocardial infarction and has dark red or brown urine, tests for both myoglobinuria and hemoglobinuria are helpful. If the patient has clinical manifestations of a myocardial infarction, the presence of myoglobinuria will be added to the data collected and nursing interventions planned (see Chapter 4). When the cause of myoglobinuria is muscle damage, nursing care must be planned based on a complete assessment of the patient and the severity of the damage. When large amounts of myoglobin are present in the blood, the kidneys may fail causing anuria.

MYOGLOBIN, BLOOD

Description

Myoglobin is a protein similar to hemoglobin found in highly oxidative muscle fibers. Injury to skeletal muscle results in the release of myoglobin.

N O R M A L R A N G E	
Adults	30–90 ng/ml

Specimen Required

A 5-ml sample of venous blood is collected in a plain collecting tube.

Preparation of the Patient

No food or fluid restrictions are needed prior to collection of the specimen.

Causes of Deviation from Normal

Serum myoglobin is used to monitor damage in myocardial infarction and to detect muscle injury or predict disease recurrence or exascerbation in polymyositis. Elevations of blood myoglobin in myocardial infarction may peak 8–12 hours after infarction occurs, and may return to normal by 12 hours. Elevations may also occur in other diseases involving damage to skeletal muscle (Table 7.3). False-positives occur when myoglobin is not excreted because of renal damage.

Nursing Implications of Abnormal Findings

Use of myoglobin monitoring for myocardial infarction needs to be accompanied by assessment and interventions specific to myocardial infarction. Careful assessment of pain levels, respiratory compromise, and cardiac monitoring are

TABLE 7.3. Causes of Elevations in Serum Myoglobin

Trauma and Ischemic Disease
Acute myocardial infarction
Muscle crushing injuries
Burns, electric shock
Muscle Exertion
Severe exercise
Convulsions
Delerium tremens
Metabolic Disorders
Alcoholic myopathy
Hypothermia
Potassium depletion
Myxedema
Muscle Wasting Diseases
Systemic lupus erythematosis
Muscular dystrophies
Infections
Tetanus
Gas gangrene

7

essential. Interventions need to parallel the symptoms present. Medical-surgical textbooks should be consulted for specific interventions.

When other causes of muscle injury are present, nursing care must be planned based on the complete assessment of the patient and appropriate interventions.

ACID PHOSPHATASE

Description

Acid phosphatase is an enzyme found primarily in the adult prostate gland. Related forms of the same enzyme are found in red cells and platelets.

N O R M A L R A N G E	
Adults and children	
1.0–4.0	King Armstrong U/dl
0.5–2.0	Bodansky or Gotman U/dl
0–1.1	Shinowara U/ml
0.1–0.73	Bessey Lowry U/ml

Specimen Required

A 5-ml sample of blood is obtained in a plain collecting tube or syringe.

Preparation of the Patient

Food and fluids are not restricted before venipuncture. When the patient has had extensive palpation or massage of the prostate gland, this should be noted on the laboratory slip because it may cause an abnormal elevation in acid phosphatase for about 24 hours.

Causes of Deviation from Normal

Elevated serum levels of acid phosphatase are most often seen in patients with metastatic carcinoma of the prostate gland. If the tumor has not extended beyond the capsule, serum levels are usually normal. Successful treatment of a metastatic tumor results in a drop in the enzyme level 3–4 days after surgery or 3–4 weeks after estrogen therapy. Minor elevations are seen in Paget's disease, hyperparathyroidism, thrombocytosis, sickle cell crisis, multiple myeloma, renal insufficiency, some liver diseases, and metastatic bone disease.

Nursing Implications of Abnormal Findings

Assessment and Interventions. Evaluation of acid phosphatase levels is helpful in assessing a patient who may have metastatic prostate cancer. When test results reveal abnormally high levels of this enzyme, nursing interventions should be planned to assist the patient if metastatic disease is diagnosed. When the diagnosis is recent, the nurse should focus on the psychosocial crisis that often occurs when a person is told cancer is present. Interventions planned for physical care depend on the extent of metastasis as well as on the planned mode of therapy.

CARCINOEMBRYONIC ANTIGEN (CEA)

Description

Carcinoembryonic antigen (CEA) is a glycoprotein which is normally shed into the lumen by gastrointestinal tract cells. It is used as a tumor-marker for carcinoma, and for some non-malignant diseases.

NORMAL RANGE

Normal values range from 0–2.5 ng/ml. For smokers, the normal values are increased to approximately 10 ng/ml.

Specimen Required

A 10-ml specimen of venous blood is required. Care should be taken to avoid hemolysis.

Preparation of the Patient

Food and fluid restrictions are not necessary.

Causes of Deviation from Normal

CEA elevations occur in a variety of cancers including gastrointestinal (esophagus, stomach, small and large intestine, rectum), pancreas, liver, lung, breast, cervix, prostate, bladder, testes, kidney, and leukemia. Non-malignant diseases which also lead to elevations in the CEA are inflammatory diseases including inflammatory bowel disease, chronic cigarette smoking, ulcerative colitis, cirrhosis of the liver, bacterial pneumonia, pulmonary emphysema, acute pancreatitis, acute renal failure, and chronic heart disease. CEA monitoring is used to assess patients' responses to treatment of the disease.

Nursing Implications of Abnormal Findings

Assessment. Patients undergoing monitoring for carcinogenic disease via CEA may have anxiety related to possible malignancy or recurrence of malignant disease. They should be assessed for other signs of anxiety and depression.

Interventions. When patients are nervous and anxious, supportive measures should be instituted to encourage the patient to use previously effective coping skills. Support from the patient's family should be encouraged. Referral to supportive therapy groups for cancer patients is often helpful to the patient and family members. Provide clear answers to questions as needed and support a hopeful environment.

PROSTATIC SPECIFIC ANTIGEN (PSA)

Description

Prostatic specific antigen is a glycoprotein normally found in the cytoplasm of prostatic epithelial cells. It is found in all males, and its level is markedly increased in patients who have prostatic cancer. It is more specific and sensitive than acid phosphatase in monitoring responses of prostatic cancer to treatment.

NORMAL RANGE	
Adult men, under 40	<2.7 ng/ml
Adult men, over 40	<4.0 ng/ml
Adult women	Absent

Specimen Required

A 2-ml venous specimen is required.

Preparation of the Patient

Food and fluids do not need to be restricted. Collection of the specimen should be done prior to palpation of the prostate.

Causes of Deviation from Normal

Increases in PSA occur in approximately 80% of patients with prostatic cancer. Patients with benign prostatic hypertrophy also experience increases in PSA. If the prostate gland is completely removed, no PSA will be detected. PSA monitoring is used to assess a patient's response to treatment.

Nursing Implications of Abnormal Findings

Assessment. Patients undergoing PSA monitoring are usually undergoing screening, diagnostic work-up, or treatment for prostate cancer. Emotional responses frequently include anger, anxiety, and depression. Assessing the patient's emotional response can provide information valuable in planning supportive therapies.

Interventions. Patients with prostatic cancer should be encouraged to use coping approaches that have helped in the past. Information should be given on support groups for men with prostatic cancer for those patients that express an interest. Clear explanations of treatment and monitoring procedures are essential. Fostering support from family members is often helpful for the patient.

URINE URIC ACID

Description

Uric acid results from the breakdown of nucleic acid, of which purine is the primary form.

NORMAL RANGE	
Adults	
Low-purine diet	200–500 mg/24 h
Normal diet	400–1000 mg/24 h
High-purine diet	≥2000 mg/24 h
Children	Consult laboratory for reference values.

Specimen Required

A 24-hour refrigerated urine specimen is required.

Preparation of the Patient

Food and fluid are not generally restricted before or during collection of the specimen. However, depending on the purpose of the test, a diet high or low in purines may be ordered before and during the collection period. (See general rules for 24-hour urine specimen collection in Chapter 1.)

Causes of Deviation from Normal

Increased levels of urine uric acid occur when increased serum uric acid (hyperuricemia) occurs. This is associated with gout, liver disease, fevers, toxemias of pregnancy, and polycythemia vera. During treatment of cancer with cytoxan chemotherapy, urine uric acid levels are greatly increased due to the destruction of cancer cells. This increase can precipitate uric acid stones if the pH is low and the urine is concentrated. Decreased levels of uric acid are found in kidney disease and are associated with decreased renal function.

Nursing Implications of Abnormal Findings

Assessment. When urine uric acid levels are increased, the nurse should assess the patient for symptoms of hyperuricemia, which include the presence of painful joints, especially in the big toe. If renal disease is present, the nurse should record and review intake and output records and note the level of irritability, edema, and consciousness status. If the patient is being treated with cytoxan drugs, the nurse should test the urine regularly for uric acid levels and note the urine pH as well.

Interventions. If the patient has gout, the nurse should position the patient to protect the painful involved joints. Dietary instruction for decreased purine content should be provided for the patient and the person who cooks for the family. Long-term medication instruction may be necessary.

If the patient is being treated with cytoxan drugs, the urine pH must be increased to prevent uric acid stone formation. This may be done by administering cranberry juice. Dilution of the urine can be maintained by providing adequate fluids.

BIBLIOGRAPHY

"Acute Renal Failure: Urine Studies." *Hospital Medicine,* 21:54 (September 1985).

Brady, S. "Urodynamics: An overview." *Urological Nursing,* 9(1):837–841 (January/March 1990).

Corbett, J.V. *Laboratory Tests and Diagnostic Procedures with Nursing Diagnoses.* Norwalk, Connecticut: Appleton and Lange, 1992.

Fischbach, F.T. *A Manual of Laboratory and Diagnostic Tests.* Philadelphia: J.B. Lippincott Company, 1992.

Frauman, A.C. "An Introduction to Physical Assessment for the Nephrology Nurse." *American Nephrology Nurses Association Journal,* 12:112–117 (April 1985).

"Hematuria: Guidelines to Laboratory Evaluation." *Hospital Medicine,* 21:42–43 (February 1985).

Ignatavicius, D.D., and M.V. Bayne. *Medical-Surgical Nursing: A Nursing Process Approach.* Philadelphia: W.B. Saunders, 1991.

Jackson, J.A. "Urinalysis: No Longer a Stepchild in the Laboratory." *Journal of Medical Technology,* 2:256–258 (April 1985).

Lazarus, J.M. "Uremia—A Clinical Guide." *Hospital Medicine,* 20:175, 176, 181–183, 187, 188 (January 1984).

Lewis, S.M., and I.C. Collier. *Medical-Surgical Nursing: Assessment and Management of Clinical Problems.* St. Louis: Mosby Yearbook, 1992.

Lybrand, M., B. Medoff-Cooper, and B.H. Munro. "Periodic Comparisons of Specific Gravity Using Urine from a Diaper and Collecting Bag." *American Journal of Maternal Child Nursing,* 15(4):238–239 (July/August 1990).

Mars, D.R., et al. "Acute Tubular Necrosis—Pathophysiology and Treatment." *Heart and Lung,* 13:194–202 (March 1984).

Paradiso, C. "Self Care Framework: A Guide for Clinical Application in the Hemodialysis Patient." *Journal of Nephrology Nursing,* 2:139–143 (May–June 1985).

Phipps, W.S., B.C. Long, N.F. Woods, and V. Cossmeyer. *Medical-Surgical Nursing.* St. Louis: Mosby Yearbook, 1991.

Ravel, R. *Clinical Laboratory Medicine.* Chicago: Year Book Medical Publishers, Inc., 1989.

Smetzer, S.C., and B.G. Ball. *Brunner and Sudarth's Medical-Surgical Nursing.* New York: J.B. Lippincott, 1992.

Wallach, J. *Interpretation of Diagnostic Tests.* Boston: Little, Brown, and Company, 1992.

Whitaker, A.R. "Acute Renal Dysfunction: Assessment of Patients at Risk." *Focus on Critical Care,* 12:12–17 (June 1985).

Widmann, F.K. *Clinical Interpretation of Laboratory Tests.* Philadelphia: F.A. Davis, 1983.

Wilson, J.D., et al. *Harrison's Principles of Internal Medicine.* New York: McGraw-Hill, 1991.

7

CHAPTER

8

Laboratory Tests of Biliary and Gastrointestinal Function

Serum Bilirubin

Urine Urobilinogen

Fecal Urobilinogen

Alkaline Phosphatase

5′ Nucleotidase

Cholinesterase

Lactic Dehydrogenase

Transaminase Enzymes
Aspartate Aminotransferase
(Glutamic-oxaloacetic
Transaminase)
Alanine Aminotransferase
(Glutamic-pyruvic
Transaminase)

Aldolase

Plasma Proteins
Total Protein
Albumin
Globulin
A/G Ratio

Coagulation Factors
Fibrinogen
Prothrombin Time

Blood Ammonia

Hepatitis Serological Tests

Cholesterol

Amylase
Serum Amylase
Urine Amylase

Serum Lipase

Lactose Tolerance Test

D-**Xylose**

Gamma Glutamyl Transpeptidase

Gastrin

Fecal Fat

Fecal Parasites (Ova and Parasites)

Fecal Occult Blood

SERUM BILIRUBIN

Description

Bilirubin is the orange-yellow bile pigment formed mainly by the destruction of old cells (Fig. 8.1). When the membranes of these cells rupture, hemoglobin is released and is phagocytized primarily in the spleen by the reticuloendothelial (RE) system. The heme portion of the molecule is converted into the green pigment biliverdin, then into bilirubin. Heme-containing proteins, such as catalase, peroxidase, myoglobin, and cytochromes, contribute to bilirubin production, as does the degradation of hemoglobin in the bone marrow. Bilirubin is then transported through the blood bound to albumin. This unconjugated bilirubin arrives at the sinusoidal surface of the liver; however, its transport into the liver cells is not completely understood. Recent studies have suggested that the rate of entry of bilirubin into liver cells is related to two acceptor-binding proteins designated "Y" and "Z". After entry into the liver cells, bilirubin is conjugated with glucuronyl transferase acid to form a more water-soluble substance that is able to pass through the glomerulus of the kidney to be excreted. The unconjugated (prehepatic) bilirubin may be distinguished from conjugated (posthepatic) bilirubin by the way it reacts with diazo reagents. Unconjugated

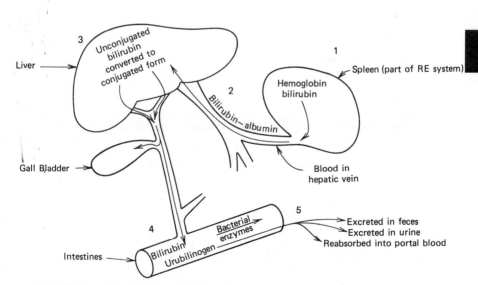

FIGURE 8.1. Bilirubin metabolism: (1) Bilirubin is produced in the RE system from hemoglobin; (2) bilirubin transported by the blood to the liver bound to albumin; (3) bilirubin conjugated with glucuronic acid to form bilirubin diglucuronide; (4) bilirubin diglucuronide converted to urobilinogen by intestinal bacterial enzymes; (5) urobilinogen excreted in feces, excreted in urine, or reabsorbed into portal blood.

bilirubin is not soluble in water; it reacts with the diazo reagent only in the presence of alcohol and is called *indirect bilirubin*. Conjugated bilirubin is water soluble and reacts without the addition of alcohol; it is called *direct bilirubin*.

N O R M A L R A N G E	
Adults and children	
Direct (conjugated)	up to 0.4 mg/dl
Indirect (unconjugated)	0.1–0.8 mg/dl
Total	0.1–1.2 mg/dl
Full-term infants	
First 24 hours	Total 2–6 mg/dl
24–48 hours	Total 6–7 mg/dl
3–5 days	Total 4–12 mg/dl
Premature infants	
First 24 hours	Total 1–6 mg/dl
24–48 hours	Total 6–8 mg/dl
3–5 days	Total 10–15 mg/dl

Specimen Required

A 5-ml sample of venous blood is obtained in a plain collecting tube or syringe.

Preparation of the Patient

Food and fluids are not usually restricted before venipuncture.

Causes of Deviation from Normal

Hyperbilirubinemia may be classified as conjugated or unconjugated. In *prehepatic unconjugated hyperbilirubinemia*, there is excessive production of bilirubin, which is attributable either to rapid hemolysis of red cells or ineffective erythropoiesis in the presence of a normal-functioning liver. Since increased amounts of bilirubin are transported to the liver, there is an increase in the amounts of conjugated bilirubin. When these amounts of conjugated bilirubin reach the intestines, there is an increase in fecal urobilinogen and urine urobilinogen; however, bilirubin is not seen in the urine. When the formation of unconjugated bilirubin exceeds the liver's capacity to conjugate and excrete it, jaundice results. The term *hemolytic jaundice* is often used to describe this condition. The serum bilirubin rarely exceeds 7 mg/dl in the adult, even in the most severe cases.

Some causes of hemolytic jaundice include sickle cell anemia, hereditary spherocytosis, Rh or transfusion incompatibility, or autoimmune hemolytic disease. It may also be caused by medications, some lymphomas, or the increased destruction of red cells or their bone marrow precursors apparent in diseases such as thalassemia or pernicious anemia. Hemolysis of red cells circulating through the heart-lung machine (used in cardiopulmonary bypass surgery) may also cause hemolytic jaundice.

There are two physiological defects that interfere with the transport of bilirubin: Gilbert's syndrome and Crigler-Najjar syndrome. In Gilbert's syndrome, a genetic defect interferes with the transport of bilirubin from the sinusoidal blood into the hepatocyte. Studies have shown that patients with Gilbert's syndrome have a deficiency of glucuronyl transferase. Crigler-Najjar syndrome is a rare congenital disorder in which there is also a deficiency of glucuronic transferase. An elevation of unconjugated bilirubin is seen in both of these disorders.

Conjugated hyperbilirubinemia consists of two types: *hepatic*, consisting of hepatocellular and hepatocanalicular hyperbilirubinemia, and *posthepatic*. In hepatocellular hyperbilirubinemia, the liver parenchyma is damaged by cirrhosis or a form of hepatitis. The liver cells swell, become disorganized, compress, and block the canaliculi. There is impairment of uptake, conjugation, and excretion of bilirubin, which results in elevated levels of both conjugated and unconjugated bilirubin. Impaired excretion of conjugated bilirubin into the intestine results in reduced levels of bile pigment in the feces and high levels of conjugated bilirubin excreted into the kidneys and appearing in the urine.

In hepatocanalicular hyperbilirubinemia (intrahepatic cholestasis), there is a defective secretion or obstruction in the flow of conjugated bilirubin within the canaliculi. This may be caused by intrahepatic disease or by hepatotoxic drugs, such as halothane, oral contraceptives, anabolic steroids, or compazine.

8

Posthepatic hyperbilirubinemia (extrahepatic cholestasis) is caused by a mechanical obstruction in the biliary tree. The most common causes are the obstruction of the common bile duct by one or more gallstones, carcinoma of the head of the pancreas that invades or compresses the pancreatic duct, and carcinoma of the ampulla of Vater. The obstruction prevents the normal flow of conjugated bilirubin into the duodenum, resulting in hyperbilirubinemia and very low levels of bilirubin in feces and urine.

Physiological jaundice may occur in the newborn and is due to increased hemolysis and slower conjugation of bilirubin by the liver. This hemolysis is normal. However, newborns have a low level of glucuronyl transferase, which slows conjugation by the liver and removal of bilirubin from the bloodstream. After 3–5 days, the bilirubin levels begin to fall and should reach normal levels within a month. Pathological jaundice will occur in newborns with an Rh incompatibility. This complication should be considered in newborns who have a high indirect bilirubin at birth that does not begin to drop within 3–5 days.

Nursing Implications of Abnormal Findings

Assessment. When serum bilirubin levels are abnormally elevated, the sclerae, mucous membranes, and skin should be assessed for jaundice. In Caucasians the skin becomes yellow or greenish-yellow. In yellow-skinned people, changes in skin tone occur but are more subtle. Brown- and black-skinned people do not show a perceptible change in skin color, so the jaundice must be observed in the sclerae and mucous membranes, particularly the posterior portion of the hard palate. In infants, jaundice may not appear until the total bilirubin is 2–4 mg. When jaundice is present the nurse must determine if it has adversely affected the person's body image. In addition, the patient with hyperbilirubinemia must also be assessed for signs and symptoms of pruritus, since the accumulation of bile salts causes severe itching. When hepatocellular or hepatocanalicular damage has caused hyperbilirubinemia, the patient should also be assessed for clinical manifestations of liver damage, such as ascites, bleeding esophageal varices, and mental confusion.

Interventions. Comfort measures are important for the patient with hyperbilirubinemia. The person with jaundice may be assured that it will disappear once the hyperbilirubinemia is treated. However, caution must be taken not to give false hope to patients who have a chronic or terminal illness. Although the severe itching that occurs is hard to control, the following palliative measures can be taken:

1. Keep the patient's fingernails short to prevent skin breakdown due to scratching.
2. Give warm or tepid baths without alkaline soap.
3. Massage the patient's skin with bland emollient creams or lotions.
4. Maintain a comfortable room temperature and advise the patient to wear loose clothing to prevent perspiration.
5. Plan diversional activities for the patient.

When a patient has severe liver damage, the nursing interventions taken will depend on the problems identified in the nursing assessment. For example, if ascites is present the nurse must place the patient in a position that does not allow fluid retention to interfere with respiration and eating. When esophageal varices are present, nursing care should focus on the possibility of massive hemorrhage and the presence of blood in the gastrointestinal (GI) tract. Mental confusion occurring in these patients requires the nurse to provide safety measures and to attempt to individualize care so that subtle changes in the patient's mental status may be identified. When posthepatic hyperbilirubinemia is present, nursing interventions depend upon the assessment of problems that accompany obstruction, such as pain and intolerance to fatty foods. If the cause is cancer, interventions related to the clinical manifestations occurring with this diagnosis must be taken. If an elevated bilirubin indicates a pathophysiological problem for which further tests are required, such as cholecystogram, nursing interventions should include patient teaching related to that procedure.

Medical treatment for an elevated indirect bilirubin in newborns depends on the clinical picture for each individual infant. The nurse can help alleviate the anxiety of new parents by explaining how the decisions are made to treat an elevated bilirubin. The parents may also need support by the nursing staff if their baby has to stay in the hospital longer than anticipated.

The most common method used to treat jaundice in the newborn is phototherapy. In severe cases of Rh incompatibility, exchange transfusions are used. A detailed discussion of these therapies may be found in maternity and pediatric nursing textbooks.

URINE UROBILINOGEN

Description

Urobilinogen is derived from the action of intestinal flora on bilirubin that has been conjugated by the liver (Fig. 8.1). Approximately 20% of this urobilinogen is reabsorbed and some is eventually excreted in the urine. For a more detailed discussion of bilirubin, see the section on Serum Bilirubin.

NORMAL RANGE

Adults and children	
2 hour	0.3–1 Ehrlich units/2 h
24-hour	0.05–2.5 mg/24 h *or* 0.5–4 Ehrlich units/24 h
Random	0.3–3.5 mg/dl *or* 0.1–1.0 Ehrlich/ml

8

Specimen Required

The specimen required depends on the laboratory requirements and the type of test performed. In some instances, only a single fresh urine specimen is required. The 2-hour specimen is more common. When possible, it should be collected between noon and four PM, when the amount of urobilinogen in the urine is highest. Occasionally, a 24-hour specimen is ordered. When urine is saved, the sample is collected in a brown bottle and protected from the light, since this can degrade bilirubin to biliverdin. If part of the specimen is lost, the test must be restarted.

Preparation of the Patient

The patient should be given the appropriate instructions about the collection of urine (see Chapter 1). A false elevation may occur when the following substances have been taken:

Amidopyrine	p-Aminosalicylic acid
Antipyrine	Salicylates
Bromsulphalein	Sodium bicarbonate
Chlorpromazine	Sulfonamides
Diatrizoate	Tetracycline
Drugs containing azo dyes	Thoradex
Epinephrine	

A note should be made on the laboratory slip when the patient has taken one of these drugs or any broad-spectrum antibiotics.

Causes of Deviation from Normal

There are several reasons for an increase in urine urobilinogen. It can occur in conditions that cause the hemolysis of red cells. In addition, elevations occur in association with increased bacterial action on the intestinal flora attributable to an increase in the number of bacteria present or a slower transit time through the intestines, as well as in association with hepatic diseases in which the reabsorption of urobilinogen into the liver is diminished.

A decrease in urine urobilinogen occurs in patients with liver disease who have posthepatic (obstructive) jaundice. A decrease can also occur when the bacterial flora are unable to act on bilirubin due to bowel sterilization or a diarrhea that leads to a decreased transit time. The decreased production of bilirubin associated with anemia may also cause a reduced urine urobilinogen. Broad-spectrum antibiotics may suppress the ability of the intestinal flora to produce urobilinogen resulting in decreased levels.

Nursing Implications of Abnormal Findings

Assessment. When assessing a patient with an elevated urine urobilinogen the nurse must remember that there are several causes for an increase. If the patient has had cardiopulmonary bypass resulting in the hemolysis of red cells, the increased urine urobilinogen should gradually diminish. If liver damage is suspected in a patient who has an increased urine urobilinogen, the patient should be observed closely for evidence of further damage, such as jaundice, lethargy, nausea, and vomiting. When a patient's urine is the color of tea or if the foam produced when the urine is shaken up has a yellow cast to it, the nurse should treat the patient as if the urine urobilinogen is elevated until laboratory data are obtained.

Interventions. If a patient with an elevated urine urobilinogen has obvious hyperbilirubinemia, the nursing interventions discussed in the section on serum bilirubin should be taken. If a change in the color of urine is the only sign that there is urobilinogen in the urine, nursing interventions should focus on the possibility that hepatic damage is present. These include small, frequent feedings if anorexia is present, rest in bed or a chair to avoid fatigue, and the prevention of dissemination of the disease until hepatitis is no longer suspected as a cause. When hemolysis of red cells is a known cause, nursing interventions depend on the degree of anemia that is present.

FECAL UROBILINOGEN

Description

Urobilinogen is present in large amounts in fecal material, since it is derived from the bacterial action of intestinal flora on bilirubin (Fig. 8.1). Approximately 80% of urobilinogen is normally excreted in the stool. For a more detailed discussion of bilirubin see the section on serum bilirubin.

N O R M A L   R A N G E
Adults and children   30–200 mg/100 g of feces   130–250 Ehrlich units/100 g of feces

Specimen Required

A stool specimen is collected and placed in a tightly covered container.

Preparation of the Patient

The patient should be given the appropriate instructions when a stool specimen is to be collected (see Chapter 1). If the patient is receiving broad-spectrum antibiotics, this should be noted on the laboratory slip.

8

Causes of Deviation from Normal

There is an increase in fecal urobilinogen when severe hemolysis of red cells has occurred. Hemolysis releases increased amounts of unconjugated bilirubin, which is conjugated by the liver and secreted into the intestinal tract. This results in increased production of urobilinogen.

    Decreases in the fecal urobilinogen are usually caused by a biliary obstruction, often a result of cancer. Hepatocellular jaundice may also cause decreases in fecal urobilinogen; however, very low levels can most often be attributed to posthepatic obstruction. Decreases in levels of fecal urobilinogen may also be caused by broad-spectrum antibiotics, which interfere with the conversion of bilirubin to urobilinogen by the intestinal flora.

Nursing Implications of Abnormal Findings

    Assessment and Interventions. When the nurse is assessing a patient with biliary obstruction or hepatocellular damage, the stool should be examined to see if it is very light or clay-colored, since this is a good indication that the fecal urobilinogen is decreased. The nurse should also try to find out when the patient first noticed the change in color, as this information may be helpful in determining how long the obstruction or damage has been present. Jaundice, dark (tea-colored) urine, and abdominal pain also occur when obstruction is present and should be looked for in the nursing assessment.

The nursing interventions taken when a patient has a decreased fecal urobilinogen should focus on problems associated with the disease process that is present. Accurate recording and reporting of the stool color is necessary. The patient needs emotional support, particularly during the diagnostic phase of the illness when it may not be known whether an obstruction is caused by a common bile duct stone that may be surgically removed or an inoperable carcinoma.

ALKALINE PHOSPHATASE

Description

Alkaline phosphatase is an enzyme synthesized primarily in the liver and in bone but also formed in the kidneys, intestines, and placenta. Most of the enzyme present in normal serum comes from bone, when osteoblasts are active. The amount present in bile comes almost entirely from the liver. Usual laboratory analysis does not differentiate the enzyme according to site of production; however, isoenzyme studies may be done to identify the tissue source. These studies are used to identify the primary site responsible for increased amounts of the enzyme in the blood. This enzyme may also be synthesized by cancer cells.

NORMAL RANGE

There are several units of measure for alkaline phosphatase. The most common are:

Adults	25–97 U/L
	1.4–4.5 Bodansky units/dl
	4–13 King-Armstrong units/dl
	0.8–2.3 Bessey-Lowry units/ml
Children	20–150 U/L
	5–14 Bodansky units/dl
	15–30 King-Armstrong units/dl
	3.4–9.0 Bessey-Lowry units/ml
Infants	50–65 U/L

Specimen Required

A 5-ml sample of venous blood is obtained in a plain collecting tube or a syringe.

Preparation of the Patient

Food and drink are usually not restricted before venipuncture. However, some medications, including oral contraceptives, can increase serum levels of alkaline phosphatase (Table 8.1). Medications should be withheld, if possible, until after blood has been drawn. Otherwise, the nurse should note on the laboratory slip the medications the patient is taking. The length of time a drug has been withheld should also be noted.

Causes of Deviation from Normal

An elevated level of alkaline phosphatase has no diagnostic value without the patient's history and physical findings. Since a large portion of this enzyme is derived from bone, abnormally high values are present when osteoblastic activity has increased. This occurs when there is bone disease, when fractures are healing, or when children's bones are growing. High levels of alkaline phosphatase are found in Paget's disease and in hyperparathyroidism with skeletal involvement. Bone metastases and osteogenic sarcoma also cause elevations in adults; moderate increases sometimes occur during pregnancy.

Measurement of alkaline phosphatase is valuable in differentiating obstructive jaundice from hepatocellular jaundice. Alkaline phosphatase levels rise with posthepatic obstruction (*obstructive jaundice*) or intrahepatic cholestasis (*hepatocanalicular jaundice*). However, levels may be normal or only slightly elevated with hepatocellular disease. Since patients with hepatitis may develop obstruction or cholestatic disease, this differentiation is not absolute.

8

TABLE 8.1. Drugs that Cause a Mild to Moderate Elevation in Alkaline Phosphatase

Allopurinol	Oral contraceptives
Antibiotics	Phenothiazine tranquilizers
Ergosterol	Procainamide
Estrogen	Propranolol
Isoniazid	Sulfonamides
Methyldopa	Tolbutamide
Methyltestosterone	

Nursing Implications of Abnormal Findings

Assessment. When a patient has an elevated alkaline phosphatase level, the nursing assessment must include the pathophysiological alteration causing the abnormal level. When the origin is liver disease, the number and severity of patient problems identified depend on the extent of liver damage. When Paget's disease causes the elevation, the musculoskeletal system must be assessed for the presence of swelling or deformity in long bone, disturbances in gait, or pain in the skull, back, or lower extremities. The nurse should remember that in some people with Paget's disease the only item of quantitative data gathered is an elevated alkaline phosphatase. The assessment of patients who have an elevated alkaline phosphatase attributable to osteogenic sarcoma or bone metastases is similar to that of other cancer patients. Attention should focus on pathological fractures and the psychological as well as physiological problems associated with fractures and persistent severe bone pain. If there is an elevated alkaline phosphatase level as a result of the osteoblastic activity that occurs with hyperparathyroidism, the patient should be assessed for the presence of bone pain, diarrhea, lethargy, irritability, kidney stones, and pathological fractures. When assessing patients with elevated alkaline phosphatase levels, the nurse must remember that slight rises might occur during the third trimester of pregnancy and growth periods in childhood and adolescence.

Interventions. When a patient has an elevated alkaline phosphatase, nursing interventions depend on the underlying disease, the severity of the clinical manifestations, and the person's psychological response to sickness. Since pain is present in many of the conditions associated with elevated alkaline phosphatase, the nurse should consider the nursing interventions for pain that may be taken. A few of these are:

1. Allow the patient to choose the method of pain relief from those that are available.

2. Reposition the patient to relieve pressure or constriction that may be aggravating the pain.

3. Plan activities that will provide distraction from the pain.

4. Attempt to provide the patient with comfortable rest periods by using relaxation techniques, massage, and breathing exercises.

5′ NUCLEOTIDASE

Description

The phosphatase enzyme 5′ nucleotidase is found throughout the body and blood. It may be assessed when alkaline phosphatase levels are elevated and there is a need to distinguish between hepatic and skeletal disease.

NORMAL RANGE

There are several units of measure for adults:
Adults
    10.6–17.5 U/L
    0–1.6 Units
    0.3–3.2 Bodansky Units
Children   Values may be lower. Consult laboratory for reference values.

Specimen Required

A 4-ml sample of venous blood is collected in a plain collecting tube or syringe.

Preparation of the Patient

There are no food or fluid restrictions before venipuncture.

Causes of Deviation from Normal

Since this enzyme originates primarily in the liver, it has been used to help diagnose liver disease, such as hepatic carcinoma, extrahepatic obstruction, and biliary cirrhosis. However, this enzyme is less sensitive than alkaline phosphatase as a measure of destructive biliary disease.

Nursing Implications of Abnormal Findings

The nursing implications are the same as for an elevated alkaline phosphatase caused by liver disease.

8

CHOLINESTERASE

Description

Cholinesterase exists in the body in two forms: acetylcholinesterase (formerly called true cholinesterase) and cholinesterase (formerly called pseudo-cholinesterase). Acetylcholinesterase is found in red cells, nerve tissue, and skeletal muscle. It rapidly hydrolyzes acetylcholine and other choline esters. It has no recognized clinical significance. Cholinesterase, which is manufactured in the liver, also breaks down acetylcholine and several other choline esters. The physiological role of cholinesterase is not well understood. The serum cholinesterase may be used to determine a patient's susceptibility to succinylcholine before major surgery or electroconvulsive therapy. It is also measured when insecticide poisoning may have occurred.

<table>
<tr><td colspan="2">N O R M A L   R A N G E</td></tr>
<tr><td>Adults and children
   Acetylcholinesterase
   (true cholinesterase)
   Cholinesterase
   (pseudocholinesterase)</td><td>3–5 IU/ml or 6–8 U/L

8–18 IU/L or 204–532 IU/dl</td></tr>
</table>

Specimen Required

A 3-ml sample of venous blood is collected in a heparinized collecting tube or syringe.

Preparation of the Patient

There are no food or fluid restrictions before venipuncture.

Causes of Deviation from Normal

An elevated cholinesterase level may be seen in association with hyperthyroidism, diabetes mellitus, or nephrotic syndrome. Decreases may be seen in several conditions, including severe infections, liver disease, malnutrition, severe anemias, shock, exposure to some insecticides, and uremia.

Nursing Implications of Abnormal Findings

Assessment and Interventions. When serum cholinesterase is assessed the results should be considered with all other data collected. There are no specific interventions, since there are several diseases in which cholinesterase levels may be altered. If the test is done before major surgery or electroconvulsive therapy and levels are found to be low, the physician should be notified. If a patient with a low cholinesterase is given succinylcholine, the nurse can expect to see a prolonged period of dyspnea and general muscle relaxation. Nursing interventions should be planned to prevent respiratory distress and bodily injury.

LACTIC DEHYDROGENASE

Description

Lactic dehydrogenase (LDH) is a cellular enzyme that contributes to carbohydrate metabolism. Specifically, it catalyzes the reversible oxidation of lactate to pyruvate. LDH is present in almost all metabolizing cells, especially in the liver, heart, kidneys, skeletal muscle, brain, and erythrocytes. It is released during tissue injury. LDH is composed of five different components (isoenzymes) that can be separated and identified by several methods, of which heat and electrophoresis are the most common. Different quantities of each isoenzyme are found in various organs and tissues. LDH_1 and LDH_2, also known as the *cardiac fraction*, are present in heart, kidneys and erythrocytes, and in small amounts in other body tissues. LDH_3 is found in the lungs, spleen, pancreas, thyroid, adrenal glands, and lymph nodes. LDH_4 and LDH_5 are the *hepatic fractions* found mainly in the liver and the skeletal muscle.

Serum levels of each isoenzyme are different. LDH_2 level is the highest, then LDH_1, LDH_3, LDH_4, and LDH_5. LDH_1 is the only isoenzyme of the five that remains stable when heated at $65°$ C for thirty minutes. This quality is used to identify what proportion of total LDH is LDH_1, and provides information useful in diagnosing cardiac disease.

N O R M A L   R A N G E

LDH

Adult	165–400 Wroblewski units/ml
	80–120 Wacher units/ml
	71–200 IU/l
Children	50–150 UI/l
Newborns	300–2000 IU/l

Normal values may vary with each laboratory and the test used.

LDH Isoenzyme Electrophoresis

Range of percent of total LDH

LDH_1	17–33
LDH_2	27–37
LDH_3	18–25
LDH_4	3–8
LDH_5	0–5

Normal values may vary with each laboratory.

8

Specimen Required

A 5-ml sample of venous blood is obtained in a plain collecting tube or syringe. When complete enzyme studies or isoenzyme analyses are to be done, a 15–30-ml sample of blood may be needed. Since the value of enzyme studies for diagnosis depends on serial analysis of enzymes, each specimen must be labeled with the time the blood was drawn. Note on the laboratory slip if the patient has received any of the following drugs:

Codeine	Mithramycin
Clofibrate	Morphine
Meperidine (Demerol)	Procainamide

Preparation of the Patient

Food and fluids are usually not restricted before venipuncture. Freezing, heating, or shaking of the blood sample should be avoided, as hemolysis of red cells releases the LDH, causing falsely elevated levels.

Causes of Deviation from Normal

Abnormal serum elevations of LDH frequently aid in the diagnosis of myocardial infarction (see Chapter 4). They are useful only as a guide in determining the severity of liver disease, because increases may accompany damage to any one of the many organs or tissues that contain this enzyme. Patients with acute or chronic viral hepatitis, toxic hepatitis, infectious mononucleosis, or liver cancer may have an increase to as high as 500–700 U/ml. Therefore, LDH levels alone do not provide enough valid information about liver damage. However, isoenzyme determinations may indicate which tissues have been damaged. Increases in LDH_1 and LDH_2 suggest myocardial infarction; an increase in LDH_3 suggests pulmonary infarction; and increases in LDH_4 and LDH_5 can reveal a liver disease such as infectious hepatitis (type A) before the clinical sign of jaundice appears. LDH_3 is also present in pheochromocytoma tissue.

Nursing Implications of Abnormal Findings

Assessment and Interventions. When assessing a patient with an elevated LDH, it is important for the nurse to evaluate this finding in relationship to the patient's clinical manifestations and any other laboratory data that have been obtained. When the LDH is elevated, the significance of this elevation in relationship to nursing care must be determined. If it appears to be an isolated finding unrelated to the clinical assessment or other laboratory data, the nurse may discuss the need for having the test repeated with the physician, because it may be a false-positive reading attributable to hemolysis of red cells. When assessing a patient with liver disease, the nurse should look at this enzyme level along with those of AST, ALT, and alkaline phosphatase. In hospitals where isoenzymes are identified by electrophoresis, the nurse will be able to determine which organ has released the LDH. Although clinical signs and symptoms are the best data used to assess patients, the nurse must not forget that the isoenzymes LDH_4 and LDH_5 may be elevated in patients with infectious hepatitis type A before clinical jaundice appears. If this occurs, nursing interventions should be planned to:

1. Prevent dissemination of the disease.
2. Encourage a high-caloric, balanced diet.
3. Provide adequate rest periods.
4. Develop a program to teach the patient and family about spread of the disease.

TRANSAMINASE ENZYMES

Description

ASPARTATE AMINOTRANSFERASE (GLUTAMIC-OXALOACETIC TRANSAMINASE)

Aspartate aminotransferase (AST) is an enzyme that contributes to protein metabolism. Specifically, it is important in the biosynthesis of amino acids because it catalyzes the reversible transfer of an amino group between glutamic and aspartic acid. The old term for this enzyme was *glutamic-oxaloacetic transaminase* (GOT). This enzyme is found in cardiac tissue, hepatic tissue, skeletal muscle, renal tissue, and cerebral tissue. When cell damage occurs, AST is released into the tissues and bloodstream.

ALANINE AMINOTRANSFERASE (GLUTAMIC-PYRUVIC TRANSAMINASE)

Alanine aminotransferase (ALT) also contributes to protein metabolism. Specifically, it catalyzes the reversible transfer of an amino group from glutamic acid to pyruvic acid to form alanine. The old term for this enzyme was *glutamic-pyruvic transaminase* (GPT).

ALT is present in high concentrations in the liver; low concentrations occur in myocardial and other tissues. Therefore, elevation of this enzyme is predictive of hepatocellular damage. For example, an elevated ALT with a mild to moderate elevation of AST indicates the presence of hepatic disease, whereas a normal ALT with elevated AST and LDH rules out hepatic origin of this enzyme.

8

NORMAL RANGE

Aspartate Aminotransferase
Adult Men	8–46 U/l
Adult Women	7–34 U/l
Children	19–28 U/l
Newborns	16–72 U/l

Alanine Aminotransferase
Adults and children	5–35 Frankel U/ml
	5–25 Wroblewski U/ml
	8–50 Karmen U/ml
	4–36 IU/l
Newborns	Up to two times adult level

Specimen Required

A 5-ml sample of venous blood is obtained in a plain collecting tube or syringe. Hemolysis should be avoided during collection of the specimen, since red cells have high concentrations of AST and ALT.

Preparation of the Patient

Food and fluids are usually not restricted before venipuncture. However, medications should be withheld until after blood is drawn if possible, because some medications increase levels of both enzymes (Tables 4.2 and 8.2). If medications cannot be withheld, note them on the laboratory slip.

If the specimen cannot be taken to the laboratory immediately, refrigerate it with a notation of the time it was drawn.

Causes of Deviation from Normal
ASPARTATE AMINOTRANSFERASE (GLUTAMIC-OXALOACETIC TRANSAMINASE)

High serum levels of AST are present in patients with acute hepatic necrosis caused by such diseases as hepatitis, infectious mononucleosis, and cirrhosis. In these conditions, the levels of AST range from 300–4000 U/ml, whereas patients with obstructive jaundice and intrahepatic cholestasis usually have elevations of less than 300 U/ml. In extreme cases of massive liver destruction the AST may be as high as 2000 U/ml.

A patient with an acute myocardial infarction also has elevated concentrations of this enzyme in the serum. Levels begin to rise 8–12 hours after the chest pain has occurred and return to normal in 3–5 days.

Nursing Implications of Abnormal Findings

Assessment. Transaminase enzymes are not absolute indicators of a specific disease in themselves; however, they aid in assessing patients with diseases of the tissues in which these enzymes are present. They must be evaluated along

TABLE 8.2. Drugs that May Cause an Increase in Alanine Aminotransferase

Antibiotics	Narcotics
Digitalis Preparations	Oral contraceptives
Flurazepam	Propranolol
Guanethidine	Rifampin
Indomethacin (Indocin)	Salicylates
Methyldopa	

with the subjective and objective data obtained from the patient, since an elevation in one enzyme does not mean that a specific disease is present. For example, AST may be elevated in the presence of myocardial damage (see Chapter 4) as well as in hepatic disease.

Interventions. When planning nursing care for patients with liver disease, the level of enzyme elevation is helpful in determining the type of liver disease present and the specific nursing interventions that should be taken. For example, if both the AST and ALT are highly elevated (between 500 and 4,000 U/ml) and the patient exhibits clinical manifestations of acute hepatic necrosis, nursing care must be planned based on that medical diagnosis. If enzyme levels do not reach the expected high elevations in the presence of a specific liver disease, the nurse must consider the possibility that the disease is beginning to resolve, that it has not yet reached its most severe level, or that the diagnosis is incorrect. If it appears that the clinical condition is worsening, signs and symptoms should be closely monitored and the eventual development of hepatic coma expected.

ALDOLASE

Description

Aldolase is a glycolytic enzyme that splits fructose-1,6-diphosphate into two triose phosphate molecules. It is used in the glycolytic breakdown of glucose. Aldolase is found in most body tissues.

8

N O R M A L R A N G E	
Adults	3.0–8.2 U/dl (Sibley Lehninger)
Men	3.1–7.5 IU/L at 37° C
Women	2.7–5.3 IU/L
Children	2.6–16.4 U/dl (Sibley Lehninger)

Specimen Required

A 5-ml sample of venous blood is collected in a plain collecting tube or syringe. The specimen should be handled carefully to avoid hemolysis. Hemolyzed blood can produce false elevations because damaged erythrocytes release aldolase.

Preparation of the Patient

Food and fluids are not restricted before venipuncture.

Causes of Deviation from Normal

Aldolase is elevated following skeletal muscle disease or injury, metastatic carcinoma, granulocytic leukemia, megaloblastic anemia, hemolytic anemia, and general tissue infarction. Elevated levels also occur in Duchenne's muscular dystrophy before clinical symptoms appear. It is also used to monitor skeletal muscle disorders such as dermatomyositis.

Nursing Implications of Abnormal Findings

Assessment and Interventions. If an elevated aldolase level is present in a young boy, the nursing assessment should include an evaluation of the following: easy fatigability, inability to keep up with his playmates, delays in motor development, and frequent stumbling or falling. An elevated creatine phosphokinase (CPK) may also occur during the early stages of this disease.

Nursing interventions will focus on the safety needs depending on the amount of gait and movement disturbances present. Patient and parent education is an important component of nursing care; it is necessary to assess the patient and family's readiness for information particularly if the patient has been recently diagnosed. The education program should include information about the disease and its expected course, special treatment methods, such as drugs or bracing, general care needs, including diet activity and rest, and any modifications that will be needed in the home setting.

PLASMA PROTEINS

Description

The *plasma proteins* formed in the liver include lipoproteins, albumin, fibrinogen, and some of the alpha and beta globulins. Plasma proteins have many functions. They participate in the transport of several constituents of the blood, including oxygen transport by hemoglobin and the transport of such substances as vitamins, lipids, hormones, and certain enzymes. They are also a source of replacement for tissue proteins that become depleted, and act as blood buffers to maintain normal acid–base balance. Plasma proteins contribute to the body's nitrogen needs and help regulate cellular activity and function. Their coagulation factors affect hemostasis and they participate in the bulk flow across capillary walls. Since plasma proteins have only a slight ability to diffuse across capillary walls, they are in low concentrations in the plasma interstitial fluid. The water concentration difference that results aids in the osmotic movement of interstitial fluid into the capillaries.

Albumin is the major component of the plasma proteins and comprises more than half of the total. Its major function is the regulation of colloidal osmotic pressure, and it is responsible for 52–68% of the total osmotic effect. It is also a transport molecule for blood constituents such as enzymes, fatty acids, hormones, bilirubin, and certain drugs.

Globulins are mainly immunological agents; but they also help maintain osmotic pressure in the vascular system. They consist of different protein fractions that are chemically unrelated. These are the *alpha 1* and *alpha 2* globulins, which consist largely of glycoproteins; the *beta globulins*, which include the low-density lipoproteins (LDL); and the *gamma globulins*, which are the immunoglobulins that participate in antibody formation. The different protein fractions can be separated by protein electrophoresis, a process in which an electric current is passed through the specimen. The fractions migrate to different fields at different rates of speed and separate into bands, which are then stained to make them visible. The fractions seen are albumin, alpha 1 globulin, alpha 2 globulin, beta globulin, and gamma globulin.

NORMAL RANGE

Adults

Protein	Range
Total protein	6.0–8.0 g/dl
Albumin	3.5–5.0 g/dl
Globulin	1.5–3.2 g/dl
Alpha 1	0.1–0.4 g/dl
Alpha 2	0.4–1.0 g/dl
Beta	0.5–1.1 g/dl
Gamma	0.5–1.2 g/dl
A/g ratio	1.5:1–2.5:1

Children

Protein	Range
Total protein	6.2–8.0 g/dl
Albumin	4.0–5.8 g/dl
Globulin	1.3–3.4 g/dl
Alpha 1	0.1–0.4 g/dl
Alpha 2	0.4–1.0 g/dl
Beta	0.5–1.0 g/dl
Gamma	0.3–1.0 g/dl

Infants

Protein	Range
Total protein	6–6.7 g/dl
Albumin	4.4–5.4 g/dl
Globulin	1.5–2.9 g/dl
Alpha 1	0.2–0.4 g/dl
Alpha 2	0.5–0.8 g/dl
Beta	0.5–0.9 g/dl
Gamma	0.3–0.8 g/dl

8

Newborns	
Protein	Range
Total protein	4.6–7.4 g/dl
Albumin	3.5–5.4 g/dl
Globulin	0.8–2.6 g/dl
Alpha 1	0.1–0.3 g/dl
Alpha 2	0.3–0.5 g/dl
Beta	0.2–0.6 g/dl
Gamma	0.2–1.2 g/dl

Specimen Required

A 5-ml sample of venous blood is obtained in a plain collecting tube or syringe.

Preparation of the Patient

If the patient has had a BSP test within 48 hours, the serum protein should be delayed for an additional 48 hours, as the BSP test may cause the serum protein levels to be falsely elevated.

Causes of Deviation from Normal

TOTAL PROTEIN

The *total protein* determination is of limited value as a diagnostic aid unless it is accompanied by serum protein electrophoresis, because the total serum protein consists of many different proteins, some of which may be elevated or depressed while others are not. In general, when total serum proteins are decreased, malnutrition, protein deprivation, hemorrhage, proteinuria, malabsorption syndrome, severe burns, open wounds, or prolonged liver insufficiency can be present. An increase in the total protein level may be caused by hemoconcentration due to dehydration, including the severe fluid volume loss occurring shortly after severe burns. Certain disease states, such as multiple myeloma, typhus, and parasitic diseases may also cause an increased total protein.

ALBUMIN

Since *albumin* constitutes a greater percentage of the total protein than globulin, changes in the albumin content affect the total protein level more than changes in globulin. Decreases in serum albumin are more common than are decreases in serum globulin and may be caused by several disease states; liver damage is one of the most common causes. Because albumin has a long half-disappearance time, complete cessation does not become apparent for several weeks. Therefore, hypoalbuminemia is more commonly associated with chronic liver disease than with conditions causing acute liver damage.

When the serum albumin level falls, colloid osmotic pressure becomes depressed, resulting in the transudation of fluid into the interstitial spaces with accompanying edema. Eclampsia, uremia, surgery, trauma, nephrotic syndrome, and protein-losing gastrointestinal disorders are conditions in which protein deprivation results in a greater rate of protein catabolism than synthesis. Hypoalbuminemia commonly occurs in hospitalized patients whose dietary intake is restricted and who do not receive protein supplements by means of hyperalimentation or tube feelings. Increased levels of albumin are caused by severe fluid losses resulting in dehydration. There are no disease states that cause an increased production of albumin.

GLOBULIN

Alpha and beta globulins do not change significantly in many disease states. *Alpha globulins* are elevated when hypoproteinemia is present. This is seen in acute and chronic liver diseases and when hepatocellular necrosis has occurred. Elevations in alpha globulins are often seen in patients with metastatic disease. *Beta globulins* are elevated in liver disease; the severity of the elevation depends upon the disease present. Disturbances in beta lipoprotein metabolism are seen in patients with fatty liver disease resulting from alcoholism and in patients with obstructive jaundice.

Low levels of gamma globulin can be attributed to congenital or acquired deficiencies. An increase in this substance occurs in chronic infection of any kind because of the increased antibody production. Nonspecific elevations may occur in chronic liver disease, with the most marked elevations occurring in postnecrotic cirrhosis and chronic active hepatitis.

8

A/G RATIO

Use of the *a/g ratio* is being abandoned with the widespread use of protein fractionation by electrophoresis. The usefulness of an a/g ratio is limited, since it gives only the proportion of the two types of protein measured. In some disease states, both the albumin and globulin are elevated, but the a/g ratio remains almost normal; in others, there may be a low ratio that might have occurred because of either an unchanged albumin with an increased globulin or a decreased albumin with a slightly decreased globulin.

Nursing Implications of Abnormal Findings

Assessment. Like other liver function tests, abnormal serum protein determinations must be assessed along with other data collected. The nurse must remember that the total protein cannot provide definitive data about the patient unless electrophoresis has also been done. In some instances, a decrease in total serum protein, in association with clinical evidence of a poor nutritional state, is helpful for the nurse when assessing malnutrition associated with a liver disease such as Laennec's cirrhosis. Although hypoalbuminemia may occur in association with several disease states, if a patient has chronic liver disease, the serum albumin indicates the severity of the illness. When all serum albumin values are plotted on a graph or flowchart, a trend toward an increase or decrease in these values can be seen. Serum globulin levels are not helpful to the nurse by themselves, but they may be useful when assessed with other data.

When albumin is lost, the colloid osmotic pressure is affected; therefore, the lower the serum albumin falls the greater the potential for ascites. Daily determinations should be made of the level of serum albumin as well as of the patient's weight and abdominal girth. Signs and symptoms of respiratory distress should be noted along with the presence of puffy eyes, and sacral and dependent edema.

Interventions. When hypoalbuminemia is associated with malnutrition, nursing interventions can be planned to treat or prevent associated problems such as lethargy, confusion, dry red skin, bleeding gums, sore red tongue, dry cornea, and muscle wasting. When large amounts of edema are present, nursing interventions should be taken to prevent massive tissue breakdowns and promote lung expansion. If a high protein diet has been ordered, the patient's food preferences should be noted. The optimal protein intake should be attained gradually, as tolerance increases slowly.

COAGULATION FACTORS

The liver plays an important role in blood coagulation by synthesizing some of the plasma factors that aid in this process. These factors include: factor I, *fibrinogen*; factor II, *prothrombin*; factor V, *proaccelerin*—serum prothrombin conversion in accelerator; factor IX, *Christmas factor*—plasma thromboplastin component; and factor X, *Stuart-Prower factor*. In addition, fat-soluble vitamin K requires bile salts produced by the liver for absorption in the gastrointestinal tract, where vitamin K is synthesized by the bacterial flora in the large intestine. Vitamin K is necessary for hepatic synthesis of prothrombin and the plasma factors. (For a more detailed discussion of blood coagulation see Chapter 3.)

Description
FIBRINOGEN

Fibrinogen (clotting factor I) is a large protein molecule that is synthesized by the liver and is present in soluble form in the plasma. It is an essential component of the blood-clotting mechanism and is converted to fibrin strands by the splitting action of thrombin during the coagulation process.

N O R M A L   R A N G E

Adults and children	200–400 mg/dl
Newborns	160–300 mg/dl

Specimen Required

Venous blood should be collected in a tube that contains the anticoagulant required by the laboratory performing the test. Sodium oxalate is the most commonly used anticoagulant, although in some instances sodium citrate may be used. The entire tube should be filled with blood.

Preparation of the Patient

Food and fluids are usually not restricted before venipuncture. Digital pressure should be maintained over the puncture site for 2–3 minutes after the procedure. The site should also be checked for further bleeding.

Causes of Deviation from Normal

Decreases in fibrinogen levels can be caused by congenital deficiencies in which: (1) no fibrinogen is present (afibrinogenemia), (2) the amount of fibrinogen is less than 100 mg/dl (hypofibrinogenemia), or (3) fibrinogen is present in normal amounts but becomes decreased when thrombin is added during clot formation (dysfibrinogenemia). Hepatic disorders can also cause decreases in fibrinogen levels, as fibrinogen is synthesized by the liver; however, fibrinogen deficiency is not a common complication, since several procoagulants are also synthesized there. Hemorrhage and disseminated intravascular coagulation (DIC) can also cause hypofibrinogenemia. There is a normal increase in fibrinogen during pregnancy. Fibrinogen levels may also increase during inflammatory diseases, multiple myeloma, cancer, uremia, and hepatitis.

8

Nursing Implications of Abnormal Findings

Assessment and Interventions. When assessing a patient with a low fibrinogen level, it is important to find out if the abnormality causing the decrease is a long-standing congenital process or an acquired deficiency. If it is congenital, nursing interventions should be related to the specific inherited defect. When hypofibrinogenemia (fibrinogenopenia) is caused by liver disease, the amount of hepatic damage is probably severe and a poor prognosis can be anticipated. Nursing interventions include continual evaluation of the patient's clinical state in anticipation of a massive bleeding episode and readiness to act quickly if one should occur. The nurse should also plan for the possibility that the patient may not recover. Plans should be made to assist the patient and family members who are aware of a poor prognosis. The nurse should also prepare for the psychological effect hemorrhage may have on the patient. The nursing care of patients with a low fibrinogen level attributable to DIC is discussed under fibrinogen degradation products in Chapter 3.

Definition
PROTHROMBIN TIME

Prothrombin (factor II) is manufactured by the liver and synthesized by a process that requires vitamin K. Prothrombin is present in normal plasma and is an inactive precursor of the coagulation process, being enzymatically converted to thrombin during clot formation. The test of prothrombin time (pro. time, PT) determines defects in the extrinsic clotting mechanism by reflecting the activity of fibrinogen (factor I), prothrombin (factor II), and factors V, VII, and X.

NORMAL RANGE

The normal range for prothrombin time is 12–14 seconds.

The prothrombin time should be assessed by comparing the patient's time to the control time that is also included in the laboratory report. When the prothrombin time is being used to determine the adequacy of anticoagulant therapy, the therapeutic range is 2–2.5 times the control time. For example, if the control time is fourteen seconds, the patient's pro. time should be approximately 28–35 seconds.

The normal range (12–14 seconds) is considered to be 100% of normal activity. Because the curve relating the percent of normal activity to the prothrombin time in seconds is not a straight line, a strict percent is not an accurate reflection of the small changes that can occur in prothrombin activity.

Specimen Required
A 5-ml specimen of venous blood is collected in a tube that contains sodium citrate or a sodium oxalate solution. The tube should be filled to capacity.

Preparation of the Patient
Food and fluids are usually not restricted before venipuncture. Several medications may affect the prothrombin time (Table 3.1). If a patient is taking one of these drugs, it should be noted on the laboratory slip. Digital pressures should be maintained over the puncture site for 2–3 minutes after the procedure. The venipuncture site should also be checked for further bleeding.

Causes of Deviation from Normal

When the prothrombin content of the blood is decreased, the prothrombin time is said to be prolonged and the clotting ability of the blood diminished. One of the most common causes of an increased prothrombin time is the presence of medically prescribed anticoagulants in the blood. The prothrombin time is used to monitor the effects of coumarin-type anticoagulants, and the dosage is adjusted depending on the test results. In general, the prothrombin time is kept within 2–2.5 times the normal range, which is equivalent to 20 or 30% of normal activity. The prothrombin time can also be prolonged if the plasma contains normal levels of most factors but lacks a few specific factors.

Because vitamin K is essential for the synthesis of prothrombin, a deficiency in, or malabsorption of, this vitamin can cause a decrease in prothrombin activity and a prolonged prothrombin time. Hepatic disease can cause a prolonged prothrombin time by interfering with the synthesis of prothrombin or with intestinal uptake of vitamin K. The hepatocellular necrosis that occurs in hepatitis and cirrhosis can interfere with prothrombin synthesis and result in a prolonged prothrombin time that can indicate the severity of the damage. A severely prolonged prothrombin time indicates that damage is extensive and the prognosis poor. On the other hand, in milder forms of the disease, the prothrombin time may be close to normal.

Obstructive jaundice also prolongs the prothrombin time because of interference with the bile salts necessary for the intestinal synthesis of vitamin K. When this interference occurs, the parenteral administration of vitamin K rapidly restores the prothrombin time to normal. This vitamin K–prothrombin time test helps to differentiate between obstructive and hepatocellular jaundice; however, it is not conclusive, as patients with obstructive jaundice may have only a slightly prolonged prothrombin time that cannot be assessed by the administration of vitamin K. The prothrombin time may also be effected by the ingestion of some drugs (Table 3.1).

Nursing Implications of Abnormal Findings

Assessment. When the prothrombin time is prolonged, the patient should be assessed for any signs of bleeding no matter how subtle. The skin and mucous membranes should be examined for petechiae, ecchymoses, or hematomas. Stools should be checked for bright red bleeding or for the black tarry appearance that occurs with the passage of old blood. The urine should be examined for hematuria and the patient observed for any signs of nosebleeds. The nurse should also observe for signs of internal hemorrhage, such as tachycardia, hypotension, confusion, disorientation, air hunger, and faintness. When the prothrombin time is abnormal because of liver disease, the nurse should be aware of the poor prognosis that accompanies this sign and should observe the patient closely for evidence of deterioration or the sudden onset of a massive hemorrhage.

8

Interventions. When a patient's prothrombin time is prolonged, the physician should be informed if a drug has been ordered that may interfere with the prothrombin level. If the prothrombin time is being monitored for anticoagulant therapy, the nurse must know what the therapeutic level for the patient is and report any significant alterations in this as soon as the data are known. If the patient is receiving daily doses of an anticoagulant, the medication should be held and the physician consulted if the prothrombin time is far beyond the therapeutic range. The patient should also be protected from trauma, particularly when on bedrest. Any person with a prolonged prothrombin time should be advised to use a soft toothbrush to prevent trauma to the oral cavity, to use an electric razor to prevent cuts while shaving, and to avoid situations that may result in bruising of tissues. Parenteral injections should be given with caution, using a small-gauge needle and applying pressure to the injection site for several minutes after administration. Rectal temperatures should not be taken because irritation to the rectal mucosa may cause bleeding.

Patients who are receiving anticoagulants for long periods of time should be given an individualized teaching plan that includes information about the bleeding tendencies associated with prolonged prothrombin time as well as medications that can affect it. When a severe bump or bruise has occurred as a result of trauma, the patient should be taught to apply ice packs to the area. Patients should also be told to inform any physician or dentist who cares for them that their prothrombin time is prolonged because of anticoagulant therapy. Patients should call their physician if they cough up or vomit any amount of bright-red blood. If gastrointestinal bleeding is or has been a problem, patients should be taught to test their stools periodically for occult blood (see Chapter 1).

BLOOD AMMONIA

Description

Ammonia is an end product of protein metabolism produced in the intestinal tract as a result of the normal digestion of protein metabolism; it is the deaminization by bacterial enzymes. The ammonia is then absorbed by the blood into the portal vein and is detoxified by the liver, where it is converted to urea and subsequently excreted by the kidneys.

NORMAL RANGE
The normal range varies depending upon the laboratory performing the test and the techniques used.

Adults	15–45 μg/dl
	11–35 μmol/L (SI Units)
Children	21–50 μ/dl
Newborns	64–107 μ/dl

Specimen Required

A 5-ml sample of venous blood is collected in a tube containing sodium heparinate. The specimen must be delivered in an iced container to the laboratory at once for immediate analysis.

Preparation of the Patient

All food and fluids except water are restricted for eight hours before collection of the specimen. Excessive amounts of dietary protein may cause abnormal values. Any antibiotics the patient is receiving should be noted on the laboratory slip, because they may cause a decrease in ammonia levels.

Causes of Deviation from Normal

Hepatocellular disease due to cirrhosis or severe hepatitis is the major cause of a rise in blood ammonia. This rise occurs because of (1) an inability of the impaired parenchymal cells to convert ammonia to urea, and (2) the development of collateral circulation from the portal vein to the inferior vena cava that shunts portal blood past the liver. Blood ammonia levels may also rise when there is excessive nitrogenous material in the intestines either from the excessive ingestion of dietary protein or the gastrointestinal bleeding that may occur in patients with severe liver disease (who have bleeding from esophageal varices or other areas of the gastrointestinal tract). Patients who have had a portal systemic surgical shunt may also have elevated blood ammonia levels. An increase in blood ammonia may be caused by Reye's syndrome.

Nursing Implications of Abnormal Findings

Assessment and Interventions. When a patient has severe hepatocellular disease, the nurse should note blood ammonia levels and assess the patient clinically to determine if hepatic coma is impending. For patients already in hepatic coma, the blood ammonia levels can assist the nurse in evaluating the severity of the coma and whether or not the patient is responding to treatment. As ammonia levels increase, the degree of hepatic coma increases. Nursing interventions should be related to the altered mental status that occurs with high levels of ammonia in the blood, such as confusion, disorientation, and changes in speech or mood. Interventions should also be related to the medical care given to decreased blood ammonia levels, such as the tap-water enemas and internal antibiotics used to promote ammonia excretion from the bowel in patients who have had gastrointestinal bleeding.

A medical-surgical text should be consulted for a more detailed discussion of the nursing care for patients with hepatic coma.

HEPATITIS SEROLOGICAL TESTS

Description

Serological tests for hepatitis are done to detect the presence of hepatitis. Viral hepatitis is caused by one of the following viruses: *hepatitis A virus* (HAV), *hepatitis B virus* (HBV), or *non-A, non-B hepatitis virus* (NANB). When any of these three viruses are present in humans, they cause similar signs and symptoms of disease; however, they have individually distinguishing characteristics (Table 8.3).

The antibodies to hepatitis A virus have been seen during the acute and convalescent phases of hepatitis. Antibodies to hepatitis B virus have been demonstrated in the general population and in patients convalescing from acute hepatitis. Antibodies have not been isolated for non-A, non-B hepatitis.

Laboratory assessment for the specific serological markers is used to determine the presence of infection with hepatitis B.

1. HB_sAg is the hepatitis B surface antigen detectable in the serum in 4–12 weeks of the initial acute stage of infection.

2. Anti-HB_c is the hepatitis B core antibody. It appears in the serum shortly after HB_sAg and is detectable for 2–16 weeks.

3. Anti-HB_s, the hepatitis surface antibody, appears during the clinical recovery period occurring approximately 5 months after exposure.

NORMAL RANGE	
Adults and children	
Hepatitis A	Negative (a positive test means an active disease state is present)
Hepatitis B (HB_sAg)	Negative (a positive test means either active hepatitis or a carrier state is present)
Hepatitis non-A, non-B	Negative

Specimen Required
A 6-ml sample of venous blood is obtained.

Note. The blood specimen should be handled as if it were capable of transmitting viral hepatitis. Universal precautions should be followed during specimen collection.

Preparation of the Patient
There are no food or fluid restrictions before venipuncture.

Causes of Deviation from Normal
Tests for hepatitis A are difficult to use because varied clinical circumstances can affect the results. When HB_sAg is present, the patient is currently infected

TABLE 8.3. Comparison of Hepatitis Viruses

Characteristics	Hepatitis A	Hepatitis B	Non-A Non-B Hepatitis
Incubation Period	30–60 days	45–160 days	14–105 days
Route of transmission	Primarily nonparenteral (fecal, oral, urine). May be parenteral	Primarily parenteral. May be non-parenteral, oral route.	Parenteral
Severity	Mild	Often severe	Mild
Antigen present	HAV	HB_cAg (core antigen); HB_sAg (surface antigen)	Nature of agent is unknown.
Corresponding antibodies	Anti-HAV	Anti-HB_c; anti-HB_s	None
Value of gamma globulin prophylaxis	Good	Good if gamma globulin has a high titer of anti-HB_s	Unknown

8

by the hepatitis B virus. HB_sAg is also present in patients with chronic hepatitis and in carriers of hepatitis B who manifest no symptoms.

Nursing Implications of Abnormal Findings

Assessment. The data collected should include the specific symptoms that caused the patient to seek health care as well as the clinical manifestations occurring at the time the test was done. The patient should also be asked about recent blood transfusions, drug usage, particularly self-administered injections, recent surgery or dental work, cuts, ear piercing, and tatooing or acupuncture. Information about exposure to persons with jaundice should also be obtained. Assessment of the patient's signs and symptoms and their response to treatment should be continuous.

Interventions. Prevention of the spread of infections is a high priority. Universal precautions should be carefully followed. Staff members and visitors should be told about the need for isolation techniques and the reasons for these procedures. Interventions should focus on the relief of symptoms. Patients who are anorexic should be offered appealing food in an attractive setting. Food and fluids should also be available to the patient throughout the day. The interventions for jaundice, a common manifestation, are discussed in detail in the section on bilirubin. Diversional activities should also be planned to prevent boredom. Patient teaching should begin before discharge from the hospital. The major focus of the plan should be to prevent the spread of infection and the importance of keeping appointments for blood tests should be stressed. The patient should be told (1) not to donate blood, (2) to avoid intimate contact (kissing and intercourse) until the blood test is negative on two consecutive tests, and (3) not to dine in restaurants until enzyme levels are near normal. A general medical-surgical textbook should be consulted for a more detailed discussion of the nursing care of hepatitis.

CHOLESTEROL

Description

Cholesterol is a steroid alcohol endogenously derived from fat metabolism. It is of great importance in the synthesis of steroid hormones, the formation of bile salts for fat digestion, and the composition of cell membranes. The cholesterol synthesized within the body is transported in the plasma as *low-density lipoproteins* (LDL) or *high-density lipoproteins* (HDL). The LDL transports cholesterol to the cells and HDL removes it. Nearly three-fourths of the total serum cholesterol is esterified by the liver and transported with LDL of blood for delivery to tissues.

N O R M A L   R A N G E
Adults   Less than 200 mg/dl

Note. There is some controversy about the normal range for blood cholesterol. It has been proposed that the normal range should be adjusted upward with age. However, it is not known whether the higher levels of blood cholesterol common in people over thirty years of age reflect a normal physiological change or a pathological process. Factors such as geographic location, diet, exercise, and stress may also affect the normal cholesterol levels.

Specimen Required

A 5-ml sample of venous blood is obtained in a plain collecting tube or syringe.

Preparation of the Patient

Food and beverage restrictions before collection of the blood sample vary among laboratories. Since the ingestion of large amounts of cholesterol during the twelve hours preceding the test may affect the results, a fasting state is often required. If no restrictions are required, the patient should be told to avoid a fatty meal for at least twelve hours before the test. A repeat test may be ordered to confirm elevated levels.

Causes of Deviation from Normal

The significance of deviations from the normal range of cholesterol is uncertain and controversial. In patients with hepatic disease, cholesterol levels are somewhat useful, since the liver esterifies approximately 70% of the circulating cholesterol. When there is biliary obstruction the total cholesterol level is elevated, but when there is hepatocellular damage it may be normal or low. When damage is great, as in severe hepatitis or cirrhosis, cholesterol levels may be markedly depressed. See Chapter 4 for a discussion of the association of cholesterol levels and heart disease.

Nursing Implications of Abnormal Findings

Assessment and Interventions. When a patient has hepatic damage, blood cholesterol levels should be assessed along with other laboratory data and the patient's clinical manifestations. The normal range of serum cholesterol is very wide, and abnormal levels are associated with many different disease states. Therefore, abnormal test results have significance only when associated with other positive signs and symptoms.

8

AMYLASE

Description

Amylase is an enzyme produced by the salivary glands and pancreas and present in the liver, muscle, adipose tissue, blood, urine, feces, semen, kidney, brain, lung, fallopian tubes, intestine, spleen, and heart. Amylase is secreted into the saliva and pancreatic juice, where its activity is extracellular. Amylase contributes to carbohydrate digestion in the gastrointestinal tract by converting starches and other complex sugars to maltose and other disaccharides.

NORMAL RANGE	
Adults	
Serum Amylase	80–150 Somogyi U/dl
	25–125 SI units/L

Urine Amylase	35–260 Somogyi U/h
	6.5–48 SI units/ hour
	260–950 Somogyi U/24 hours
Children	
Serum Amylase	60–160 Somogyi U/dl
	111–296 SI units/L
Urine Amylase	Not usually done. Consult laboratory for reference values.

Specimen Required

SERUM AMYLASE

A 5-ml sample of venous blood is obtained in a plain collecting tube or syringe.

URINE AMYLASE

A 2-, 12-, or 24-hour urine specimen is ordered. An accurately timed specimen should be collected. The 24-hour specimen must be iced.

Preparation of the Patient

SERUM AMYLASE

Since the administration of glucose can cause a decrease in serum amylase, the patient should fast for at least one hour, preferably two, before the blood specimen is drawn. Administration of intravenous fluids containing glucose can also decrease serum amylase levels and produce unreliable serum determinations. Several drugs may cause elevated serum amylase levels if taken within twenty-four hours before the sample is drawn. These include narcotic drugs (Demerol, morphine, codeine, etc.), Talwin, Indocin, Urecholine, methyl choline, and diatrizoate. A notation should be made on the laboratory slip if the patient has received any of these medications.

URINE AMYLASE

The patient should be instructed to void and discard the specimen before the timed collection period. A container should be provided for urine collection. See Chapter 1 for further information about 24-hour urine collections. The same drugs listed above may cause elevated urine amylase levels. A notation should be made on the laboratory slip if the patient has received any of these medications.

Causes of Deviation from Normal

The most common cause of elevated serum and urine amylase levels is pancreatitis. In acute pancreatitis the serum amylase level rises sharply as soon as four hours after the onset of the disease. Levels can rise to as high as 2000 Somogyi units and then decline rapidly, even though active inflammation may still be present. Urine amylase levels rise within several hours of the serum levels and remain elevated for about a week after an acute attack. The way in which pancreatic enzymes are activated in acute pancreatitis is still not known. Enzymes are presumed to escape into the interstitial tissue and peritoneal cavity. Reflux of duodenal contents through the sphincter of Oddi is a possible cause. The amylase level may also rise in chronic pancreatitis; however, elevations are not as high as in acute pancreatitis and at times may be within normal limits. Carcinoma of the pancreas causes elevations in serum amylase in approximately one-third of patients.

Amylase may also be elevated in diseases other than those involving the pancreas. Perforated peptic ulcer, empyema of the gallbladder, intestinal obstruction, ruptured ectopic pregnancy, and peritonitis are also possible causes. Diseases of the salivary glands, particularly mumps, also cause elevated amylase levels.

Low amylase values have been found in patients with serum protein loss, such as in congestive heart failure, gastrointestinal cancer, fractures, pleurisy, and intestinal obstruction.

Nursing Implications of Abnormal Findings

Assessment. The nursing assessment of a patient with an elevated amylase level depends on the cause of the elevation. If acute pancreatitis is present, assessment of the patient for degree of pain and possibility of impending shock is of primary concern. Infection and fluid and electrolyte disorders also occur with acute pancreatitis and should be included in the assessment. If chronic pancreatitis is the cause of an elevated amylase level, the nursing assessment should include not only the physical manifestations of the disease but also the ability of the patient and family to deal with this chronic illness on a long-term outpatient basis. If the patient with an elevated amylase has a carcinoma in the area of the pancreas, gallbladder, or common bile duct, the nursing assessment is similar to that done for all patients with cancer; particular attention should be given to the rapidly fatal nature of this type of cancer.

Interventions. Nursing interventions are closely related to the cause of the elevated amylase. Pain control is often the primary problem, as pain may become unbearable if acute pancreatitis is present. Pain medications should be administered before the pain becomes intolerable. If morphine has been ordered, the nurse may request a change of narcotics, as morphine tends to constrict the sphincter of Oddi. Positioning is important for patients with pain from pancreatitis, and the side-lying position with the knees and back flexed is often the most comfortable. Splinting the abdomen with a pillow may also help relieve the pain. Nursing interventions should also relate to the medical therapy, such as the monitoring of vital signs of patients in shock and the care

8

of patients with nasogastric tubes and intravenous therapy when nothing by mouth is ordered.

In general, nursing interventions for patients with chronic pancreatitis focus on assisting the patient to live with the disease outside of an acute-care setting. When a patient has chronic pancreatitis, the nurse is still concerned with the patient's pain, although nursing interventions focus on the chronicity of pain, prevention of narcotic addiction, and attempts to decrease stimulation of pancreatic enzymes. Inadequate nutrition should also be dealt with by means of diet teaching focusing on foods that promote minimal gastric and pancreatic secretions. The usual diet prescribed is composed of frequent feedings of bland low-fat, high-carbohydrate, and high-protein foods. Patients should also be taught to avoid alcohol, caffeine, and overeating, as all may increase pancreatic secretions.

SERUM LIPASE

Description

Pancreatic lipase is an enzyme that influences the digestion of fat in the small intestine. Bile salts, lecithin, and cholesterol emulsify ingested fat into tiny globules, increasing the surface area of the fats. Lipase then acts on the surface of the small fat droplets by catalyzing the splitting of the bonds linking fatty acids and the first and third carbon atoms of glycerol, producing free fatty acids and 2-monoglycerides.

NORMAL RANGE	
Adults	20–180 IU/L
Children	20–136 IU/L
Infants	9–105 IU/L

Note: Consult laboratory for reference values as methods vary among laboratories.

Specimen Required

A sample of venous blood is collected in a plain collecting tube or syringe. The amount collected varies between 5–10 ml, depending on the laboratory that performs the test.

Preparation of the Patient

Some laboratories require blood to be drawn after the patient has been fasting, as it is not known if food interferes with this test. If a patient has taken cholinergics, narcotics, or protamine during the twenty-four hours before the sample is drawn, it should be noted on the laboratory slip, since these substances may cause falsely elevated readings.

Causes of Deviation from Normal

The most common cause of elevation of serum lipase levels is acute pancreatitis. It begins to rise 24–48 hours after the onset of the disease and remains elevated for one week after the acute period. Although serum lipase levels occasionally rise in patients with chronic pancreatitis, this does not occur frequently enough to be of diagnostic significance. The same is true for patients with pancreatic carcinoma.

Nursing Implications of Abnormal Findings

Assessment and Interventions. Since acute pancreatitis is the most common cause of an elevated serum lipase, the nursing assessments and interventions are the same as those discussed in the section on amylase for patients with acute pancreatitis.

LACTOSE TOLERANCE TEST

Description

The *lactose tolerance test* is performed to determine if there is a deficiency of the enzyme lactase in the small intestine of individuals who have an intolerance to milk and milk products. If lactase is not present, lactose will not be converted to glucose and galactose to be absorbed into the blood stream.

8

N O R M A L   R A N G E
Adults and children

Normal lactose tolerance 20–50 mg/dl rise over the fasting glucose level

Lactase deficiency (lactose intolerance) <20 mg/dl rise over fasting glucose level

Specimen Required

At the beginning of the test, a 5-ml sample of venous blood is collected in a tube containing an oxalate anticoagulant. A mixture of 50 g–100 g of lactose in 200–300 ml of water is administered during a 5–10 minute period. Additional blood specimens are obtained in thirty minutes and one, two, and three hours after the administration of lactose.

Preparation of the Patient

Food and fluid should be restricted for at least eight hours prior to the test. Since patients may have sudden severe abdominal cramping and diarrhea, they should be told that this response may occur and should be directed to the nearest bathroom.

Causes of Deviation from Normal

An absence of or a decline in the digestive enzyme lactase will result in lactose intolerance which results in gastrointestinal discomfort and diarrhea following the ingestion of milk and milk products.

Nursing Implications of Abnormal Findings

Assessment and Interventions. The nursing assessment of patients with a lactose intolerance should include a dietary history with a focus on the patient's tolerance to milk and milk products. When lactose intolerance is present, patients will report abdominal cramping, discomfort, and diarrhea following their ingestion. Once the diagnosis of lactose intolerance is made, the patient should be told to either avoid dairy products or use lactose free milk. They should also be told the importance of taking calcium supplements if an assessment of their dietary intake reveals an inadequate amount of daily calcium intake.

D-XYLOSE

Description

The *D-xylose test* is an indirect measure of intestinal absorption and is an important test for malabsorption. It is used to differentiate interogenous steatorrhea or sprue-type diseases from pancreatic steatorrhea, as pancreatic enzymes are not required for absorption of D-xylose.

N O R M A L R A N G E	
Adults	
Blood	25–40 mg/dl in two hours
Urine	3.5 g in 5 hours
Children	
Blood	30 mg/dl/hour
Urine	16–33% of the dose in 5 hours

Specimen Required

A 3-ml sample of venous blood is obtained in a plain collecting tube or syringe two hours after the oral administration of D-xylose. All urine voided during the testing period should be saved. A final urine specimen is collected five hours after the test was started, added to the collection bottle, and sent to the laboratory.

Preparation of the Patient

All food and fluids should be withheld from the patient after midnight of the day of the test. The patient is asked to void and the urine is discarded just before the test begins. A dose of 25 g of D-xylose dissolved in 250 ml of water is given orally to adults, followed by another 250 ml of water. Children are given 0.5 g of D-xylose per pound of body weight up to 25 g, with the amount of water adjusted accordingly. The time should be recorded on the patient's record. The patient is given no other fluids or food and must remain on bedrest until the test is completed.

Causes of Deviation from Normal

A decrease in D-xylose absorption occurs in cases of interogenous steatorrhea associated with malabsorption diseases such as sprue and celiac disease. Occasionally, an abnormal urinary D-xylose excretion occurs in myxedema, diabetic neuropathic diarrhea, rheumatoid arthritis, or alcoholism. The cause is not known, and the abnormal results are of no diagnostic value. If the patient has taken aspirin, indomethacin (indocin), or atropine it should be noted on the laboratory slip as these medications may cause abnormal test results.

8

Nursing Implications of Abnormal Findings

Assessment. Patients who have a decrease in D-xylose absorption should be assessed for the presence of other signs and symptoms of malabsorptive disorders. These include malnutrition, weight loss, diarrhea, bulky and frothy stools, weakness, easy fatigability, amenorrhea, bleeding problems, and the clinical manifestations that accompany the malabsorption of vitamins, minerals, and proteins, as well as fat. It is also helpful to determine the patient's normal dietary habits, including attempting to list all of the foods eaten containing gluten and lactose.

Interventions. Nursing interventions should be planned based on symptoms exhibited, such as planned rest periods for fatigue and weakness, suggesting the use of a soft-bristled tooth brush to avoid bleeding, avoiding bumps and bruises, and applying pressure after giving parenteral medications. In addition, nursing care should be planned according to the patient's diagnosis and medical-care plans. Plans for altering dietary intake should be made if the cause for malabsorption is related to foods, particularly those containing gluten. A dietitian should be contacted to begin diet teaching, and the nurse should provide continuous reinforcement of teaching about diet restrictions. Patients and/or families should be taught to read the labels on canned or packaged foods and to call or write food manufacturers when in doubt. Patients who have celiac sprue should also be given the names of food companies that manufacture gluten-free flour.

GAMMA GLUTAMYL TRANSPEPTIDASE

Description

Gamma glutamyl transpeptidase (glutamyl transpeptidase, glutamyl transferase, GGT) is an enzyme that catalyzes glutamyl groups to polypeptides or amino acids. It is found in large quantities in the kidneys and in small amounts in the liver, pancreas, and prostate. The amount of enzyme derived from the liver is the most clinically significant and is considered to be the source of normal serum activity.

N O R M A L R A N G E	
Adults	
Men*	4–23 IU/l
Women	3.5–13 IU/l
Children	3.5–13 IU/l
Newborns	5 times higher than children
*Levels are higher in men because of amounts found in the prostate.	
Since normal values may vary, consult laboratory for reference values.	

Specimen Required

A 10-ml sample of venous blood is collected in a plain collecting tube or syringe.

Preparation of the Patient

There are no food or fluid restrictions before collection of the specimen. Alcohol and anticonvulsant medication can cause elevations. Note on laboratory slip if these substances have been taken by the patient.

Causes of Deviation from Normal

This enzyme is elevated in hepatobiliary disorders even when there is minimal damage. It is a particularly sensitive test for alcoholic liver disease and the enzyme is mildly elevated at all times in chronic alcoholism. It is not as useful in the diagnosis of specific liver disease as are other enzymes. This enzyme is elevated in acute pancreatitis, cholecystitis, cholelithiasis, hepatocarcinoma, cirrhosis, and cases of barbiturate use.

Nursing Implications of Abnormal Findings

Assessment and Interventions. Since this enzyme may be elevated when there is a small amount of liver damage as well as in several other medical problems, nursing implications of elevated levels are minimal. When an elevation is present in a patient with several manifestations of alcoholism, nursing care should include the possibility that the patient is an alcoholic. A psychosocial assessment to determine events surrounding chronic alcohol abuse should be done when the nurse is involved in rehabilitation of an alcoholic. Gamma glutamyl transpeptidase levels are helpful objective data about recent alcohol ingestion, and nursing interventions can be planned using this information.

GASTRIN

Description

Gastrin is a hormone secreted by the endocrine cells in the antrum of the stomach. The secretion of gastrin is inhibited by high concentrations of acid. When there is a decrease in acidity, such as after ingestion of a protein meal, gastrin is released. This stimulates hydrochloric acid secretion, which, when high, eventually inhibits gastrin secretion, completing a negative feedback control mechanism.

N O R M A L   R A N G E

The normal range for adults for serum gastrin is <300 pg/ml.

8

Specimen Required

A 5–10-ml specimen of venous blood is obtained in a plain collecting tube or syringe.

Preparation of the Patient

All food and fluids except water, should be withheld for twelve hours before the test.

Causes of Deviation from Normal

The two primary causes of increased gastrin secretion are (1) diseases in which gastric production is reduced, such as stomach cancer or pernicious anemia, and (2) the growth of an autonomous tumor that produces excess gastrin, such as those found in Zollinger-Ellison syndrome.

Nursing Implications of Abnormal Findings

Assessment and Interventions. Gastrin levels should be assessed in association with other clinical data obtained, since the primary causes of elevations in this hormone have two separate etiologies. Interventions for the patient with increased gastrin level associated with pernicious anemia include patient teaching about the primary disease and the importance of following through on prescribed treatments, such as taking regular injections of vitamin B_{12}.

The nursing-care plan for patients with gastric cancer should include goals for long-term comfort and patient education about the progress of the disease and what to expect.

When Zollinger-Ellison syndrome is the cause of the elevation of gastrin levels, nursing interventions should focus on trying to alleviate signs and symptoms, such as discomfort associated with the gastritis and diarrhea that often accompany this illness. The necessity of strict adherence to the diet should be emphasized since these patients may succumb to the adverse effects of the excessive release of gastrin.

An increase in gastrin may also be seen in several other diseases including peptic ulcers, chronic atrophic gastritis, cirrhosis of the liver, and end-stage renal disease.

FECAL FAT

Description

A *fecal fat test* is done to determine if there is any excess fat in the stools (steatorrhea). The sources of fecal fat are the diet (the largest portion), gastrointestinal secretions, cellular desquamation, and colonic flora. Normally, the fat that enters the small bowel is acted upon by pancreatic lipase and conjugated bile salts. In the complete absence of bile or pancreatic juice, fat escapes into the stool roughly in proportion to the amount in the diet.

NORMAL RANGE

Adults and children
Total fat   <5 g/24 h
             10–25% of the weight of the dry matter

Specimen Required

A stool sample weighing at least 5 g is collected. The number of days stool is collected varies with each institution and the desire of the physician; however, at least three days of stool collection is most common.

Preparation of the Patient

The patient is placed on a normal or standard diet containing 100 g of fat per day for at least three days before the sample is collected. Specific instructions for the collection of stool specimens are provided in Chapter 1.

Causes of Deviation from Normal

Steatorrhea can be caused by one of several problems in fat absorption, all known as disorders of malabsorption. These include: (1) *celiac sprue,* which is characterized by malabsorption, lesions in the small intestinal mucosa, and sensitivity to gluten and gluten breakdown products; (2) *pancreatic insufficiency* attributable to diseases such as chronic pancreatitis, cystic fibrosis, and neoplasms, which cause gradual destruction and disappearance of pancreatic acinar cells and in some instances islet-cell tissue; (3) *bile-salt deficiencies,* which lead to abnormal bacterial proliferation of the small bowel, or a bile-salt deficiency caused by liver and biliary-tract disease in which there is impaired digestion of fat; and (4) *malabsorption of fat* attributed to such causes as subtotal gastrectomy, diabetes mellitus, Zollinger-Ellison syndrome, or regional enteritis.

Nursing Implications of Abnormal Findings

Assessment. Patients who have an abnormal amount of fat in their stools should be assessed for the presence of other signs and symptoms of malabsorptive disorders. These include malnutrition, weight loss, diarrhea, bulky, frothy stools, weakness, easy fatigability, amenorrhea, bleeding problems, and the clinical manifestations that accompany the malabsorption of vitamins, minerals, and proteins as well as fat. It is also helpful to determine the patient's normal dietary habits, including attempting to list all the foods eaten containing gluten and lactose.

Interventions. Nursing interventions should be planned based on symptoms exhibited, such as planned rest periods for fatigue and weakness, suggesting the use of a soft-bristled tooth brush to avoid bleeding, avoiding bumps and bruises, and applying pressure after giving parenteral medications. In addition, nursing care should be planned according to the patients' diagnosis and medical-care plans. Plans for altering dietary intake should be made if the cause for malabsorption is related to foods, particularly those containing gluten. A dietitian should be contacted to begin diet teaching, and the nurse should provide continuous reinforcement of teaching about diet restrictions. Patients should be taught to read the labels on canned or packaged foods and call or write the manufacturers when in doubt. Patients who have celiac sprue should also be given the names of food companies that manufacture gluten-free flour.

8

FECAL PARASITES (OVA AND PARASITES)

Description

The examination of feces for parasites is done to determine if either parasites or their eggs are present in the gastrointestinal tract.

NORMAL RANGE

It is not unusual for some individuals to harbor harmless parasites; however, parasites that cause pathological problems are normally not present in feces of adults and children.

Specimen Required

The size of specimen needed and the methods of collection of fecal material depend on the type of ova and parasites that are suspected. In some instances the stool that is collected may be either held at room temperature until delivery to the laboratory or placed in a refrigerator. It is best to ask the laboratory for the appropriate procedure to be used for each type of parasite. The physician should be consulted if the written order does not specify the type of organism that is suspected.

Preparation of the Patient

There are no food restrictions for the examination of feces for the presence of ova or parasites. However, oily cathartics should not be given. Specific instructions for stool collection are given in Chapter 1.

Causes of Deviation from Normal

There are many parasites prevalent in different parts of the world that can infect man. Some of the the more common ones are listed in Table 8.4.

Nursing Implications of Abnormal Findings

Assessment. When a patient has a parasitic infection, the nurse must do a physical assessment to determine if there are any clinical manifestations that require specific nursing care. An evaluation of the skin around the anus is important to determine if the patient has been scratching and if there are any infected lesions. It is also important to determine if there is any pulmonary involvement when an organism that invades lung tissue, such as roundworm, has been identified. The extent of nausea, vomiting, and diarrhea must also be identified and the patient assessed for hydration, particularly if the patient is a child who has been ill at home for several days. The nurse should also gather

TABLE 8.4. Common Gastrointestinal Parasites

Parasite	Geographic Distribution	Portal of Entry	Source
Pinworm (*Enterobius vermicularis*)	Cosmopolitan	Mouth, anus	Autoinfection anus-to-mouth or via a fomite
Large roundworm (ascariasis)	Cosmopolitan	Mouth	Eggs from soil-contaminated food
New world hookworm (American uncinariasis)	Warm, moist climates	Mouth, skin	Fecal-contaminated soil
Old world hookworm (ancylostomiasis)	Cosmopolitan	Mouth, skin	On surface of sandy soil
Whipworm (*Trichuris trichiura*)	Cosmopolitan	Mouth	Eggs from soil-contaminated food
Trichinella spiralis (causing trichinosis)	Cosmopolitan	Mouth	Ingestion from infected raw or partially cooked pork or pork products
Entamoeba histolytica	Tropics, occasionally temperate zones	Mouth	Food or water contaminated with feces of an infected person
Tapeworm (costodes)	Cosmopolitan (tapeworms of different types can be found worldwide)	Mouth	Partially cooked fresh-water fish, partially cooked beef and pork, and eggs contaminating food and water

8

data about the individual's community environment as well as the amount of travel the patient has done to areas where parasites are found.

Interventions. Nursing interventions should be related to the physical manifestations caused by the organism and the prevention of reinfection after treatment. If a child is infected with organisms that deposit eggs around the anus, tight-fitting diapers or pants should be used to prevent scratching. Fingernails should be cut short and the use of mittens considered to prevent the lodging of eggs under the fingernails when excessive scratching occurs. Hand washing after urinating or defecating should also be emphasized. If a bacterial infection is present, dressings and medications should be applied on time and the patient taught how to care for the affected areas at home. Pulmonary care must be planned based on the nursing assessment of lung function. Plans for fluid replacement should be made if dehydration is a problem, and the medical plan for the treatment of diarrhea and electrolyte imbalance should be discussed with the physician.

A teaching plan should be developed that includes medication instruction, with special emphasis placed on the dangers of overdose. This is particularly important when the patient desires to get rid of the infestation quickly. The patient should be told that the presence of parasites does not imply uncleanliness and mothers should be encouraged not to feel guilty about a child's infestation. The teaching plan should include information about ways to prevent reinfestation, such as careful cleansing of toilet seats, bedding, underclothing, and linens used to wash and dry the anal region, if eggs are deposited in the perianal area. Patients and families should be told about the source of infestation and how to prevent reinfestation. The geographical distribution of the organism should be discussed, particularly if the infected person is a frequent traveler. For some infections, treatment for the entire family is carried out, with individual doses of medication determined by body weight. The importance of administering the dose to each family member should be stressed.

FECAL OCCULT BLOOD

Description
When blood coming from the gastrointestinal tract is so changed by the digestive process that is not recognized as blood on visible inspection, it is said to be occult.

NORMAL RANGE

Normally there is no occult blood in the feces of adults or children. Negative reactions for occult blood are often referred to as *guaiac negative*, since guaiac preparation is often used in the testing procedure.

Specimen Required

In most situations a random stool is used. However, a 3-day fast from meat, fish, and poultry may be required before a stool specimen is collected. Three specimens are generally collected, and more than one area of each specimen is tested. More than one specimen is examined because intermittent bleeding is present in most gastrointestinal lesions.

Preparation of the Patient

In most instances there is no specific preparation for the patient. When a false-positive test for occult blood is suspected, the patient may be placed on a meat-, poultry-, and fish-free diet, since these foods have been known to cause false-positive results. Specific instructions for the collection of stool specimens are discussed in Chapter 1.

Causes of Deviation from Normal

The causes of occult blood are numerous. Minimal abrasions of the nasopharynx and oral cavity can cause small amounts of blood to enter the gastrointestinal tract. Blood from the stomach and small intestines, which often comes from malignant tumors or ulcers, can also be the cause of occult blood in the stool. Drugs such as salicylates, steroids, organic iron, rauwolfia derivatives, colchicine, and indomethacin can result in a positive test for occult blood. A false negative may be caused by large doses of vitamin C.

Nursing Implications of Abnormal Findings

Assessment. When a patient has occult blood in the stool the main focus of the nursing assessment of physiological status is the patient's bleeding. Particular attention should be paid to the oronasopharynx, since bleeding in this area may be the source of the occult blood. The patient should be asked if tooth brushing results in bleeding gums, which might be the cause. The nurse should be alert to signs and symptoms of a slowly developing anemia, such as fatigue, pallor, irritability, and tachycardia (see Chapter 2 for further discussion of anemia), as well as the clinical manifestations of a sudden massive hemorrhage, which might occur if a slowly bleeding peptic ulcer perforated, a malignant tumor eroded a major blood vessel, or esophageal varices began to bleed. A review of the drugs the patient is taking is also an important part of the assessment, since medication might be the source of the bleeding. A common rule for assessment of stools is if they are black or contain occult blood it is an indication of upper-gastrointestinal bleeding and when bright-red blood is apparent there is active bleeding in the lower portion of the gastrointestinal tract. This generalization is helpful but not absolute as bright-red blood from above the pyloris can appear in the stools of individuals with rapid peristalsis.

Interventions. Nursing interventions depend on the cause and seriousness of the gastrointestinal bleeding. When the bleeding has resulted in a severe ane-

8

mia, rest periods must be provided to lower the patient's oxygen requirements, and the patient must be protected from chilling or burns because of the poor peripheral circulation. Skin care should also be a major nursing intervention because of decreased oxygenation to the tissues causing rapid skin breakdown. If the occult blood is caused by medication therapy, the patient should be informed of this complication. If the cause is salicylates, the nurse should suggest the patient choose another drug without this substance. If the drug causing the problem cannot be discontinued, plans should be made for the patient to take the medication with meals, if possible, to reduce gastric irritation. The nurse should also perform interventions related to the specific disease causing the bleeding.

BIBLIOGRAPHY

Ahtone, J., and J. Maynard. "Laboratory Diagnosis of Hepatitis B." *Journal of the American Medical Association*, 249:2067–2069 (April 1983).

Byrne, C.J., D.F. Saxton, P.K. Pelikan, and P.M. Nugent. *Laboratory Tests: Implications for Nursing Care.* Menlo Park: Addison-Wesley, 1986.

Cello, J.P. "Diagnostic Approaches to Jaundice." *Hospital Practice*, 17:49–60 (February 1982).

Centers for Disease Control. "Update: Universal Precautions for Prevention of Transmission of Human Immunodeficiency Virus, Hepatitis B Virus, and Other Bloodborne Pathogens in Health-Care Settings." *Morbidity and Mortality Weekly Report*, 37:377–382, 387–388 (June 24, 1988).

Centers for Disease Control. "Guidelines for Prevention of Transmission of Human Immunodeficiency Virus and Hepatitis B Virus to Health-Care and Public-Safety Workers." *Morbidity and Mortality Weekly Report*, 38:1–37. (Supplement No. S-6). (February 1989).

Centers for Disease Control. "Recommendations for Preventing Transmission of Human Immunodeficiency Virus and Hepatitis B Virus to Patients During Exposure-Prone Invasive Procedures." *Morbidity and Mortality Weekly Report*, 40:1–9 (Recommendations and Reports) (July 12, 1991).

Davenport, H.W. *Physiology of the Digestive Tract.* Chicago: Year Book Medical Publishers, 1976.

Dickson, E.R., R.S. Koff, S.M. Sabesin, and B.W. Shaw. "Acting on Abnormal Liver Findings." *Patient Care*, 21:50–53, 57 (March 30, 1987).

Dickson, E.R., R.S. Koff, S.M. Sabesin, and B.W. Shaw. "Which Tests for Liver Disease?" *Patient Care*, 21:124–127, 131 (April 15, 1987).

Dougherty, W.M. "Serum Bilirubin." *Nursing 82*, 12:138–139 (November 1982).

Gannon, R.B., and K. Pickett. "Jaundice." *American Journal of Nursing*, 83:404–408 (March 1983).

Henry, J.B. *Clinical Diagnosis and Management by Laboratory Methods*. Philadelphia: W.B. Saunders Co., 1991.

Ignatavicius, D.D., and M.V. Bayne. *Medical-Surgical Nursing: A Nursing Process Approach*. Philadelphia: W.B. Saunders, 1991.

Kasanof, D. "When to Act on Unexpected Test Results." *Patient Care*, 12:14–17 (January 1978).

Lewis, M. "What Bilirubin Tests Can Tell You." *RN*, 48:85–88 (March 1985).

Lewis, S.M., and I.C. Collier. *Medical-Surgical Nursing: Assessment and Management of Clinical Problems*. St. Louis: Mosby Yearbook, 1992.

Luckman, J., and K.C. Sorensen. *Medical-Surgical Nursing: A Psychophysiological Approach*. Philadelphia: Saunders, 1987.

Munn, N.E. "When the Bile Duct is Blocked." *RN*, 52:50–56 (January 1989).

Phipps, W.S., B.C. Long, N.F. Woods, and V. Cossmeyer. *Medical-Surgical Nursing*. St. Louis: Mosby Yearbook, 1991.

Ravel, R. *Clinical Laboratory Medicine*. Chicago: Year Book Medical Publishers, 1989.

Roberts, A. "Senior Systems-18." *Nursing Times*, 83:51–55 (September 2, 1987).

Sacher, R.A., and R.A. McPherson. *Widmann's Clinical Interpretation of Laboratory Tests*. Philadelphia: F.A. Davis, 1991.

Smetzer, S.C., and B.G. Ball. *Brunner and Sudarth's Medical-Surgical Nursing*. New York: J.B. Lippincott, 1992.

Vander, A.J., J.H. Sherman, and D.S. Luciano. *Human Physiology: the Mechanisms of Body Function*. New York: McGraw-Hill Publishing Co., Inc., 1990.

Vyas, G.N. "Effective Use of Hepatitis Tests." *Patient Care*, 24:82–85 (February 28, 1990).

Wilson, H., et al. *Harrison's Principles of Internal Medicine*. New York: McGraw-Hill Publishing Co., Inc., 1991.

8

CHAPTER

9

Laboratory Tests of Metabolic and Endocrine Disorders

Vitamins
Vitamin A
Vitamin D
Vitamin E
Vitamin C
Vitamin B$_1$
Vitamin B$_2$
Vitamin B$_5$
Vitamin B$_6$
Folic Acid
Vitamin B$_{12}$

Carotenoids

Creatinine Height Index

Nitrogen Balance

Prealbumin

Retinol-Binding Protein

Serum Transferrin

Ferritin

Urine Urea Nitrogen

Glucagon

Glucose

Glucose, Capillary Blood

Glucose Tolerance Test

Lactose Tolerance Test

Glycosylated Hemoglobin and Hemoglobin A$_{1C}$

Urine Glucose

Urine Ketones

Insulin, Serum

Triiodothyronine and Thyroxine
Hyperthyroidism
Hypothyroidism

Thyroid-Stimulating Test

T$_3$ Resin Uptake (Triiodothyronine T$_3$RU)

Calcitonin

Urine Catecholamines and Vanillylmandelic Acid

Urine Chlorides

Urine Steroids

Urine Porphyrins and Porphobilinogen

Urine Phenylpyruvic Acid

VITAMINS

Description
VITAMIN A

Vitamin A, also called *retinol*, is one of the fat-soluble vitamins (Table 9.1). Its specific function takes place in the retina of the eye (thus the name retinol), where it functions in visual adaptation to light and dark. Vitamin A also has a generalized function in epithelial tissue, growth, development of the teeth, and endocrine function. Primary food sources of vitamin A are liver, kidney, cream, butter, egg yolk, and some green and yellow vegetables that contain carotene, the precursor of vitamin A. A large amount of ingested vitamin A is stored in the liver.

NORMAL RANGE	
Adults	20–80 μ/dl
	65–275 IU/dl
Children	Consult laboratory for reference values.
Infants	15–60 μ/dl

TABLE 9.1. Vitamins

Fat-soluble vitamins
A (retinol)
D (calciferol)
E (tocopherol)
K (menadione)[a]
Water-soluble vitamins
C (ascorbic acid)
B-complex
    B_1 (thiamine)
    B_2 (riboflavin)
    B_5 (niacin, nicotinic acid)
    B_6 (pyridoxine)
    Pantothenic acid[a]
    Lipoic acid[a]
    B_7 (biotin)[a]
    Folic acid
    B_{12} (cobalamin)

[a] Not measured by present laboratory methods.

9

Specimen Required

A 15-ml specimen of venous blood is collected in a plain collecting tube or syringe. The specimen should be protected from light once collected, since vitamin A absorbs light. Send to the laboratory immediately.

Preparation of the Patient

Food and fluids are withheld for 10–12 hours before venipuncture.

Causes of Deviation from Normal

Decreased levels of vitamin A are caused by (1) inadequate dietary intake, (2) poor intestinal absorption due to lack of bile or a defective absorbing surface, or (3) inadequate conversion of carotene to vitamin A. Decreases are associated with kidney infections, liver disease, sprue, cystic fibrosis, fat malabsorption problems, alcoholism, and chronic small intestinal disease. Levels lower than 10 μg/dl are associated with deficiency symptoms, including eye damage. Serial measurements are used to evaluate the response to refeeding during treatment of malnutrition. Increased levels of vitamin A are associated with excessive intake of vitamin A supplements or the hyperlipidemia and hypercholesterolemia of uncontrolled diabetes mellitus.

Nursing Implications of Abnormal Findings

Assessment and Interventions. The nurse should carry out a nutritional assessment for all patients with decreased levels of vitamin A (Table 9.2). One of the earliest signs of vitamin A deficiency is night blindness or the inability to see in dim light. Interventions should include improved patient ingestion of foods rich in vitamin A, administration of supplemental vitamins, if ordered, and improved nutritional intake (Table 9.3).

Description

VITAMIN D

Vitamin D is a fat-soluble vitamin, also called *cholecalciferol*. It causes normal mineralization of bone which prevents rickets in children and osteomalacia in adults. Working in conjunction with parathyroid hormone, it prevents hypocalcemic tetany. It only occurs naturally in a few foods including liver, egg yolk, butter, cream, and fish liver oils. Another source of vitamin D occurs when the skin is exposed to ultraviolet light. This exposure causes a derivation of cholesterol found in the skin to convert to cholecalciferol. Therefore, dietary requirements for vitamin D are only needed when there is no exposure to sunlight or to another source of ultraviolet light.

N O R M A L R A N G E	
Adults	20–76 pg/ml
Children	Consult laboratory for reference values.

TABLE 9.2. Nursing Guidelines for Assessment of Nutritional Status

Physical findings	Dietary information
Body frame	Response to nutritional intake
Weight changes	Appetite
Weight–height ratio	Food tolerances
Condition of hair, skin, nails	Taste changes
Muscle mass and fat stores	Allergies
Triceps skinfold thickness	**Nutritional intake**
Mid–upper-arm circumference	Protein intake
Arm-muscle circumference	Caloric intake
Symptoms	Vitamin and mineral intake
Anorexia	**Nutritional needs**
Nausea	Basal metabolic needs
Vomiting	Presence of acute illness
Cachexia	**Complications**
Diarrhea	Draining wounds
Inability to swallow (dysphagia)	Infections

Specimen Required

A 10-ml specimen of venous blood is collected in a plain collecting tube or syringe.

Preparation of the Patient

Foods and fluids are not restricted before venipuncture. Medications that may alter test results include corticosteroids and anticonvulsants, which may lower serum levels by inhibiting formation of metabolites to vitamin D. If these medications are being administered, this should be noted on the laboratory slip.

Causes of Deviation from Normal

Vitamin D deficiency is most often seen in patients with metabolic disorders including malabsorption and inadequate activation of vitamin D precursors. Chronic renal failure is also associated with vitamin D deficiency as is inadequate intake, as in cases of malnutrition.

Nursing Implications of Abnormal Findings

Assessment and Interventions. The nurse should carry out a nutritional assessment for all patients who have potential nutritional deficiency diseases (Table 9.2). The focus for detecting vitamin D deficiency includes assessment of the ability to see in dim light or to adapt to changes in light from daylight to darkness. Interventions should include improved

9

TABLE 9.3. Nursing Interventions to Improve Nutritional Status

General guidelines
Maintain accurate intake and output records.
Refer to dietitian for diet counseling.
Prepare teaching plan for special diets or alternate feeding techniques.
Alter nutritional intake based on patient's response.

Oral feeding
Provide pleasant meal environment.
Remove hospital equipment from room.
Straighten room and bedclothes.
Prepare food for patient to eat.
Allow sufficient time before removing tray.
Carry out personal hygiene before meals.
Refresh mouth with mouthwash.
Wash hands and face.
Provide meal supplements as needed and ordered.

Enteral Feeding
Position patient to prevent aspiration.
Verify location of tube with each feeding.
Flush tube with water before and after intermittent feedings.
Administer feeding slowly.
Hold feedings if residual is over 100 ml.

Parenteral Feeding
Maintain steady infusion rate.
Verify patency of catheter within vein.
Use aseptic technique with dressing changes.

patient ingestion of foods rich in vitamin D and a supplemental vitamin as ordered.

Description
VITAMIN E

Vitamin E, also known as *tocopherol*, is a required dietary essential, but its specific functions are not clear. Vitamin E functions as a biological antioxidant, entrapping free radicals found in the body. It also helps to stabilize cell membranes and coenzyme Q. It is widely distributed in food; wheat germ, vegetable oil, and their products form the richest sources.

N O R M A L R A N G E	
Adults	20–76 pg/ml
Children	Consult laboratory for reference values.

Specimen Required

A 10-ml specimen of venous blood is collected in a plain collecting tube or syringe.

Preparation of the Patient

Foods and fluids are not restricted before venipuncture.

Causes of Deviation from Normal

Vitamin E deficiency is most frequently seen in response to profound malnutrition or when enteral or parenteral nutrition without vitamin E is the only source of intake.

Nursing Implications of Abnormal Findings

Assessment and Interventions. The nurse should carry out a nutritional assessment for all patients who have potential nutritional deficiency diseases (Table 9.2). Patients at high risk for vitamin E deficiency include premature infants and patients with extreme malnutrition, fat malabsorption, or liver disease. If patients are on a diet high in polyunsaturated fats, the need for vitamin E increases. Interventions include encouraging an adequate intake of foods rich in vitamin E for patients susceptible to deficiencies. Vitamin E replacement therapy needs to be used and explained to the patient.

9

Description
VITAMIN C

Vitamin C (*ascorbic acid*) is a water-soluble vitamin (Table 9.1) that is easily absorbed from the small intestine. Absorption can be hindered by a lack of hydrochloric acid or by bleeding in the gastrointestinal tract. Vitamin C provides the body with the intercellular cementing substance needed to build supportive tissue and is thus required to build and maintain bone matrix, cartilage, dentin, collagen, and connective tissue. Vitamin C is necessary for firm capillary walls; it functions in the formation and maturation of hemoglobin and red cells, and it is associated with protein metabolism. Primary food sources include citrus fruits, tomatoes, cabbage, sweet potatoes, white potatoes, and green and yellow vegetables. Other sources include berries, melon, guava, and pineapple.

N O R M A L   R A N G E
Adults   0.6–2.0 mg/dl Children   Consult laboratory for reference values.

Specimen Required

A 10-ml sample of venous blood is collected in a tube containing glycolytic inhibitor.

Preparation of the Patient

Food and fluids are restricted for 12 hours before collection of the specimen.

Causes of Deviation from Normal

Decreases in vitamin C levels are primarily caused by a lack of intake, as the body has no means of synthesizing the substance. Scurvy, which occurs with long-term deficiency, is characterized by easy bruising, pinpoint peripheral hemorrhages, bone and joint hemorrhage, easy bone fracture, poor wound healing, and friable, bleeding gums. Depletion of vitamin C from the body occurs rapidly during wound healing and infectious processes because of a tenfold increase in daily requirements during such conditions. Additional vitamin C is needed during growth periods, pregnancy, and any major body stress. Increases in vitamin C suggest excessive ingestion of vitamin C in amounts far above that required for recommended daily allowances. Excess vitamin C does not accumulate in the body, but is converted to oxalate and excreted through the kidneys.

Nursing Implications of Abnormal Findings

Assessment and Interventions. When a patient has decreased vitamin C levels, the nurse should assess other nutritional parameters (Table 9.2) and observe for hemorrhaging in peripheral areas and joints. Wound healing may be a problem while replacement therapy is taking effect, and the patients should be protected from potential infections by scrupulous medical asepsis during wound care. Oral hygiene is required if bleeding gums are present. Patients with bruises, large wounds, and infections and stress are at risk of developing vitamin C deficiency and should be observed carefully for changes in these conditions. Nursing interventions for improved nutritional intake should be implemented (Table 9.3).

Description
VITAMIN B₁

Vitamin B$_1$ (*thiamine*) is a water-soluble vitamin (Table 9.1) absorbed in the acid medium of the proximal duodenum. It is stored in only small amounts and is continually excreted in the urine. Thiamine functions as a coenzyme in carbohydrate metabolism and is essential for the prevention of beriberi. Primary food sources of thiamine are lean pork, beef, liver, whole or enriched grains, and legumes; eggs, fish, and a few vegetables are sources as well.

N O R M A L   R A N G E

Thiamine levels in the body may be measured through urinary excretion in a 24-hour urine sample. Results are expressed in terms of creatinine excretion.

Age	Thiamine *μg/g* creatinine
Adults	66
Pregnant women	
Trimester 2	55
Trimester 3	50
Children	
1–3 yr	176
4–6 yr	121
7–9 yr	181
10–12 yr	181
13–15 yr	151

Thiamine can also be analyzed in serum. The normal range for serum thiamine is 1.6–4.0 mg/dl.

9

Specimen Required

If thiamine is being measured in the urine, a complete 24-hour urine specimen is collected in a plain collecting bottle. Refer to Chapter 1 for the procedures involved in collecting a 24-hour urine specimen. If the serum specimen is ordered, 10 ml of blood is collected in a heparinized collecting tube or syringe.

Preparation of the Patient

Foods and fluids are not restricted before or during collection of either the urine or blood specimen.

Causes of Deviation from Normal

Deficiency in thiamine is seen in chronic alcoholism, anorexia, vomiting, diarrhea, postoperative conditions, dietary insufficiency, hyperthyroidism, and prolonged diuretic therapy.

Nursing Implications of Abnormal Findings

Assessment and Interventions. If a decrease in thiamine occurs, the nurse should assess the patient for (1) gastrointestinal manifestations, such as anorexia, severe constipation, and indigestion, (2) nervous-system manifestations, such as diminished reflexes, general apathy, fatigue, prickly pain sensations, and paralysis, and (3) cardiovascular manifestations, such as weakened pulse, peripheral vasodilation, peripheral edema, and cardiac failure. A standard nutritional assessment should be carried out as well (Table 9.2). The nurse should provide for adequate thiamine intake, through either normal food sources or vitamin supplements. If weakness and cardiovascular manifestations are present, the nurse should protect the patient from falls and monitor symptoms regularly in order to detect early cardiovascular complications. Interventions to improve nutritional intake should be implemented (Table 9.3).

Description

VITAMIN B$_2$

Vitamin B$_2$ (*riboflavin*) is a water-soluble vitamin (Table 9.1) that is absorbed from the upper section of the small intestine by combining with the phosphorus in the intestinal mucosa. It is stored in limited amounts in the liver and kidneys. Riboflavin is a coenzyme in protein metabolism and combines with phosphorus to form coenzymes essential for tissue respiration. The primary food sources of riboflavin are milk, organ meats, enriched cereals, and some vegetables. Because riboflavin is water-soluble and destroyed by heat, retention during cooking is fostered by use of covered containers and by limiting water used and cooking time.

NORMAL RANGE

Riboflavin levels are measured through urinary excretion in a 24-hour urine sample. Results are expressed in terms of creatinine excretion.

Age	Riboflavin µg/g creatinine
Adults	80
Pregnant women	
Trimester 2	120
Trimester 3	90

Children	
1–3 yr	500
4–6 yr	300
7–9 yr	270
10–15 yr	200

Specimen Required

A 24-hour urine specimen is collected in a plain collecting bottle. Refer to Chapter 1 for the procedures involved in collecting a 24-hour urine specimen.

Preparation of the Patient

Food and fluid restrictions are not needed before or during collection of the specimen.

Causes of Deviation from Normal

Decreases in riboflavin are found in cases of protein/calorie malnutrition and in association with deficiencies in other B vitamins. People susceptible to deficiencies in riboflavin include those who have (1) eaten a diet composed of inexpensive, high-starch foods, (2) gastrointestinal disorders or chronic illnesses in which special diet and limited digestion occur, (3) undergone extensive surgical procedures, or (4) extensive burns. Riboflavin decreases may also be seen during stress, growth periods, pregnancy, and lactation.

9

Nursing Implications of Abnormal Findings

Assessment and Interventions. When a patient has decreased levels of riboflavin the nurse should carry out a standard nutritional assessment (Table 9.2) and administer supplements as ordered. Interventions to improve nutritional intake should be implemented (Table 9.3).

Description

VITAMIN B$_5$

Vitamin B$_5$ (*niacin, nicotinic acid*) is a water-soluble vitamin (Table 9.1) that is related to its precursor, the amino acid tryptophan. Niacin functions with riboflavin in the cellular coenzyme systems that convert proteins and fats to glucose and then oxidize glucose to release energy within the cell. The primary food sources of niacin are meat, peanuts, beans, and peas. Corn and rice are poor sources unless enriched.

NORMAL RANGE

Niacin is measured through urinary excretion in a 24-hour urine sample. Results are expressed in terms of creatinine excretion.

	Niacin mg/g creatinine
Adults	≥1.6
Pregnant women	
Trimester 1	≥1.6
Trimester 2	≥2.0
Trimester 3	≥2.5
Children	Consult laboratory for reference values.

Specimen Required
A 24-hour urine specimen is collected in a plain collecting bottle. Refer to Chapter 1 for the procedures involved in collecting a 24-hour urine specimen.

Preparation of the Patient
Food and fluid restrictions are not needed before or during collection of the specimen.

Causes of Deviation from Normal
Decreases in niacin levels are caused by malnutrition and are usually found in association with other vitamin deficiencies. The niacin-deficiency disease, called *pellagra*, causes neurological symptoms such as weakness and lassitude, anorexia, indigestion, and various skin eruptions. Exposed skin may develop a dark, scaly dermatitis. Continued neurological involvement may result in confusion, apathy, disorientation, and neuritis.

Nursing Implications of Abnormal Findings
Assessment and Interventions. When a patient has a decrease in niacin, the nurse should carry out a thorough nutritional assessment and continue to monitor nutritional parameters regularly (Table 9.2). The nurse should provide a safe environment so that falls and injury can be prevented. Nursing interventions to improve nutritional intake should be implemented (Table 9.3).

Description
VITAMIN B$_6$

Vitamin B$_6$ (*pyridoxine*) is a water-soluble vitamin (Table 9.1) absorbed from the upper portion of the small intestine. Pyridoxine functions as a coenzyme in protein, carbohydrate, and fat metabolism. Primary food sources are yeast, wheat, corn, liver, kidney, and other meats. It is fairly prevalent in foods.

N O R M A L R A N G E	
Adults	3.6–18.0 ng/ml
Children	Consult laboratory for reference values.

Specimen Required

A 7-ml specimen of venous blood is collected in a tube containing EDTA.

Preparation of the Patient

Food and fluid restrictions are not required before collection of the specimen.

Causes of Deviation from Normal

Decreases in vitamin B$_6$ are caused by malnutrition. During pregnancy and lactation, vitamin B$_6$ deficiencies with or without symptoms may also occur; decreases occur in patients receiving isoniazid, a known antagonist of pyridoxine.

Nursing Implications of Abnormal Findings

Assessment and Interventions. The nurse should assess the patient with decreased pyridoxine levels for signs of neurological involvement as well as the usual measures of nutritional assessment (Table 9.2). If neurological involvement is present, the nurse should protect the patient from injury and provide precautions during seizures. The patient is likely to demonstrate other vitamin deficiencies as well, so the nurse should expand the assessment to include all the major vitamins. If the patient has tuberculosis and is being treated with isoniazid, the nurse should design a patient-teaching plan that explains the reasons that supplementation of high doses of pyridoxine are necessary. Nursing interventions for improved nutritional intake should be implemented (Table 9.3).

9

Description
FOLIC ACID

Folic acid (*folate*) is a water-soluble vitamin (Table 9.1) absorbed from the small intestine and stored primarily in the liver. Folic acid is involved in the synthesis of purines and pyrimidines and is essential for DNA formation. It is also needed for normal red cell multiplication and maturation. Folic acid can be formed by intestinal bacteria or may be made available to the body through ingestion of foods which contain it. The body can store only limited amounts of folic acid; thus, serum levels are easily influenced by dietary factors. Primary food sources are milk, eggs, yeast, liver, leafy vegetables, and fruits.

NORMAL RANGE

Adults	5.9–21.0 ng/ml
Children	Consult laboratory for reference values.

Specimen Required
A 7-ml sample of venous blood is obtained in a plain collecting tube or syringe.

Preparation of the Patient
Instruct the patient to fast for 12 hours or more prior to the collection of the specimen.

Causes of Deviation from Normal
Causes of folic acid deficiency include (1) inadequate dietary intake, which results in megaloblastic anemia, (2) defective absorption of folic acid associated with malabsorption syndromes, (3) inadequate utilization during administration of folic acid antagonists, such as methotrexate, antimalarial drugs, and alcohol, and (4) increased requirements for folic acid for pregnant women and infants.

Nursing Implications of Abnormal Findings
Assessment. A decrease in folic acid level must be evaluated in conjunction with all other nutritional data collected (Table 9.2). A nutrition history should be included in the assessment when the patient is a child, a pregnant woman, or an elderly person, since chances of dietary deficiency are greater among these groups of people. Any folic acid antagonists the patient might be taking should be recorded.

Interventions. The nurse has a primary role in the care of patients who have folic acid deficiency because of poor dietary intake. Patient education should be the primary focus of the nursing-care plan. Interventions should be planned to evaluate the patient's diet, where and when meals are eaten, and the adequacy of finances to purchase and prepare nutritious food. A meal plan should be developed with the patient using a realistic approach to the patient's life style.

Plans for altering dietary intake should be made for patients who have defective absorption of folic acid and for those patients for whom the cause of malabsorption is related to gluten foods. A dietitian should be contacted to begin diet-teaching and the nurse should provide continuous reinforcement of diet restrictions. Patients should be taught to read the labels on canned or packaged food to determine their vitamin content and should be encouraged to call or write the manufacturers when inadequate information is provided. Vitamin supplements are needed for persons who do not eat fresh, uncooked vegetables and fruits, for infants fed milk diets exclusively, and for patients on long-term parenteral feeding. Nursing interventions for improved nutritional intake should be implemented (Table 9.3).

Description

VITAMIN B₁₂

Vitamin B_{12} (*cobalamin*) is a water-soluble vitamin (Table 9.1). The absorption of B_{12} from the small intestine is made possible by two gastric secretions, *hydrochloric acid* and a mucoprotein enzyme called the *intrinsic factor*. Vitamin B_{12} functions in protein metabolism and in the utilization of fat and carbohydrate. It has a well-established role in the formation of red cells. The primary food sources of vitamin B_{12} are animal foods.

N O R M A L R A N G E	
Adults	150–900 pg/ml
Children	130–785 pg/ml

9

Specimen Required

A 7-ml sample of venous blood is collected in a tube containing EDTA.

Preparation of the Patient

Instruct the patient to fast for 12 hours before the test. Note on laboratory slip if patient is taking colchicine, neomycin, para-aminosalicylic acid, or phenytoin, as these may alter test results.

Causes of Deviation from Normal

Decreases in serum levels of vitamin B_{12} can be caused by malnutrition in association with many vitamin deficiencies and by lack of either hydrochloric acid or the intrinsic factor. This latter pathology results in pernicious anemia. Deficiencies may also be found in patients who have malabsorption as a result of small bowel disorders, inadequate dietary intake, or metabolic changes associated with certain malignancies, hyperthyroidism, and pregnancy. Treatment with intramuscular vitamin B_{12} is needed to bypass the digestive system and provide sufficient B_{12} for normal red cell production.

Nursing Implications of Abnormal Findings

Assessment and Interventions. When a patient has a decrease in serum levels of vitamin B_{12}, the nurse should carry out a standard nutritional assessment (Table 9.2). The patient should be observed for cardiovascular complications if the decrease is of long duration and has interfered with red cell production. A teaching plan may be needed to educate the patient about the long-term need for replacement therapy. Nursing interventions for improved nutritional intake should be implemented (Table 9.3).

CAROTENOIDS

Description

Carotenoids are a group of compounds that are precursors of vitamin A. The normal absorption of dietary fat is essential for the absorption of carotenoids in the intestine.

N O R M A L R A N G E	
Adults	40–300 μg/dl
Children	40–130 μg/dl

Specimen Required

A 5-ml sample of venous blood is collected and placed in a collecting tube with a substance that prevents hemolysis.

Preparation of the Patient

The specimen should be obtained while the patient is fasting from food or fluids other than water.

Causes of Deviation from Normal

Decreased serum levels of carotenoids can be caused by lack of carotene in the diet or by disturbances in lipid absorption from the intestines resulting in steatorrhea. Liver disease and illnesses accompanied by high fever are also causes of low serum levels.

Increased serum carotenoid levels can be caused by hyperlipidemia, diabetes mellitus, hypothyroidism, or the excessive dietary intake of carotene, particularly the ingestion of a large number of carrots.

Nursing Implications of Abnormal Findings

Assessment and Interventions. Since serum carotenoid levels are usually obtained in conjunction with other laboratory tests ordered to determine the presence of a particular disease process, nursing care is not specific for this test. See laboratory tests discussed for specific diseases, such as fat malabsorption (Chapter 8), diabetes mellitus (Chapter 9), and hypothyroidism (Chapter 9).

When the nurse determines that poor dietary habits cause a decrease or increase in carotenoids, diet teaching should be planned to help the patient understand the need for a well-balanced diet.

CREATININE HEIGHT INDEX

Description

The *creatinine height index* is a comparison of 24-hour urine creatinine excretion with a standard amount established for normal adult males and females. The creatinine height index is expressed as a percentage. Creatinine available for excretion is dependent upon the extent of skeletal muscle catabolism. Therefore, it provides an estimate of changes in body muscle mass. The validity of the creatinine height index as a nutritional parameter is undergoing continued study.

NORMAL RANGE	
Adults	
Normal	>60%
Marginal nutritional depletion	40–60%
Severe nutritional depletion	<40%
Children	Consult laboratory for reference values.

9

Specimen Required

A 24-hour urine specimen is required.

Preparation of the Patient

Food and fluids are not restricted before or during the collection period. Refer to Chapter 1 for the procedure for collecting a 24-hour urine specimen. Accurate, timed, 24-hour urine collection is essential for reliable test results.

Causes of Deviation from Normal

Under conditions of normal renal function and sufficient fluid intake, active muscle tissue releases a constant amount of free creatinine at a steady rate proportional to the muscle mass. Creatinine excretion decreases simultaneously with a decrease in muscle mass. Chronic wasting diseases such as cancer, tuberculosis, chronic obstructive pulmonary disease, AIDS, and Crohn's disease cause a decrease in the creatinine height index. However, if a patient has renal disease or renal involvement, test results will be inaccurate, because of decreased ability of the kidney to handle normal creatinine output. The creatinine height index decreases in a patient with one of these chronic wasting diseases when the patient is in a state of protein/calorie malnutrition.

Nursing Implications of Abnormal Findings

Assessment and Interventions. Nursing assessment of patients with decreases in creatinine height index should include other assessments of nutritional status, such as weight changes, dietary intake, and the occurrence of anorexia, nausea, vomiting, and diarrhea. If protein/calorie malnutrition is diagnosed, either enteral or parenteral nutrition is likely to be ordered. Continued nutritional assessment of patients on such a feeding regimen is a priority. Interventions for the patient should include carrying out safe enteral or parenteral nutrition. When patients are on oral feedings, the nurse should (1) provide a physical environment conducive to eating, (2) schedule treatments that necessitate exposure of body excretions or discharges so that they do not overlap feeding times, and (3) provide for basic hygiene before meals. Other assessment and interventions should focus on the underlying pathological condition that produced the malnutrition.

NITROGEN BALANCE

Description

Nitrogen balance is the difference between the daily intake and the daily output of nitrogen in the body. When intake is greater than output, a positive balance exists. When output is greater than intake, a negative balance exists. Nitrogen is an end product of protein metabolism; thus, nitrogen balance indicates the daily status of body protein.

When growth occurs and new tissue protein is being formed, nitrogen is retained by the body for the synthesis of new tissues, and the body is in a state of positive nitrogen balance, also referred to as *anabolism.* When malnutrition, major trauma, infection, or other causes of tissue breakdown are present, nitrogen excretion exceeds the intake, and a state of negative nitrogen balance, or *catabolism,* occurs. In normal healthy individuals, the rate of catabolism and the rate of anabolism are in equilibrium and a nitrogen balance of zero is present.

During pregnancy, growth, healing, or recovery from illness, a positive nitrogen balance is expected.

Measurement of total nitrogen balance involves meticulous evaluation of all nitrogen intake (oral, enteral, and parenteral) and all nitrogen output (urinary, fecal, dermal, and other). This is accomplished in controlled research settings or metabolic units. In the usual clinical setting, methods for measuring nitrogen balance involve stool analysis for nitrogen content (described here) and, more frequently, urine urea nitrogen determination (discussed under urine urea nitrogen).

NORMAL RANGE

Adults	<2 g/24 h
Children	Consult laboratory for reference values.

Specimen Required

A 24-hour specimen of stool is the minimal requirement for analysis. Frequently, a 3-day specimen is used to allow for daily variations in stool pattern.

Preparation of the Patient

No food or fluid restrictions are needed before or during the test period. However, all protein intake during the test period should be accurately recorded so that calculation of nitrogen intake will be possible. The measurement of the protein in the diet is generally done by the dietitian, and the nursing responsibility is to record accurately the amount of protein in the diet that was ingested. The proper method of stool collection should be taught to the patient, so that the entire specimen is collected (Chapter 1).

Causes of Deviation from Normal

Negative nitrogen balance occurs in patients who are using up protein stores in the body and breaking down body muscle mass. Protein catabolism occurs in cancer, tuberculosis, Crohn's disease, AIDS, and any muscle-wasting disease. It also occurs during weight loss in obese patients. Positive nitrogen balance, or a surplus of nitrogen intake over nitrogen output, occurs when patients are recovering from disease or gaining weight. This can occur during the healing phase of burns or during recovery from massive trauma, microbiological injury, or acute inflammatory conditions. Positive nitrogen balance also occurs in patients receiving enteral or parenteral hyperalimentation for malnutrition states.

9

Nursing Implications of Abnormal Findings

Assessment and Interventions. When a patient is in negative nitrogen balance, the nurse should assess other nutritional parameters (Table 9.2), such as dietary intake, daily weight, and the occurrence of anorexia, nausea, vomiting, and diarrhea. Interventions depend on the underlying pathology involved. When a patient is in positive nitrogen balance, the same nutritional parameters should be used for assessment, in addition to accurate recording of the daily intake of oral foods, enteral nutrition, or parenteral fluids. Interventions should focus on the specific pathology involved.

PREALBUMIN

Description

Prealbumin is a serum carrier protein that functions as a transport for about one-third of the active thyroid protein thyroxine, and is referred to as *thyroxine-binding prealbumin* (TBPA). It also functions as a carrier protein for *retinol-binding protein* (RBP), the specific protein for vitamin A alcohol transport. All RBP is bound to TBPA in a 1:1 ratio in the bloodstream. The concentration of the TBPA–RBP complex is known to decrease drastically in the acute stages of protein malnutrition and to return to normal during nutritional rehabilitation. TBPA is sensitive to influences that change the protein status of the body and will decrease as body protein decreases. The biological half-life of TBPA is only 2.5–3 days (as compared to 4–8 days for transferrin and 20 days for albumin). Because of this, prealbumin may indicate the body's response to calorie and protein therapy for protein/calorie malnutrition earlier than either plasma albumin or total protein level.

N O R M A L R A N G E	
Adults	20–50 mg/dl
Children	Consult laboratory for reference values.

Specimen Required

A 5–7-ml specimen of venous blood is collected in a heparinized collecting tube or syringe.

Preparation of the Patient

Foods and fluids are restricted for 12 hours before collection of the specimen. If enteral or parenteral nutrition is being administered, notation to that effect should be made on the laboratory request slip. The specimen should not be drawn from a vein in which parenteral nutrition, albumin, or blood products are being administered.

Causes of Deviation from Normal

Decreased levels of prealbumin are found in protein/calorie malnutrition, cirrhosis, hepatitis, stress, inflammation, hyperthyroidism, cystic fibrosis, and surgical trauma. An increase to normal range will be seen in a patient who responds positively to refeeding. Administration of corticoids results in an increase in serum prealbumin levels.

Nursing Implications of Abnormal Findings

Assessment and Interventions. If a patient has a decreased serum prealbumin level, the nurse should assess other nutritional parameters (Table 9.2). The nurse should expect this test to be used in patients receiving enteral and parenteral nutrition therapy. The nurse should plan to provide increased amounts of high-protein foods and arrange for a pleasant environment during mealtime (Table 9.3). The patient's food preferences should be relayed to the dietary department and a dietary consultation made, if necessary. If either parenteral or enteral nutrition is ordered, safe techniques should be used, and the patient's response to the treatment noted and recorded.

RETINOL-BINDING PROTEIN

Description

Retinol-binding protein (RBP) is a protein synthesized by the liver and released in association with vitamin A. RBP, along with prealbumin, is a transport protein for vitamin A in the bloodstream. RBP is sensitive to dietary changes and has a very short biological half-life of only 12 hours (as compared to 2.5–3 days for prealbumin, 4–8 days for transferrin, and 20 days for albumin). Because of this short half-life, it is vulnerable to a number of normal or pathological influences, and is not as sensitive an indicator of the progress of refeeding treatment as prealbumin or transferrin. For example, factors such as intravascular changes, interstitial transfer of fluids, and state of hydration can influence plasma concentrations. However, RBP does give indications of response when conducted along with tests of other serum proteins.

9

NORMAL RANGE	
Adults	3.0–6.0 mg/dl
Children	Consult laboratory for reference values.

Specimen Required

A 7-ml specimen of venous blood is collected in a plain collecting tube or syringe.

Preparation of the Patient

Foods and fluids are restricted for 12 hours before collection of the specimen. If enteral or parenteral nutrition is being administered, notation to that effect should be made on the laboratory request slip. The specimen should not be drawn from a vein in which parenteral nutrition, albumin, or other blood products are being administered.

Causes of Deviation from Normal

RBP is deficient when the liver is unable to synthesize protein. Decreases are found in cases of protein/calorie malnutrition, liver disease, such as hepatitis and cirrhosis, hyperthyroidism, and cystic fibrosis. Decreases may be helpful in the early detection of subclinical malnutrition. An increase in RBP may indicate increased protein synthesis during enteral and parenteral nutrition therapy.

Nursing Implications of Abnormal Findings

Assessment and Interventions. When a patient has a decrease in RBP, the nurse should assess other parameters of nutritional status (Table 9.2). Continued evaluation of RBP is likely to be carried out during the treatment of malnutrition diseases. The usual treatment for decreased RBP is to increase the dietary protein intake. The nurse should assist the patient who is able to swallow in increasing ingestion of protein-containing foods. Interventions should focus on improving nutritional status (Table 9.3).

SERUM TRANSFERRIN

Description

Transferrin (*siderophilin*) is a plasma glycoprotein whose main function is to transport iron in the bloodstream. Each molecule of transferrin can bind two molecules of iron. Over 99% of the serum iron is bound to transferrin, and this acts as a cushion to buffer large amounts of iron that would be toxic to the body if circulating in a free state. Transferrin may also play a role in transport of trace elements. In addition, it has been associated with bacteriostasis, since it prevents release of trivalent iron, which is necessary for bacterial survival and replication. For example, patients with congenital atransferrinemia have died of sepsis.

Because it is a hepatically synthesized transport protein, transferrin has been used as an indicator of nutritional status. It has a half-life of 4–8 days. Levels of transferrin vary widely among patients with obvious malnutrition, so it is generally compared with other nutritional parameters in the evaluation of subclinical malnutrition.

N O R M A L   R A N G E

Direct measurement by radial immunodiffusion

Adults   200–400 mg/dl
Children   Consult laboratory for reference values.

Estimated values calculated from total iron-binding capacity (TIBC) are used in settings where radial immunodiffusion is not routinely available. One formula developed by Blackburn is as follows:

$$\text{Transferrin} = (\text{total iron-binding capacity} \times 0.8) - 43$$

This calculation tends to overestimate transferrin concentration by 10–20%; thus, modification of the formula by institutions for the specific patient population being tested may be necessary. Normal values for estimated transferrin levels are as follows:

Adults   250–350 mg/dl
Children   Consult laboratory for reference values.

Specimen Required

A 5-ml specimen of venous blood is collected in a plain collecting tube or syringe.

9

Preparation of the Patient

Foods and fluids are restricted for 12 hours before collection of the specimen. If enteral or parenteral nutrition is being administered, a note should be made on the laboratory request slip. The specimen should not be drawn from a vein in which parenteral nutrition, albumin, or other blood products are being administered.

Causes of Deviation from Normal

Elevations in serum transferrin occur in cases of chronic blood loss, hypoxia, iron deficiency, and pregnancy. Transferrin has a half-life of 4–8 days, and its serum level falls rapidly in patients who are catabolic and receiving only dextrose solutions intravenously. Decreases in serum transferrin occur in cases of chronic infections, iron overload, liver disease, protein malnutrition, pernicious anemia, and protein-losing enteropathies. Decreases indicate a decreased protein store in the body. Normal levels can be restored readily with refeeding.

Nursing Implications of Abnormal Findings

Assessment and Interventions. When a patient has changes in serum transferrin, the metabolic status of the body is affected; thus, assessment should include other nutritional parameters (Table 9.2). The nurse should expect to carry out regular re-evaluation of serum transferrin as the nutritional problem is identified and treated. The patient should be prepared for these additional tests. Decreases in serum transferrin levels indicate a low protein store that interferes with the body's ability to heal. The patient should be protected from potential infection by means of medical aseptic techniques and isolation from other patients who have infections. Nutritional intake of a well-balanced diet should be encouraged and interventions to improve nutritional status should be carried out (Table 9.3). If nutritional support is ordered via enteral or parenteral feeding, the nurse should follow the procedures for safe administration and observe and record the patient's response to feeding.

FERRITIN

Description

Ferritin is a major iron-storage protein produced in the liver, spleen, and bone marrow. It may also be produced by inflamed tissue and tumor cells. Serum ferritin reflects the amount of iron stored in body tissues.

NORMAL RANGE	
Adults	
Male	20–250 ng/ml
Female	
Premenopausal	12–200 ng/mL
Postmenopausal	25–155 ng/mL
Children	
Newborn	20–200 ng/mL
1 month	200–550 ng/mL
2–12 months	30–200 ng/mL
1–16 years	8–140 ng/mL

Specimen Required

A 7-ml sample of venous blood is obtained in a plain collecting tube or syringe. A notation should be made on the laboratory slip if the patient is taking iron supplements.

Preparation of the Patient

Food and fluids are not restricted before venipuncture.

Causes of Deviation from Normal

Serum ferritin levels are increased in several conditions including inflammation, liver disease, such as cirrhosis, hepatitis and cancer of the liver, as well as several malignancies such as leukemia, lymphoma, breast cancer, Hodgkins disease, and metastic tumors; all anemias except those associated with iron deficiency also increase the levels. Iron overload, which occurs with hemochromatosis and hemosiderosis, also results in elevated serum ferritin levels. There is a decrease in serum ferritin levels before iron stores are depleted. Iron deficiency also causes a deficiency in serum ferritin.

Nursing Implications of Abnormal Findings

Assessment. When there is an increase or decrease in serum ferritin, nursing care depends on the specific cause of the abnormal value. Premenopausal women should be asked about their menstrual and pregnancy history since a decrease is common in women during both. Patients with low levels should be observed for pallor, weakness, fatigue, dizziness, sensitivity to cold, and acute or chronic bleeding. If a low serum ferritin level is associated with nutritional deficiencies, a diet history should be taken that includes an assessment of the patient's knowledge of a well-balanced diet and the ability and willingness to follow such a diet. When there is an increase in serum ferritin, a medical-surgical nursing textbook should be consulted for specific nursing care.

Interventions. See interventions under iron.

9

URINE UREA NITROGEN

Description

Urea nitrogen is one of the nitrogenous end products of protein metabolism. The amount of urine urea nitrogen (UUN) excreted in a 24-hour period is used as an index for the amount of nitrogen excreted as a result of body catabolism. UUN constitutes 90% of the total nitrogen lost in the urine and also comprises 90–95% of the total nitrogen loss from the body. Thus, UUN provides a valuable measure to compute nitrogen balance. Calculations of nitrogen balance from UUN include a factor of 4 to account for the nitrogen lost through the skin, feces, and any other sources. The formula for nitrogen balance using UUN is as follows:

$$\text{Nitrogen intake (in grams)} - (\text{urine urea nitrogen} + 4) = \text{nitrogen balance (in grams)}$$

N O R M A L   R A N G E
Adults 6.0–17.0 g/24 h
Children Consult laboratory for reference values.

Specimen Required

At least one 24-hour urine specimen is needed. Accuracy of the estimate is increased when a mean of the results from 3–4 consecutive days is used.

Preparation of the Patient

Food and fluids are not restricted before the test period. During the test period, an accurate protein intake record is necessary. It should be recorded in "grams-of-protein" intake so the intake of nitrogen may be calculated.

Causes of Deviation from Normal

Increased nitrogen loss occurs in protein-wasting diseases such as malnutrition and cachexia. Decreased nitrogen loss occurs in patients who are recovering from injury, burns, or a major illness, or are increasing protein stores in the body.

Nursing Implications of Abnormal Findings

Assessment and Interventions. Urine urea nitrogen levels are used primarily to determine appropriate nutritional therapy for patients. Additional tests are needed to determine the underlying cause of an abnormality. The nurse should include assessment of other nutritional parameters (Table 9.2). Nursing interventions should focus on the specific problems presented by the patient and on the underlying disease pathology. General nursing interventions for patients with negative nitrogen balance due to excessive nitrogen loss are aimed at ensuring nutritional intake by means of safe parenteral nutrition techniques, appropriate administration of enteral nutrition, or provision of small, frequent oral feedings.

GLUCAGON

Description

Glucagon is a hormone secreted from the alpha cells of the islets of Langerhans in the liver. Within the liver glucagon promotes glucose production and controls glucose storage. It is secreted in response to hypoglycemia and inhibited by insulin and somatostatin. Normally, the coordinated release of glucagon, insulin, and somatostatin provides an adequate and constant level of blood glucose, a constant fuel supply for cellular metabolism.

NORMAL RANGE	
Adults	75–150 pg/ml
Children	Consult laboratory for reference values.
Newborns	Consult laboratory for reference values.

Specimen Required

A venous blood sample of 10 ml is collected in a chilled heparinized or EDTA container. The sample is immediately placed on ice and sent to the laboratory. Failure of icing and immediate analysis may affect the test results.

Preparation of the Patient

Food and fluids are restricted for 10–12 hours before the test. Fasting time needs to be noted, since prolonged fasting can lead to elevation of glucagon levels. Withhold insulin, catecholamines, and other drugs that could influence test results and note on the laboratory slip. To prevent elevations in glucagon from exercise or stress, the patient should be relaxed and recumbent for thirty minutes before the test.

Causes of Deviation from Normal

Increased levels of glucagon are found in diabetes mellitus, acute pancreatitis, glucagonoma, and uremia. The kidneys play an important role in the metabolism of glucagon; elevated fasting levels occur in patients with renal failure. For patients with diabetes mellitus, elevated glucagon levels return to normal when diabetes control occurs. Increased levels of glucagon are also associated with extreme exercise and in trauma patients. Decreased levels of glucagon occur with pancreatic disease. This may include inflammations of the pancreas, neoplastic disease of the pancreas, or surgical removal of the organ.

Assessment and Interventions. The nursing assessment and related interventions for deviations in blood glucagon depend on the cause of the elevation or decrease. For patients with diabetes mellitus, thorough assessment and interventions are in order, and described below under glucose. Medical-surgical textbooks should be consulted for patients suffering from other pathologies.

9

GLUCOSE

Description

Glucose, measured as fasting blood sugar or 2-hour postprandial blood sugar, is the form in which sugar circulates in the bloodstream and is oxidized by all body cells to provide energy for cellular metabolism. It is a simple sugar, or monosaccharide, and is the predominant form of carbohydrate in the human body. Ingested carbohydrate consists of disaccharides, such as starches or cereals and grains. Other important dietary sources include sugars, such as fructose and pentoses found in fruits; lactose, found in milk and milk products; and sucrose, from sugar cane or sugar beets. When digested, these forms of carbohydrate are reduced to glucose, which is then absorbed through the gut, circulated in the bloodstream, and stored by the liver. Blood glucose levels are regulated by two hormones, glucagon and insulin. In a fasting state, blood glucose levels drop, stimulating the release of the hormone glucagon. Glucagon stimulates release of glucose from the liver to raise the level of blood glucose to normal. Following ingestion of food, blood glucose levels rise rapidly. Insulin, a hormone secreted by the beta cells of the pancreas, allows glucose molecules to move out of the bloodstream and into the liver and other body cells.

N O R M A L   R A N G E

Normal serum glucose levels vary according to the length of time from the ingestion of food and the type of food ingested.

Fasting		
Adults	70–110 mg/dl	
Newborns	30–80 mg/dl	
Children	60–100 mg/dl	
2-Hour Postprandial Glucose Serum Level		
Adults	>70 mg/dl and <145 mg/dl	
Children	>70 mg/dl and <145 mg/dl	

Random glucose measurements can be taken at any convenient time. Normal levels for random glucose determinations have not been standardized, but measurements below 70 mg/dl or above 145 mg/dl are considered abnormal and indicate a need for further testing.

Specimen Required

A 5–10-ml venous blood sample is needed. Serum or plasma is generally used for the analysis. Because glucose undergoes changes at room temperature, the specimen should be analyzed within 30 minutes of collection or preserved with sodium fluoride, which will prevent glycolysis for approximately 48 hours. Peripheral blood may be used for rapid analysis by reagent strips. This method is discussed under peripheral blood glucose.

Preparation of the Patient

For a fasting blood sugar, the patient should be instructed to refrain from all eating for at least 12 hours before the test. If the patient is a diagnosed diabetic receiving medication, the insulin or oral hypoglycemic should be held until after the blood has been drawn. The patient may have water before the test, but no other liquids are permitted. After the test, if no additional blood specimens are ordered, the patient may eat and drink and the insulin or oral hypoglycemic is administered.

A patient who is having a 2-hour postprandial blood glucose level should eat a high-carbohydrate diet for 2–3 days before the test. The patient should fast the night before the test and then eat a meal with at least 75 grams of carbohydrate, such as milk, cereal, fruit, and toast. The time the patient finishes eating should be noted and the blood specimen drawn exactly two hours later. Instruct the patient not to smoke and to avoid strenuous exercise after eating and before the blood specimen is drawn.

Random glucose determinations may be done at any convenient time without special patient preparation. Blood glucose levels drawn during the administration of intravenous glucose solutions do not accurately reflect the blood glucose status.

Causes of Deviation from Normal

The most common cause of elevated blood glucose level (hyperglycemia) is diabetes mellitus (Table 9.4). In this condition, blood glucose levels are persistently elevated. Two major types of diabetes are recognized. *Insulin-dependent diabetes* (type I) involves the patient's need for insulin in order to prevent ketosis. If this type of diabetes is untreated or out of control, the blood glucose level can rise dangerously high and may be accompanied by ketoacidosis. Treatment generally involves diet regulation and the administration of insulin. In type II, or *insulin-independent diabetes*, hyperglycemia occurs even though insulin appears to be present. Ketoacidosis and ketonuria do not occur, and the problem appears to be one of insulin resistance. This type of diabetes is generally treated with diet alone or in combination with oral hypoglycemics. Approximately 10–15% of the total population of persons with diabetes mellitus have Type I, or insulin-dependent diabetes mellitus; 85–90% have Type II, or non-insulin-dependent diabetes mellitus.

Mild hyperglycemia is associated with a number of other conditions besides diabetes mellitus (Table 9.4). In conditions in which steroids, catecholamines, or thyroxine (a growth hormone) are elevated, the liver is stimulated to increase secretion of glucose into the bloodstream. As this increased secretion persists, elevated blood glucose levels can occur. During intravenous hyperalimentation, blood glucose levels rise because of the concentrated glucose solutions being administered. Diuretic therapy can lead to elevated blood glucose levels by producing hypokalemia, which in turn decreases the release of insulin

9

TABLE 9.4. Causes of Hyperglycemia

Mild—serum glucose 120–130 mg/dl
  Acute stress
  Cushing's disease
  Diabetes mellitus
  Diuretic therapy
  Hyperthyroidism
  Intravenous hyperalimentation
  Pheochromocytoma
  Steroid elevations
  Tumors or inflammations of the pancreas
Moderate—serum glucose 300–500 mg/dl
  Diabetes mellitus
Marked—serum glucose over 500 mg/dl
  Hyperglycemia without acidosis
  Nonketotic hyperglycemia
  Uncontrolled diabetes with ketoacidosis

from the pancreas. Tumors and inflammation of the pancreas can cause destruction of the cells that produce insulin and can result in elevated blood glucose levels.

Hypoglycemia, a blood glucose level below 50 mg/dl, is encountered far less frequently than is hyperglycemia. Patients with diagnosed diabetes mellitus may have hypoglycemic attacks if too large a dose of insulin or oral hypoglycemics is administered. These attacks can occur when treatment is begun or when medication dosages are increased or may be associated with the peak action time of the medication. Exercise can lower blood sugar as well. This occurs in diabetic patients during unexpected and unplanned exercise periods. Other causes of hypoglycemia include exposure to severe cold, prolonged fever, and malnutrition.

Although they are rare, other instances of hypoglycemia may occur in association with pancreatic insulin-secreting tumors or decreases in pituitary or adrenocortical function.

Nursing Implications of Abnormal Findings

Assessment. The nursing assessment of a patient with an elevated blood glucose level depends on the cause of the elevation. In patients with diabetes mellitus, assessment should include a thorough health history. The nurse should note whether there is an occurrence of diabetes mellitus in other family members. Laboratory assessment should include urine glucose and ketone levels. Some patients may complain of the classic signs of polyuria, polydipsia, polyphagia, and weight loss. These symptoms are associated with type I diabetes. In type II diabetes, patients are more likely to be overweight and to complain of fatigue and hunger.

Assessment of a patient with hyperglycemia who is already being treated for diabetes mellitus should include the following: a diet history, exploration of the methods the patient uses to administer insulin or oral hypoglycemics, and observations for other diabetic complications, such as skin infections, urinary-tract infections, and vaginitis.

Assessment of patients who have hyperglycemia but who do not have diabetes mellitus should be specific to the suspected cause of the problem, such as the rate and concentration of intravenous hyperalimentation being administered or the presence of steroid therapy or steroid diseases.

In assessing patients with hypoglycemia, the nurse should note first whether the patient is a diagnosed and treated diabetic. The patient should be assessed for changes in level of consciousness and in urine glucose levels. The patient may complain of sweating, nervousness, a fast pulse, and a headache. If the blood glucose level drops to 50 mg/dl, loss of consciousness with or without convulsions may occur.

Interventions. If hyperglycemia or hypoglycemia occurs in a patient with diabetes mellitus, the nursing care plan should include patient education on dietary changes, skin and foot care, urine and blood testing for glucose and ketones, insulin administration (if ordered), oral hypoglycemic administration (if ordered), and symptoms of hyperglycemia and hypoglycemia. Psychosocial support should be provided for the newly diagnosed diabetic, who needs to adjust to major lifelong changes. If another condition, such as steroid therapy or intravenous hyperalimentation, has caused the hyperglycemia, the patient may need to be taught to check urine glucose levels at home after hospital discharge. Medical follow-up for all patients with hyperglycemia is needed and should be encouraged.

If a patient has a hypoglycemic attack, the nurse should intervene immediately to administer glucose orally. A 50% injectable glucose solution should be available for the medical treatment of an unconscious patient. Treatment of hypoglycemia is urgent, as brain damage may occur if decreased serum glucose levels persist. Patients with diabetes mellitus should be taught to observe for the clinical manifestations of hypoglycemia and to treat them with ingestion of a simple carbohydrate.

Additional nursing interventions depend on the stage of disease and the specific patient's needs. Consult general medical-surgical textbooks for specific nursing care.

9

GLUCOSE, CAPILLARY BLOOD

Description
Glucose, as measured in capillary blood collected from a finger, earlobe, or heel stick, is a test used most commonly in patients with diabetes mellitus. The technology available for this analysis has provided an easier method for monitoring blood glucose that does not require a venipuncture. Capillary blood glucose measurements are replacing urine glucose testing as a method of monitoring control and adjusting daily needs for diet, insulin, and exercise. Capillary blood glucose monitoring can be used at the bedside to provide timely and accurate measurements for rapid administration of appropriate therapy. This method is also used by patients for self monitoring responses to therapy.

NORMAL RANGE

Two methods are available for peripheral blood glucose analysis. A strip containing the drop of blood is either inserted into a digital monitor or meter where the level of glucose is registered, or a color-sensitive strip containing a drop of blood is compared to a color-coded chart.

Fasting Capillary Blood Glucose
Adults   70–110 mg/dl
Children   60–100 mg/dl
Newborns   30–80 mg/dl
2-Hour Postprandial Capillary Blood Glucose
Adults   >70 mg/dl and <145 mg/dl
Children   >70 mg/dl and <145 mg/dl

Specimen Required
Following cleansing of the fingertip, a sterile lancet is used to collect a drop of capillary blood on the appropriate paper strip.

Preparation of the Patient
For a fasting blood sugar, the patient should be instructed to refrain from all eating for at least 12 hours before the test. If the patient is a diagnosed diabetic receiving medication, the insulin or oral hypoglycemic should be held until after the blood specimen has been collected. The patient may have water before the test, but no other liquids are permitted. After the test, if no additional blood specimens are ordered, the patient may eat and drink and the insulin or oral hypoglycemic is administered.

A patient who is having a 2-hour postprandial blood glucose level should eat a high-carbohydrate diet for 2–3 days before the test. The patient should fast the night before the test and then eat a meal with at least 75 grams of carbohydrate, such as milk, cereal, fruit, and toast. The time the patient finishes eating should be noted and the blood specimen obtained exactly 2 hours later. Instruct the patient not to smoke and to avoid strenuous exercise after eating and before the blood specimen is drawn.

Random glucose determinations may be done at any convenient time without special patient preparation. Blood glucose levels drawn during the administration of intravenous glucose solutions do not accurately reflect the blood glucose status.

Causes of Deviation from Normal

Capillary blood glucose determinations are used predominantly to detect deviations in blood sugar control in patients with diabetes mellitus. Thus, normal ranges are defined within the individual patient's tolerance for hyperglycemia and hypoglycemia. Adjustments in diet, insulin dosage, and exercise are implemented from plans prescribed by the physician. Gross abnormalities are generally followed up by a venous blood glucose test, since they may herald the need for physician intervention. The growing use of bedside capillary blood glucose monitoring has produced a number of regulatory issues to ensure accurate results. The Joint Commission of Accreditation of Healthcare Organizations has published standards for decentralized laboratory procedures that require competancy validation of personnel performing these tests. Both the laboratory and the unit personnel share responsibility for developing procedures that provide quality control checks each time it is performed, developing methods to detect and correct problems, and maintaining accurate records that document appropriate quality control procedures and test results.

9

Nursing Implications of Abnormal Findings

Assessment. The nursing assessment of a patient with an elevated capillary blood glucose should include a comparison of the findings with the normal range for the individual patient, and a history of recent diet, insulin, and exercise. Assessment should also include other factors that could precipitate hyperglycemia, such as a systemic infection or vaginitis. For hypoglycemia, the assessment should include what hypoglycemic agents (oral or insulin) have been administered and at what times, and what dietary intake has occurred. The patient should be assessed for changes in consciousness, vital signs, and headache. Changes in behavior should be noted. When patients are doing their own capillary blood glucose monitoring, the nurse should assess the patient's ability to conduct the test accurately.

Interventions. If capillary blood glucose levels are either above or below the normal range for the individual patient, interventions related to the patient's specific plan should be implemented. This may include adjustments in diet, insulin, or exercise, depending on the physician's orders. When patients are doing their own peripheral blood glucose monitoring, they should be instructed on how to collect the specimen and use the digital monitor or color-coded chart. Actions to take when abnormal findings occur should be included, and specific instructions should be given as to when to notify the nurse or physician about abnormalities.

GLUCOSE TOLERANCE TEST

Description

The *glucose tolerance test* measures serum glucose levels at timed intervals after ingestion of a specified amount of glucose. This test may be done for several reasons. If a patient's fasting blood sugar and postprandial blood sugar tests are abnormal, the glucose tolerance test may be done to describe more definitively the diabetic condition present. If a patient's fasting blood sugar and postprandial blood sugar tests are normal but the patient has a family history that strongly suggests diabetes, is obese, has recurrent skin infections, such as abscesses, or has a history of delivering large babies, stillbirths, or premature labor, the glucose tolerance test is performed to determine whether diabetes is present.

N O R M A L R A N G E	
Adults	
Fasting blood sugar	70–100 mg/dl
30 minutes	155 mg/dl
60 minutes	165 mg/dl
2 hours	140 mg/dl
3 hours	80 mg/dl
Children	Consult laboratory for reference values.
Urine should be negative for glucose at each time period.	

Specimen Required

At the beginning of the test, fasting blood and urine specimens are obtained. A concentrated oral glucose mixture, either 1/75 g of glucose per kilogram of body weight, or a standard 100 g is administered, and additional blood specimens are obtained 30 minutes and 1, 2, and 3 hours after the glucose administration. These specimens are timed precisely, and if urine glucose is being evaluated it must be obtained at the same time.

Preparation of the Patient

The patient should eat a normal diet with the addition of high carbohydrates for 3 days before the test. During these 3 days, the patient should discontinue the following medications: hormones (including birth-control pills), hypoglycemic agents, diuretics, nicotinic acid, and salicylates. The patient should fast from all foods and fluids except water for 12 hours before the test. Neither insulin nor oral hypoglycemics should be taken before the test. If simultaneous urine specimens are ordered, the bladder should be emptied before the start of the test and urine specimens should be obtained simultaneously with each blood specimen. The patient may be given water during the test. Following the test, the patient may eat and drink, and insulin or oral hypoglycemics can be administered.

Causes of Deviation from Normal

If the patient has insulin-dependent diabetes (type I), the glucose tolerance test will show abnormally high glucose levels throughout the test period. If insulin-independent diabetes (type II) is present, the 2-hour specimen will be elevated with or without other abnormal specimens (Fig. 9.1).

Nursing Implications of Abnormal Findings

Assessment and Interventions. The nursing implications of abnormal glucose tolerance test results are discussed in the section on blood glucose.

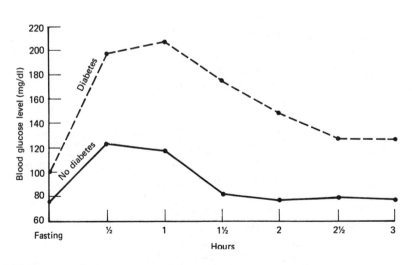

FIGURE 9.1. Glucose Tolerance Test Curves

LACTOSE TOLERANCE TEST

Description

Lactase is a disaccharide enzyme secreted by the small intestine. It is responsible for splitting lactose into two monosaccharides, *glucose* and *galactose*. These sugars are then absorbed through the wall of the intestinal tract.

N O R M A L   R A N G E

Results of lactose tolerance are measured in terms of response of blood glucose levels and/or stool analysis.

Adults	Serum glucose levels rise more than 200 ml/dl over fasting within 15–60 minutes after lactose ingestion. Stool analysis shows normal pH (7–8) and low glucose content.

Specimen Required

At the beginning of the test a fasting blood glucose is drawn; then, a concentrated load of lactose, 50 g in 400 ml of water for the average adult, is administered. Blood glucose samples are drawn at 30, 60, and 120 minutes after giving the loading dose. A stool sample, if requested, is collected five hours after the loading dose of lactose is given. Blood samples should be iced and sent to the laboratory for immediate analysis. Specify the time of the collection on the laboratory slip.

Preparation of the Patient

Food and fluids are restricted for 8 hours before the test. The patient needs to be instructed not to exercise strenuously before the test. Water may be administered during the test after the loading dose of lactose is administered.

Causes of Deviation from Normal

A lack of increase in blood glucose following administration of the loading lactose dose illustrates a lack of lactase, the enzyme required for digestion of lactose. Lactase, is more commonly absent in patients of black and Asian ethnicity than in other patient groups. Lactose intolerance sometimes develops with age.

Nursing Implications of Abnormal Findings

Assessment and Interventions. The nursing implications of abnormal lactose intolerance relate to the elimination of lactose from the diet. The nurse should observe for signs of lactose intolerance such as abdominal cramps, bloating, flatulence, nausea, and watery diarrhea. If diabetes mellitus is present, assessment and interventions discussed under blood glucose need to be implemented.

GLYCOSYLATED HEMOGLOBIN AND HEMOGLOBIN A_{1c}

Description
Normal hemoglobin is modified by glycosylation in a high glucose environment. After six months of age, 90% of the hemoglobin is classified as *hgb A*, and this group contains three components that have glucose attached: A_{1a}, A_{1b}, and A_{1c}. *Hgb A_{1c}* is the most abundant of the three types, and is sometimes used for the test. Some laboratories measure only *hgb A_{1c}*, while others measure all the hgb A and call the test *glycosylated hemoglobin*. The differentiation is important because the normal values for the combined three types are always higher than the normal value for hgb A_{1c} alone. Glycosylated hemoglobin remains stable for several weeks and can be used as a long term indicator of carbohydrate blood levels. This test is useful as a means of evaluating a diabetic patient's response to the management of the disease.

NORMAL RANGE	
Hemoglobin A_{1c}	
Adult, non-diabetic	2.2–4.8%
Child, non-diabetic	1.8–4.0%
Diabetic, good control	2.5–5.9%
Diabetic, fair control	6.0–8.0%
Diabetic, poor control	>8.0%
Glycosylated Hemoglobin (Includes A_{1a}, A_{1b}, and A_{1c}	
Adult, non-diabetic	4.0–7.0%
Child, non-diabetic	4.0–7.0%
Diabetic, good control	<7.6%
Diabetic, fair control	7.6–8.9%
Diabetic, poor control	>8.9%

9

Specimen Required
A 5–10-ml specimen of venous blood is collected in a test tube or syringe containing EDTA.

Preparation of the Patient

Food and fluid restrictions are not required before collection of the specimen.

Causes of Deviation from Normal

Changes in levels of glycosylated hemoglobin are used to evaluate long-term response of diabetic patients to management of the disease. Increased levels reflect an increase in serum glucose for an extended period of time, from 2 weeks to 3 months. Test results are *not* affected by recent diet, exercise, insulin, or oral hypoglycemics.

Nursing Implications of Abnormal Findings

Assessment and Interventions. Diabetic patients with elevations of glycosylated hemoglobin levels should be assessed for history of diet, exercise, and use of insulin or oral hypoglycemic agents. Assessment should include adherence of the patient to the prescribed diabetic treatment plan. Modifications of the plan are likely to be made by the physician, and the nurse should explain and discuss them with the patient. The nurse should clarify the patient's understanding of the treatment planned and arrange for periodic measurement of glycosylated hemoglobin as follow-up evaluation.

URINE GLUCOSE

Description

Urine normally contains no glucose. When the blood glucose level exceeds the renal threshold for the reabsorption of glucose, some glucose remains in the urine. Renal threshold levels vary among individuals, but an average of 180 mg/dl of blood glucose is associated with glucose in the urine. In diabetics this can rise to much higher levels.

NORMAL RANGE

Normally, urine tests for glucose are negative. However, normal individuals who have eaten a meal very high in concentrated carbohydrates can have transient glucosuria. Pregnancy may also cause transient glucosuria. Urine glucose test results are reported in percentage of glucose or in number of pluses; that is, one plus (+), two plus (++), and so forth. A variety of products are available to test urine glucose levels. Differences in percentages and pluses for different products illustrated in Table 7.1 indicate the need to report urine glucose levels as percentages as well as product-specific results. TesTape and Diastix are specific for glucose, whereas the reducing-agent products measure all reducing substances. If the specimen is rated using a color chart, evaluate results in a good light and make sure the chart is specific to the product being used.

Specimen Required

A fresh urine specimen of at least 15 ml is required. A sequence of timed specimens during the day is frequently ordered; for example, a fasting morning specimen, specimens taken from 30–60 minutes before lunch and dinner, and a bedtime specimen. If the tests on the urine specimen are not done immediately, the specimen should be stored in the refrigerator or kept cool until transported to the laboratory.

Because a urinary glucose determination represents a lag time of at least 20 minutes from the serum glucose level, the collection of a second-voided specimen has been recommended as the most accurate reflection of serum glucose levels in the urine. The bladder is emptied 30–60 minutes before the specimen is due, and a second-voided specimen is collected 30 minutes later. Some physicians prefer to have both specimens analyzed; however, the second specimen is believed to be more reflective of current blood glucose status. Present studies of first- and second-voided specimens have not revealed significant differences. However, study samples may not have included adequate numbers of unstable diabetics or may have included diabetics with neurological bladders, who cannot completely empty the bladder.

Preparation of the Patient

Food and fluids are restricted overnight for 8 hours before collection of a fasting urine specimen. If a double-voided specimen is collected, the bladder should be emptied 30–60 minutes before the time the specimen is ordered. The patient may have a glass of water after the first specimen is collected to ensure adequate urine formation for the collection of the second-voided specimen.

Causes of Deviation from Normal

The most common cause for the presence of glucose in the urine is diabetes mellitus. As blood glucose levels rise above the renal threshold level, the urine glucose level rises as well. The higher the urine glucose level, the higher the blood glucose level. Urine glucose can also be present in patients who receive intravenous hyperalimentation with a high glucose concentration.

9

Nursing Implications of Abnormal Findings

Assessment. When a diabetic patient has glycosuria, the same urine specimen used for glucose testing should be assessed for ketone bodies. In carrying out the glucose test, the nurse must make sure that the directions are followed exactly and that the products used have not deteriorated. If urine glucose levels are high, the patient should be assessed for other indications of hyperglycemia, including peripheral blood glucose levels, acetone breath, drowsiness, abdominal cramps, Kussmaul respirations, and decreased muscle tone and reflexes. These symptoms should be reported to the physician for treatment. The patient's history should include recent, unusual emotional distress, since such episodes can increase release of glucocorticoids, adding additional glucose to the serum. The patient should also be assessed for infection and fever, which can also trigger release of serum glucose from epinephrine and cortisol secretion. If the patient is a diabetic receiving treatment, the nurse should determine whether the patient has been taking the prescribed insulin or oral hypoglycemic and whether the prescribed diet has been followed.

If urine glucose is present in a patient who is not a diagnosed diabetic, the nurse should determine whether the patient has received high-carbohydrate intravenous hyperalimentation or has had an unusually highly concentrated carbohydrate meal.

Interventions. If the patient with urinary glucose is a diabetic, the nurse should implement a teaching program for the patient that includes urine testing and other pertinent self-care information. Since diabetes mellitus requires lifelong adaptations and changes in daily routine, emotional support should be provided by the nursing staff as well as by the family. For patients who are on hyperalimentation and who have urinary glucose, the nurse may be responsible for adding insulin to the hyperalimentation solution. For all patients with urinary glucose, perineal hygiene after urination should be carried out, since residual glucose on the perineal tissues may lead to inflammations, vaginitis, and urinary-tract infections.

URINE KETONES

Description

Ketones are composed of acetone, keto hydroxybutyric acid, and acetoacetic acid. These products result from fatty acid metabolism and are normally completely metabolized by the liver.

NORMAL RANGE

Normally there are no ketone bodies in the urine.

Specimen Required

A small amount of freshly voided urine is required, since reagent strips are used for measurement. A note should be made on the laboratory slip if the patient is taking any of the drugs which may interfere with urine ketones (Table 9.5).

Preparation of the Patient

Food and fluids are restricted for 8 hours before collection of fasting urine specimens. If double-voided specimens are being used for glucose and ketone determination, the patient's bladder should be emptied 30–60 minutes before

TABLE 9.5.	Drugs that May Cause a False Positive for Urine Ketone Bodies

Levodopa	Phthalein compound (BSP or PSP)
Pyridium	Ether
Isopropyl alcohol	Insulin
Metformin	Paraldehyde

the time the specimen is ordered, and a second specimen should be collected at the specified time. The patient may have a glass of water after the first specimen is collected to ensure adequate urine formation for the second specimen.

Causes of Deviation from Normal

Ketones collect in the body and are eliminated via the urinary tract during abnormal fat and protein metabolism. Ketonuria is most common in unregulated diabetes mellitus with ketoacidosis, but can also occur in patients with cachexia, febrile diseases, excess exposure to cold, starvation, and strenuous exercise. As ketoacidosis increases, ketone levels in the urine increase.

Nursing Implications of Abnormal Findings

Assessment. The patient with ketonuria should be assessed for other evidence of ketoacidosis, such as acetone breath, elevated temperature, poor skin turgor, dry mucous membranes, electrolyte imbalances, nausea, vomiting, and Kussmaul respirations. The presence of infection should be noted, and the nurse should anticipate follow-up blood ketone analysis. Intravenous fluids and insulin should be administered carefully, and the patient's responses should be observed.

Interventions. The diabetic patient with ketoacidosis is generally a type I insulin-dependent diabetic who needs to adjust to lifelong adaptations of diet and exercise. Nursing interventions should include teaching the various aspects of diabetes care and should be geared to the individual patient's needs and resources.

9

INSULIN, SERUM

Description

Insulin is a hormone secreted by the beta cells of the islets of Langerhans in the liver. Insulin regulates the metabolism and transport of carbohydrates, amino acids, and lipids. Normally, insulin reaches its peak levels after meals. Because glucose directly stimulates insulin release, serum glucose levels are frequently measured at the same time as serum insulin levels.

N O R M A L   R A N G E

Adults   6–24 uU/ml (35–145 pmol/L)
Children   Consult laboratory for reference values.
Newborns   3–20 uU/ml

Specimen Required

A 7–10-ml venous blood sample is needed. The insulin sample should be packed in ice and sent to the laboratory for immediate analysis. If blood glucose is collected at the same time, it should be sent along with the blood insulin sample.

Preparation of the Patient

Foods and fluids are restricted for 10–12 hours prior to the test. All medications that influence test results must be held as well. The patient should be relaxed and recumbent for 30 minutes before the test, since exercise, stress, and agitation can affect insulin levels. Glucose should be kept at hand and the patient watched for hypoglycemia, since this pretest fast may precipitate a hypoglycemic response.

Causes of Deviation from Normal

Both insulin and glucose levels are needed for test result interpretation. High insulin and low glucose levels after a significant fast suggest *insulinoma*. For patients who are insulin-resistant diabetic, insulin levels are increased. For patients who are non-insulin-resistant, insulin levels are decreased. Patients who are on adrenocorticotropic hormones, steroids, thyroid supplements, and epinephrine, hyperglycemia occurs, along with an increase in insulin level.

Nursing Implications of Abnormal Findings

Assessment and Interventions. The nursing assessment and related interventions for increases in serum insulin depend on the cause of the increase. The most common increase is related to diabetes mellitus, and assessment and interventions for this are discussed in the glucose section. Textbooks on medical-surgical nursing should be consulted for patients with other diagnoses.

TRIIODOTHYRONINE AND THYROXINE

Description

Iodine is a trace element concentrated primarily in the thyroid gland. It is essential to the synthesis of thyroid hormone, which stimulates metabolism and is needed for normal growth and development. Ingested iodides are absorbed from the gastrointestinal tract and cleared from the bloodstream by the thyroid gland. In this gland one iodine atom is incorporated into an amino acid, tyrosine, to form *monoiodotyrosine*, which then incorporates another iodine atom to form *diiodotyrosine*. *Triiodotyrosine* (T_3) is formed when diiodotyrosine condenses with monoiidotyrosine. *Thyroxine* (T_4) is formed when diiodotyrosine condenses with itself. In serum, 90–95% of the thyroid hormone material found is T_4, whereas the remainder is primarily T_3. About 99% of circulating serum thyroid hormone is reversibly bound to serum proteins.

Iodine intake is derived primarily from seafood. Since the average American diet contains an inadequate amount of iodine, iodized salt is the primary dietary source of iodine.

NORMAL RANGE

Iodine is found in serum in several forms.

Adults
    Triiodothyronine (T_3)   75–195 ng/dl
    Thyroxine (T_4)   6–12 μg/dl
Children   Consult laboratory for reference values.
Newborns
    Triiodothyronine (T_3)   180–240 ng/dl
    Thyroxine (T_4)   7.8–23 μg/dl

9

Specimen Required

A 5–10-ml sample of venous blood is required. Serum is used for the analysis.

Preparation of the Patient

Many substances can lower or raise normal iodide levels. The more common of these substances are summarized in Table 9.6. These are restricted for a week before the test. If this restriction is contraindicated, the substance taken should be noted on the laboratory slip that accompanies the specimen.

TABLE 9.6. Factors Influencing T_3 and T_4 Levels

T_3-Decreasing Factors	T_3-Increasing Factors
ACTH	Cardiac Arrhythmias
Antithyroid drugs	Chronic obstructive pulmonary diseasse
Estrogens	Dextrothyroxine
Liver disease	Dicumarol
Menstruation	Heparin
Oral contraceptives	Liver disease
Pregnancy	Metastatic cancer
Sulfonylureas	Methadone
Thiazide diuretics	Nephrosis
	Penicillin
	Prednisone
	Salicylates

T_4-Decreasing Factors	T_4-Increasing Factors
Cortisone	Diethylstilbestrol
Heparin	Estradiol
Lithium	Estrogen
Prednisone	Oral contraceptives
Reserpine	Pregnancy
Sulfonamides	Progestine
Tolbutamide	

Causes of Deviation from Normal

Hyperthyroidism, or overactivity of the thyroid gland, leads to increases in serum T_3 and T_4 levels, as does exophthalmic goiter, in which there appears to be an autoimmune etiology and a thyroid-stimulating factor. Other causes include toxic goiter, associated with multiple toxic thyroid nodules that produce excessive thyroxine, and malignant tumors of the thyroid tissue.

Hypothyroidism, or decreased functioning of the thyroid gland, is classified as primary or secondary hypothyroidism. The primary disease may be caused by an idiopathic atrophy of the thyroid gland, an inflammatory autoimmune disease known as Hashimoto's thyroiditis, or inadvertent surgical removal of the thyroid gland. Secondary hypothyroidism is caused by a decreased secretion of thyroid-stimulating hormone from the pituitary gland.

Hypothyroidism in newborn infants with resulting low levels of thyroxine will result in neurological impairment, growth deficits, and mental retardation (cretinism). Neonatal screening for hypothyroidism is generally done via thyroxine blood levels, since clinical and radiological criteria are not valid in the newborn. Early diagnosis can lead to initiation of appropriate therapy, and prevent neurological defects and improve intellectual and physical progress.

Nursing Implications of Abnormal Findings
HYPERTHYROIDISM

Assessment. When the patient has an increase in levels of T_3 or T_4 or both, the metabolic activity is usually increased. The nurse should watch for nervousness, agitation, irritability, and insomnia. The respiratory and heart rates will be increased, as will the bowel sounds. The legs, hands, and eyes should be examined carefully for peripheral and periorbital edema.

Interventions. Increases in metabolic activity lead to increases in the patient's heat tolerance. When diaphoresis is present, the nurse should arrange frequent clothing and bedding changes and frequent cool baths or showers. Creation of a quiet and non-stressful environment will assist the patient in trying to rest, a difficult task because of marked hyperactivity and insomnia resulting in extreme fatigue. Increased dietary intake of both calories and bulk is needed to combat weight loss and increased stool frequency.

HYPOTHYROIDISM

Assessment. Patients with hypothyroidism have vague complaints of fatigue, lethargy, increased need for sleep, increased sensitivity to cold, and inability to concentrate. Menstrual periods may decrease in frequency or stop. Constipation is a frequent complaint. The skin may be rough and dry and the nails brittle. Swelling of the hands, feet, and eyelids may occur, and the thyroid gland itself may be enlarged. The temperature will be low, as will the pulse rate and blood pressure.

Interventions. The environment provided for a patient with hypothyroidism should have a warm stable temperature to help the patient cope with sensitivity to cold. Periods of activity should be interspersed with rest periods to allow for patient fatigue and lack of energy. Dry skin should be attended to by reducing use of soap and applying lanolin and other skin creams. Treatment involves thyroid replacement therapy, and thus a teaching plan should include information about self-administration of medication, the need for frequent monitoring with diagnostic tests, and regular follow-up by the physician. Because the patient may be sluggish and forgetful until the treatment is effective, the teaching plan should include written instructions and the informing of a family member or significant other. Parents of newborn infants with hypothyroidism must be taught about the critical necessity of replacement therapy and medical check-ups to monitor progress and prevent mental and physical retardation.

9

THYROID-STIMULATING TEST

Description

The *thyroid-stimulating test* measures the response of the thyroid gland to the administration of a given amount of thyroid-stimulating hormone (TSH). Response is measured by the amount of iodine uptake by the thyroid gland and the amount of protein-bound iodine in the blood. The test is used to differentiate primary thyroid disease from secondary thyroid disease caused by deficiency of the pituitary gland.

NORMAL RANGE

In normal individuals, the serum thyroxine level and the radioactive iodine uptake by the thyroid gland are increased within 8–10 hours after administration of TSH. If primary thyroid disease is present, no response occurs. If pituitary deficiency of TSH is present, radioactive iodine uptake by the thyroid gland increases by at least 10%.

Specimen Required

A 5–10-ml specimen of venous blood is required. Radioactive uptake of iodine by the thyroid gland is measured by means of radioactive scanning procedures carried out in the diagnostic radiation laboratory.

Preparation of the Patient

Iodine intake is restricted for 1 week before the test. On the morning of the test, the patient receives an intravenous injection of thyroid-stimulating hormone, plus radioactive iodine either by injection or by capsule. Blood specimens are collected at specified intervals designated by the laboratory and the patient is taken to the diagnostic radiation laboratory at a specified hour for the scanning procedure. Specimen collection may continue for 24 hours.

Causes of Deviation from Normal

Increased amounts of TSH are found in patients with untreated hypothyroidism or with Hashimoto's thyroiditis. If radioactive iodine uptake is increased in the thyroid gland, secondary hypothyroidism from pituitary deficiency of TSH is present.

Nursing Implications of Abnormal Findings

Assessment and Interventions. The nurse should observe the patient for indications of hypothyroidism, such as fatigue, poor skin turgor, and weight gain. Interventions depend on the degree of illness present. A medical-surgical textbook should be consulted for specific interventions.

T_3 RESIN UPTAKE (TRIIODOTHYRONINE T_3RU)

Description

The T_3 resin uptake test is used to measure the amount of thyroid hormone in the blood. A specific amount of radioactive-tagged T_3 and resin is added to a sample of the patient's blood. Thyroid hormone is carried in the blood by thyroid-binding globulin (TBG). The greater the amount of thyroid hormone present in the blood, the fewer sites on TBG available to bind with additional hormone. The resin uptake test measures the amount of T_3 that is left over and not bound to the TBG in the blood sample.

NORMAL RANGE	
Adults	25–35% uptake of T_3 by the resin
Children	Generally not done

Specimen Required

A 5-ml specimen of venous blood is required.

Preparation of the Patient

There are no food or fluid restrictions required. The test is done on a sample of blood taken from the patient, and no radioactive material is injected into the patient. This test can be performed on patients who are taking food or medications with iodine or who have received an iodine X-ray medium. However, factors influencing T_3 and T_4 levels, as indicated in Table 9.5, can interfere with this test as well.

9

Causes of Deviation from Normal

Decreased levels of T_3 resin uptake are seen in hypothyroidism, such as cretinism and myxedema, during pregnancy, thyroiditis, and cirrhosis of the liver. Increased levels of T_3 are seen in hyperthyroidism, protein malnutrition, malignancies, metastatic carcinoma, uremia, liver disease, nephrotic syndrome, and myasthenia gravis.

Nursing Implications of Abnormal Findings

Assessment and Interventions. See thyroxine for nursing care of the patient with hypothyroidism and hyperthyroidism. Consult medical-surgical textbooks for other pathological conditions.

CALCITONIN

Description

Calcitonin is a hormone secreted to the "C" cells of the thyroid gland. It is active in regulating the number and activity of osteoblasts. Calcitonin is secreted in response to high blood calcium levels and may control abrupt changes in blood levels.

N O R M A L   R A N G E

Basal values
    Adult Men   <19 pg/ml
    Adult Women   <14 pg/ml
After provocative testing with 4-hour calcium infusion
    Adult Men   <190 pg/ml
    Adult Women   <130 pg/ml
After provocative testing with pentagastrin infusion
    Adult Men   <110 pg/ml
    Adult Women   <30 pg/ml

Specimen Required

Two fasting serum specimens of 10 ml each are obtained initially. Additional specimens are obtained if provocative testing is conducted.

Preparation of the Patient

Food and fluids are held overnight before the test is administered.

Causes of Deviation from Normal

Elevated serum calcitonin levels in the absence of hypocalcemia typically indicate medullary carcinoma of the thyroid. Occasionally increased calcitonin levels may be due to ectopic calcitonin production by oat-cell carcinoma of the lung or by breast carcinoma.

Nursing Implications of Abnormal Findings

Assessment and Interventions. Elevated calcitonin levels may be indicative of thyroid carcinoma. The patient will need to be prepared for surgical and radiation approaches to cancer treatment. Specific interventions should be reviewed in medical-surgical textbooks and specific care plans developed.

URINE CATECHOLAMINES
AND VANILLYLMANDELIC ACID

Definition

Urine catecholamines include epinephrine, norepinephrine, metanephrine, and normetanephrine. These substances are secreted by the adrenal medulla and excreted from the body via the kidneys. Because vanillylmandelic acid (VMA) is a metabolic by-product of the degradation of urine catecholamines, it is evaluated at the same time.

N O R M A L   R A N G E

Adults
Vanillylmandelic acid	up to 9 mg/24
Total catecholamines	100 μg/24 h
Epinephrine	100–230 μg/24 h
Norepinephrine	100–230 μg/24 h
Metanephrine	24–96 μg/24 h
Normetanephrine	12–288 mg/24 h
Dopamine	65–400 ug/24 h
Children	Consult laboratory for reference values.

Specimen Required

A 24-hour urine specimen is required for evaluation of catecholamines and VMA. This is necessary because of diurnal variations that result in decreased output during sleep hours. The procedure for collection of an accurate 24-hour urine specimen is outlined in Chapter 1.

Preparation of the Patient

A number of medications may affect the levels of both catecholamines and vanillylmandelic acid. Therefore, any drugs administered during the collection period should be noted on the collection slip. Restrictions before and during the collection period vary from one hospital to another, but they generally include elimination of coffee, tea, bananas, cocoa products, vanilla products, and aspirin for 3 days before and during the specimen-collection period. Timed specimens are frequently difficult to collect, and the nurse should make the procedure a high priority in the patient's care so accuracy in specimen collection is ensured. The container to be used, which is generally provided by the laboratory, should contain approximately 10 ml of concentrated

9

hydrochloric acid so a pH of 2.0–3.0 can be maintained during the collection period.

Causes of Deviation from Normal

This test is carried out primarily for the adult diagnosis of pheochromocytoma, a benign tumor of the adrenal medulla and of neuroblastoma and ganglioneuroblastoma in children. The organ secretes abnormally high amounts of both epinephrine and norepinephrine, which leads to hypertension. An increase in catecholamine levels also occurs after vigorous exercise. False-positive results are associated with drugs and diet (Table 9.7). Decreases in catecholamine levels are rare, nonpathogenic, and nonsignificant.

Nursing Implications of Abnormal Findings

Assessment. Since a series of 24-hour urine tests may be needed once an increase in urine catecholamines has occurred, the patient's ability to continue to collect specimens accurately should be assessed. The patient should be observed for signs and symptoms of hypertension and blood pressure recorded at least three times a day. Additional evaluations should include other vasomotor changes, such as headache, perspiration, palpitation, and tremors. A high blood glucose level and a high basal metabolic rate (BMR) may occur as well.

Interventions. When pheochromocytoma has been diagnosed, nursing interventions are related to preparation of the patient for surgery and recording and reporting any hypotensive reactions to antihypertension medications that occur.

If abnormally high urine catecholamine levels are attributable to a condition

TABLE 9.7.   Substances that Affect Urine Catecholamine and VMA Levels

Drugs	Diet
Ascorbic acid	Bananas
Aspirin	Chocolate
Chlorpromazine	Citrus fruits
Declomycin	Coffee
Erythromycin	Tea
Hydralazine	Vanilla
Isuprel	
Mandelamine	
Methyldopa	
Quinine	
Tetracycline	
Vitamin B complex (large doses)	

other than pheochromocytoma, nursing interventions depend on the cause of the high value.

URINE CHLORIDES

Description

Chloride is the primary anion found in the extracellular fluid. Urine chloride results from elimination of excess body chloride via the renal tubules. Chloride is indirectly regulated by aldosterone, which causes reabsorption of sodium by the kidney. As each sodium ion is reabsorbed, a chloride or a bicarbonate ion is reabsorbed as well. Chloride is also found in gastric secretions as hydrochloric acid.

NORMAL RANGE

The normal range of urine chloride is 110–250 mEq/24 h. The normal range of urine sodium chloride is 10–20 g/24 h.

Specimen Required

A 24-hour urine specimen is collected in a plain collecting bottle.

Preparation of the Patient

Food and fluid restrictions are not required before or during the collection period.

9

Causes of Deviation from Normal

Decreased levels of urine chloride are associated with Addison's disease, in which aldosterone levels are decreased. Decreased urine chloride levels also occur with malabsorption syndrome, diarrhea, diaphoresis, pyloric obstruction, prolonged gastric suction, and emphysema. Increased levels of urine chloride are found in cases of dehydration, starvation, salicylate overdose, and in patients taking mercurial and chlorthiazide diuretics.

Nursing Implications of Abnormal Findings

Assessment and Interventions. The nurse should observe the patient with urine chloride imbalance for indications of other fluid and electrolyte problems, daily weight changes, intake and output changes, skin turgor, and the condition and appearance of the tongue and urine. Nursing interventions depend on the disease and symptoms presented.

URINE STEROIDS

Description

Urine steroids include three groups of substances: *17-ketosteroids* (17-KS), *17-ketogenic steroids* (17-KGS), and *17-hydroxycorticosteroids* (17-OHCS). All three types of substances are formed within the adrenal cortex and are eliminated from the body via the kidneys. The 17-KS group includes specific chemical configuration involving 19 carbon atoms and a ketone group at C-17. These 17-KS substances are composed primarily of metabolic products derived from testicular androgens. The 17-KGS group includes steroids with 21 carbon atoms and a hydroxyl group at C-17. The 17-KGS' are composed of glucocorticoid derivatives and pregnanetriol. The 17-OHCS group includes steroids with 21 carbon atoms and a dihydroxyacetone side chain. The 17-OHCS group includes aldosterone and several metabolites from glucocorticoids.

NORMAL RANGE	
17-Ketosteroids	
Men	7–25 mg/24 h
Women	5–15 mg/24 h
Infants	<1 mg/24 h
Children	
1–3 years	<2 mg/24 h
3–6 years	<3 mg/24 h
7–10 years	<4 mg/24 h
10–12 years	<5 mg/24 h
17-Ketogenic Acids	
Men	5–20 mg/24 h
Women	5–20 mg/24 h
Children	Consult laboratory for reference values.
17-Hydroxycorticosteroids	
Men	1–10 mg/24 h
Women	1–10 mg/24 h
Children	Consult laboratory for reference values.

Specimen Required

A 24-hour urine specimen is required.

Preparation of the Patient

Food and fluids are not restricted before or during the collection of the specimen. A number of medications may influence the results; if they cannot be discontinued before the test, the nurse should check with the laboratory before collecting the specimen. Medications being administered should be noted on the laboratory slip. To minimize interfering effects, physical and emotional stress should be avoided during the collection period.

Causes of Deviation from Normal

Increases in 17-KGS levels occur in cases of adrenal hyperplasia and in patients who have had surgery, extensive burns, or infections. Elevation of all steroids occurs in Cushing's syndrome, eclampsia, acute pancreatitis, and adrenocorticotropic hormone (ACTH) therapy. When both 17-OHCS and 17-KGS are elevated, the adrenal cortex is functioning at increased levels. This can be attributable to tumors, cancer, or adrenogenital syndrome. Decreases in 17-KS and 17-KGS levels occur in Addison's disease, hypopituitarism, and cretinism.

Nursing Implications of Abnormal Findings

Assessment. When a patient has elevated urine steroid levels, the nurse should watch for increases in body weight, particularly of the trunk. The patient may complain of recent weight gain, changes in secondary sexual characteristics, decreased menses and libido, and physical weakness and irritability. The patient's family may report these changes. The nurse should note whether the patient has had long-term steroid therapy.

For patients with decreased urine steroids, the nurse should observe for muscle weakness; gastrointestinal symptoms, including nausea, vomiting, anorexia, and weight loss; increased skin pigmentation; and fluid and electrolyte changes. These patients are generally thin and may be drowsy or irritable.

Interventions. The patient with increased urine steroid levels caused by hyperfunction of the adrenal cortex may be undergoing a variety of diagnostic tests. The nursing care plan should include teaching the patient the importance of saving all urine during these tests. The nurse must plan for emotional support, adapting to the frequent mood swings that are common in these patients. Insomnia may be a problem, and nursing interventions should include measures to promote a relaxed, comfortable environment. Because of the patient's susceptibility to infection, the nurse should protect the patient and use strict medical aseptic techniques. Catheterization should be avoided, if possible. Precautions should be taken to prevent skin injury by means of careful handling and patient positioning. If surgery is planned, postoperative care should include measures to prevent fluid and electrolyte problems and infectious complications.

Patients with decreased urinary steroid levels due to hypofunction of the adrenal cortex have a reduced ability to cope with stress. The care plan for these patients should include orientation to the usual physical routines. The patient should be informed about diagnostic testing and provided with adequate rest periods. Dehydration may be a problem and can be minimized by provision of a variety of fluids. If addisonian crisis occurs, the nurse needs

9

to provide emergency measures for dehydration, hypovolemia, and hypotension.

URINE PORPHYRINS AND PORPHOBILINOGEN

Description
Porphyrins and *porphobilinogen* are precursors of hemoglobin formation. Small excesses are excreted in the urine and feces.

N O R M A L R A N G E	
Adults	
Porphobilinogen	2 mg/24 h
Porphyrins	50–300 mg/24 h
Children	Consult laboratory for reference values.

Specimen Required
A 24-hour urine specimen is required.

Preparation of the Patient
Food and fluids are not restricted before or during the specimen collection period.

Causes of Deviation from Normal
Increased levels of porphyrins and porphobilinogens occur in a group of diseases referred to as the *porphyrias*, which are hereditary metabolic diseases. Increases are also sometimes seen in cases of liver disease, lead poisoning, and pellagra.

Nursing Implications of Abnormal Findings
   Assessment and Interventions. The urine of patients with increased porphyrins and porphobilinogen has a characteristic reddish-black tinge. Depending on the specific porphyria present, the patient may have abdominal pain and leukocytosis. Symptoms may be brought on by ingestion of alcohol, barbiturates, or other central nervous system depressants detoxified by the liver, and vary according to the underlying disease present; the nurse should plan assessments of and interventions for the problems confronting the patient.

URINE PHENYLPYRUVIC ACID

Description

To test for the disease *phenylketonuria* (PKU), the level of phenylpyruvic acid in the urine and the level of phenylalanine in the blood are measured. These substances accumulate in patients with PKU because of the hereditary deficiency of a liver enzyme needed to convert the amino acid phenylalanine to tyrosine.

N O R M A L   R A N G E

The urine normally contains no phenylpyruvic acid. The normal range of phenylalanine in the blood is less than 4 mg/dl.

Specimen Required

A 5–10-ml specimen of venous blood is required for serum phenylalanine measurement. For measurement of phenylpyruvic acid in the urine, a reagent strip is dipped into freshly voided urine or pressed against a wet diaper.

Preparation of the Patient

There are no food or fluid restrictions before collection of the specimens. The blood test is performed 24 hours after the newborn has ingested protein, or at least 3 days after birth. Urine testing is done from 4–6 weeks after birth.

Causes of Deviation from Normal

Elevations of blood phenylalanine levels and urine phenylpyruvic acid are indications of incomplete metabolism of phenylalanine. The most common cause of this defect is the hereditary disease phenylketonuria, in which the necessary liver enzyme for phenylalanine metabolism is absent. Premature infants may have a positive test because of incomplete liver development. Repeat testing on these infants is necessary.

9

Nursing Implications of Abnormal Findings

Assessment. If an elevation of serum phenylalanine or urine phenylpyruvic acid occurs, the results of several specimens for both tests are needed to eliminate the possibility of false-positive results. If the diagnosis of PKU is established, the nurse should assess the patient for any indications of mental retardation and any unusual urine odors. Dietary intake should be recorded, specifically including protein foods ingested.

Interventions. The treatment for PKU involves the restriction of all phenylalanine in the food. This amino acid appears in all meat products and other protein foods. Teaching the parents and eventually the patient what foods must be omitted is an essential nursing intervention. If the disease is untreated, the nurse should use information about the occurrence of mental retardation in a positive manner to reinforce the importance of the special diet. Genetic counseling for the parents and eventually for the patient is recommended.

BIBLIOGRAPHY

Brucker, M.C., et al. "What's New in Pregnancy Tests." *Journal of Obstetric, Gynecologic and Neonatal Nursing*, 14:353–359 (September–October 1985).

Corbett, J.V. *Laboratory Tests and Diagnostic Procedures with Nursing Diagnoses.* Norwalk, Connecticut: Appleton and Lange, 1992.

Donohue-Porter, P. "Insulin Dependent Diabetes Mellitus—Educating the Diabetic Person Regarding Diabetes and Infections." *Nursing Clinics of North America,* 20:191–198 (March 1985).

Fischbach, F.T. A *Manual of Laboratory and Diagnostic Tests*. Philadelphia: J.B. Lippincott Company, 1992.

Green, W.L. "Screening for Thyroid Disease in the Clinical Laboratory." *Journal of Medical Technology* 1(10):747–751, October, 1984.

Hamera, E., V. Cassmeter, K.A. O'Connell, G.T. Weldon, T.M. Knapp, and J.L. Kyner. "Self-Regulation in Individuals with Type II Diabetes." *Nursing Research* 37(6):363–367, November/December, 1988.

"Hypothyroidism: Diagnostic Value of T4 and TSH Assessment." *Hospital Medicine, 21*:190 (July 1985).

Ignatavicius, D.D., and M.V. Bayne. *Medical-Surgical Nursing: A Nursing Process Approach*. Philadelphia: W.B. Saunders, 1991.

Lewis, S.M., and I.C. Collier. *Medical-Surgical Nursing: Assessment and Management of Clinical Problems*. St. Louis: Mosby Yearbook, 1992.

Lockwood, D., et al. "The Biggest Problem in Diabetes: Diet Related Issues." *Diabetes Educator, 12*:30–33 (Winter 1986).

McCarthy, J.A. "The Continuum of Diabetic Coma." *American Journal of Nursing, 85*:878–882 (August 1985).

McFadden, H.E. "The Ups and Downs of Diabetic Coma." *American Journal of Nursing, 85*:881 (August 1985).

Newman, R.H. "Bedside Blood Sugar Determinations in the Critically Ill." *Heart and Lung* 17(6):667–669, November, 1988.

Phipps, W.S., B.C. Long, N.F. Woods, and V. Cossmeyer. *Medical-Surgical Nursing*. St. Louis: Mosby Yearbook, 1991.

Ravel, R. *Clinical Laboratory Medicine*. Chicago: Year Book Medical Publishers, Inc., 1989.

Safras, M., et al. "Thyrotoxicosis and Graves Disease." *Hospital Practice*, 20:33–42, 46, 48, 49 (March 1985).

"Self Monitoring of Blood Glucose: Consensus Statement." *Diabetes Care 13* (Supplement 1):41–45, January 1990.

Shatsky, F. "Blood Chemistry Considerations for Parenteral Nutrition." *Nutrition Support Services*, 6:25–27 (June 1986).

Smetzer, S.C., and B.G. Ball. *Brunner and Sudarth's Medical-Surgical Nursing*. New York: J.B. Lippincott, 1992.

Walker, E.A., D.J. Paduano, and H. Shamoon. "Quality Assurance for Blood Glucose Monitoring in Health-Care Facilities." *Diabetes Care 14*:1043–1049, 1991.

Wallach, J. *Intepretation of Diagnostic Tests*. Boston: Little, Brown, and Company, 1992.

Whitehouse, F.W. "Diabetes Mellitus: Current Concepts on Proper Management." *Hospital Medicine*, 22:231–234, 237–239, 243–244 (May 1986).

Wilson, J.D., et al. *Harrison's Principles of Internal Medicine*. New York: McGraw-Hill, 1991.

9

Laboratory Tests of Infectious Diseases and Allergic Reactions

Alpha₁-Antitrypsin Test

Antinuclear Antibody Test

Antistreptolysin O
(Streptozyme,
Streptodornase B)

Blood Culture

Carcinoembryonic Antigen
Assay

Cold Agglutinins

Coombs' Antiglobulin

C-Reactive Protein Test

Hemagglutination Inhibition
Test (HIA, Rubella Antibody
Test, Passive Hemagglutination
[Rubacell], Enzyme Linked
Immunosorbent Assay
[Elisa])

Cytomegalovirus Antibody

Heterophile Antibody Test
(Mono-Spot, Mono-Screen,
Epstein Barr Virus Test)

Legionnaire's Antibody Test

Lyme Disease Antibody Test

Lupus Erythematosus
Cell Test

Rheumatoid Factors

Syphilis Serology Tests

Torch Test

HIV Antibody to Human
Immunodeficiency Virus

Vaginal Smear

Vaginal Culture

Papanicolaou Smear
(Pap Smear)

Urine Culture

ALPHA₁-ANTITRYPSIN TEST

Description

Alpha₁-antitrypsin, an alpha globulin, is a serum protein produced by the liver. It inhibits the release of proteolytic enzymes (proteases) and has a broad inhibitory spectrum. Alpha$_1$-antitrypsin has been specifically associated with inactivation of endoprotease released by dying cells. A deficiency of alpha$_1$-antitrypsin has been associated with the accumulation of endoproteases released from dead lung tissue allowing destruction of alveolar tissue and leading to the development of emphysema.

N O R M A L R A N G E	
Adults	80–226 mg/dl
Children	Similar to adults
Newborns	145–270 mg/dl

Specimen Required

A 5-ml sample of venous blood is collected in a plain collecting tube or syringe.

Preparation of the Patient

A patient who has an elevated serum cholesterol or triglyceride should fast from food and fluids (except water) from midnight.

Causes of Deviation from Normal

Increases in alpha$_1$-antitrypsin in the blood are associated with inflammatory conditions, necrosis, and some infections. Both surgery and exercise can lead to temporary elevations. During pregnancy, increases up to 100% of normal may be seen. Oral contraceptives and food ingestion including cholesterol and triglycerides can cause temporary elevations of alpha$_1$-antitrypsin.

Decreases in alpha$_1$-antitrypsin are associated primarily with emphysema and chronic obstructive pulmonary disease. In addition, decreases have been seen in patients with liver disease, malnutrition, and nephrotic syndrome.

10

Nursing Implications of Abnormal Findings

Assessment and Interventions. Patients with decreases in alpha$_1$-antitrypsin may be developing emphysema or have physiological changes already related to emphysema. These patients need to be assessed for respiratory problems and taught to avoid further lung irritation from smoking, air pollution, and infections.

Because elevations in alpha$_1$-antitrypsin are found in many inflammatory conditions and are influenced by nonpathogenic conditions, they are not as helpful in identifying specific nursing interventions.

ANTINUCLEAR ANTIBODY TEST

Description
Antinuclear antibodies (ANAs) are immunoglobulins that react with the nuclear components of leukocytes. They are usually from the IgM class but may be from the IgG or IgA classes of immunoglobulins. This test is used to determine the presence of certain autoimmune diseases and is strongly associated with systemic lupus erythematosus (SLE).

N O R M A L   R A N G E

Normally, there are no ANAs present in the blood. Titers of between 1:10 and 1:20 are considered positive; however, individual laboratory norms should be checked. Fluorescent staining techniques to reveal nuclear patterns are used to identify specific diseases (Table 10.1).

Specimen Required
A 5-ml sample of venous blood is collected in a plain collecting tube or syringe.

TABLE 10.1. Specific Diseases Associated with ANA Fluorescent Nuclear Staining Patterns

Pattern	Diseases
Diffuse or homogeneous	Systemic lupus erythematosus
Nucleolar	Scleroderma
	Sjögren's syndrome
	Systemic lupus erythematosus
	Rheumatoid arthritis
Peripheral or marginal	Sjögren's syndrome
	Scleroderma
	Dermatomyositis
Speckled	Scleroderma
	Raynaud's disease
	Sjögren's syndrome
	Polymyositis

TABLE 10.2. Drugs that Affect the Antinuclear Antibody Test

Acetazolamide	Phenytoin
Hydralazine	Procainamide
Isoniazid	Streptomycin
Methyldopa	Tetracycline
Oral contraceptives	Trimethadione
Para-amino salicylic acid	Thiazides
Penicillin	

Preparation of the Patient

There are no food or fluid restrictions before venipuncture. Several drugs may cause false-positive results (Table 10.2). If the patient is receiving any of these drugs, it should be noted on the laboratory slip.

Causes of Deviation from Normal

Autoimmune immunoglobulins, produced by the body against one or more nuclear antigens from leukocytes, are found in a number of collagen diseases, the most common of which is systemic lupus erythematosus (SLE). If the ANA test is negative or normal, SLE is not present. A positive test also occurs in scleroderma, dermatomyositis, rheumatoid arthritis, and hypersensitive states. Fluorescent nuclear staining techniques are used to differentiate these diseases (Table 10.1). Other diseases in which positive results may occur include myasthenia gravis, leprosy, infectious mononucleosis, malignancy, Hashimoto's disease, and some liver diseases associated with autoimmunity or viral infections.

Nursing Implications of Abnormal Findings

Assessment. When a positive ANA test occurs and SLE is present, the patient should be assessed for the presence of generalized signs and symptoms such as chills, low-grade fever, aching joints, weakness and fatigue, malaise, loss of appetite, and weight loss. Scaly rashes, alopecia, hyperpigmentation of the skin, and ulcerations of the mouth and pharynx should also be noted. All physiological systems should be assessed carefully as this disease can affect all of them. The nurse should also be aware of psychological or emotional problems that can occur. Nursing assessment may vary as other collagen diseases are present.

Interventions. In general, nursing interventions for SLE depend on the system involved and the clinical manifestations that occur. Rest is important during the active phase of the illness. Activities should be spaced to provide rest

10

periods, and patients should be advised to keep regular hours and avoid becoming fatigued. Plans should be made to provide emotional support as needed. A teaching program should include information about the insidious nature of the disease, its pattern of exacerbations and remissions, and the side effects of prescribed medications, particularly steroids and other antiinflammatory agents. Consult general medical-surgical textbooks for nursing interventions in other diseases.

ANTISTREPTOLYSIN O (STREPTOZYME, STREPTODORNASE B)

Description
The *antistreptolysin* O (ASO) test (also referred to as the streptozyme, streptodomase-B, and ASLO test) is done to determine the presence of antibodies against streptolysin. *Streptolysin*, an antigen that hemolyzes red cells, is a streptococcal enzyme secreted by group-A beta-hemolytic streptococci. It appears in the blood from 1–5 weeks after infection with the streptococcus and peaks at 4–6 weeks. Elevations may continue for months.

NORMAL RANGE	
Age	Range
Adults	up to 160 Todd units/ml
Children	
6 months–2 years	up to 50 Todd units/ml
2–4 years	may be 160 Todd units/ml ⎫ Depending on
5–12 years	may be 200 Todd units/ml ⎭ degree of exposure

Specimen Required
A 10-ml sample of venous blood is collected in a plain collecting tube or syringe.

Preparation of the Patient
There are no food or fluid restrictions before venipuncture. If the patient has had antibiotic therapy, this should be noted on the laboratory slip, as it may cause inaccurate low levels. Subsequent testing is advisable 1–2 times a week for 4–6 weeks following infection.

Causes of Deviation from Normal
Elevated ASO titers indicate a recent infection with group-A beta-hemolytic streptococcus or recent exposure to the organism without signs or symptoms

of infection. Elevated ASO levels are found in 80% of patients with acute rheumatic fever, 75% of poststreptococcal glomerulonephritis patients, and 90% of patients with streptococcal pharyngitis; however, only 25% of patients with streptococcal pyoderma (skin infections) have elevated levels. False-positive results can occur in patients with increased beta lipoproteins.

Nursing Implications of Abnormal Findings

Assessment and Interventions. An elevated ASO titer usually indicates that a streptococcal infection is present, but results of the test are not useful in identifying the type of infection. Test results must be assessed along with the clinical manifestations exhibited by the patient. When a high titer is present in a healthy person, information about possible contacts with infected people should be gathered.

Nursing interventions should relate to the disease present. Current nursing textbooks should be consulted for information about the care of patients with rheumatic fever, glomerulonephritis, streptococcal pharyngitis, and streptococcal pyoderma, since these are the diseases most often associated with high ASO titers.

BLOOD CULTURE

Description

A blood culture is used to identify the microorganisms causing bacteremia or septicemia. It is ordered when a patient has a sudden rise in temperature accompanied by chills, increased pulse rate, and a general feeling of malaise. Results of the culture are used to prescribe appropriate treatment.

> ### N O R M A L   R A N G E
>
> Normally there are no organisms cultured from blood.

10

Specimen Required

A 5–15-ml sample of venous blood is collected in a syringe. Bacterial invasion of the bloodstream tends to be episodic. Repeated collection of three or more blood culture samples is done at approximately 30-minute intervals within a 24-hour period. Each blood specimen is collected in a special kit that provides one container for aerobic organisms and one container for anaerobic organisms. The specimen should be sent to the laboratory immediately. Chapter 1 outlines in more detail the required procedures.

Preparation of the Patient

Foods and fluids are not restricted before or during collection of the specimen. The blood culture sample should be obtained before any antibiotic therapy is given so the causative organism can be identified. If therapy has been ongoing, the antibiotics being given should be identified on the laboratory slip. Since the blood specimen must be drawn through the skin, which is contaminated with organisms, careful preparation of the skin is important. The patient should be prepared to have several specimens drawn.

Causes of Deviation from Normal

Organisms can enter the bloodstream from a number of infectious foci. Susceptible patients include the young, the debilitated, the aged, and patients who are immunosuppressed. Patients receiving antibiotics, steroids, or parenteral hyperalimentation are also at risk. The most common site of entry is through the urinary tract. Other areas include the lungs, the hepatobiliary tract, the endocardium, the central nervous system, the peritoneal cavity, skin wounds, burns, indwelling arterial and venous lines, and the gastrointestinal tract. Septicemia may cause as high as 12–20% mortality, especially in the populations at risk. Gram-negative sepsis is not uncommon and is found frequently in large medical centers and university hospitals. One positive culture of an organism usually found on the skin is frequently considered a contaminated culture rather than a positive one. However, the possibility of the organism being a pathogen exists, especially in debilitated or immunosuppressed patients.

TABLE 10.3. Pathogens Commonly Found in Blood Culture

Organism	Gram Stain	Morphology
Bacteria		
Pseudomonas aeruginosa	Negative	Rod
Escherichia coli	Negative	Rod
Klebsiella pneumoniae	Negative	Rod
Staphylococcus aureus	Positive	Cocci
Staphylococcus epidermis	Positive	Cocci
Enterobacteria sp.	Negative	Rod
Corynebacterium sp.	Positive	Rod
Clostridium sp.	Positive	Rod
Serratia sp.	Negative	Rod
Fungi		
Candida sp.	(Not applicable)	(Not applicable)

Some of the most commonly cultured organisms associated with septicemia are listed in Table 10.3.

Nursing Implications of Abnormal Findings

Assessment. When a patient has a positive blood culture, the nurse should assess the patient for clinical manifestations of infection. The temperature should be monitored, wounds observed for drainage, urine inspected for indications of cloudiness, and the respiratory tract examined for signs of either upper or lower respiratory tract involvement. The patient should be observed for indications of an acute septicemic episode, including chills, fever, and a rapid pulse. When these manifestations occur, another blood culture should be drawn if ordered, as the organisms are likely to be multiplying in the bloodstream during such an episode. The patient's history should be reviewed for indications of recent infections that may be the source of the septicemia.

Interventions. When a patient has a positive blood culture, the nurse should implement appropriate precautionary measures to prevent the spread of pathogens. These measures vary depending on the nature of the organism and its ability to spread. The patient with septicemia is very ill and requires increased physical and mental rest as well as nutritional support, since increases in temperature cause large increases in the body's metabolic demands. The patient should be encouraged to eat the high-protein, high-caloric foods that are ordered. Dehydration may also occur from diaphoresis or diarrhea. The nurse should offer small amounts of fluids frequently and evaluate intake–output ratios for indications of problems. Additional measures depend on the body systems involved in the infectious process and may include nursing activities that assist the patient in mobilizing respiratory secretions, oral hygiene, safe handling of secretions and drainage, or measures to decrease local inflammatory symptoms. Arterial or venous lines may need to be removed if they are a potential source of the infection. When removed, the lines may be cultured as well in order to more clearly delineate the contaminating source.

10

CARCINOEMBRYONIC ANTIGEN ASSAY

Description

The *carcinoembryonic antigen* (CEA) is present in embryonic tissue. When cancer occurs, this antigen is released into the bloodstream in large amounts. The CEA assay is a nonspecific test used to evaluate treatment in patients with colon or pancreatic carcinoma. It is not used for diagnosis, because elevated CEA titers may occur in the presence of other gastrointestinal diseases. However, it is valuable in assessing the response to cancer treatment. It may also be used to monitor the treatment response in patients with cancer of the stomach, lung, breast, head and neck, and ovary.

N O R M A L   R A N G E
Adults   2.5–3.0 mg/ml Children   Consult laboratory for reference values.

Note. Levels for normal are increased in smokers.

Specimen Required
A 7–10-ml sample of venous blood is collected in a plain collecting tube or syringe.

Preparation of the Patient
There are no food or fluid restrictions before venipuncture. This test should not be performed on patients who have received heparin during the preceding 2 days.

Causes of Deviation from Normal
There are several diseases that cause an elevation of CEA levels. These include disorders of the gastrointestinal tract, cirrhosis, heart disease, emphysema, bronchitis, and several types of cancer. However, elevated CEA assay is most commonly associated with colon, rectal, and pancreatic cancer, and is the test used to assess a patient's response to therapy for these types of cancer.

Nursing Implications of Abnormal Findings
Assessment and Interventions. When a CEA test has been performed on a patient suspected to have cancer, the results must be looked at along with other clinical manifestations. However, test results should be used in assessing the results of medical therapy. A fall indicates successful treatment, whereas a rise indicates that the carcinoma has recurred or grown larger.

Nursing plans for emotional support of the patient and family and for patient education about the success of therapy may be guided by CEA rises or falls in the patient with colon, rectal, or pancreatic cancer who is receiving therapy. Patients who are showing a rise in CEA levels need emotional support because of the recurrence of tumor. The patient who has had successful results of treatment can be encouraged to look forward to a lessening of symptoms.

COLD AGGLUTININS

Description
Cold agglutinins are antibodies that cause agglutination (clumping) of red blood cells at refrigerator temperatures of 0–10° C. They are present in small amounts in healthy people.

Adults and children
Normally there is a minimal number of cold agglutinins. Titers of 1:32 or higher are abnormal.

Specimen Required

A 5–10-ml specimen of venous blood is obtained in a plain collecting tube or syringe at 37° C, placed in water at 37° C, and immediately transferred to the laboratory.

Preparation of the Patient

There are no food or fluid restrictions before venipuncture.

Causes of Deviation from Normal

A high cold agglutination titer is seen in 60–65% of patients with mycoplasmal pneumonia, particularly during the acute phase of the illness. Cold agglutinin levels may also be elevated in mononucleosis, lymphoid neoplasms, malaria, frostbite, Raynaud's syndrome, scleroderma, multiple myeloma, pulmonary embolism, influenza, and anemia. Elevations also occur in congenital syphilis, cirrhosis, and in the elderly.

Nursing Implications of Abnormal Findings

Assessment. Although the cold agglutinins are elevated in several diseases, this test is most commonly performed on patients who have atypical pneumonia. It is particularly helpful because of the insidious onset of atypical pneumonia and its general symptoms of infection rather than the severe respiratory-tract symptoms that occur with other pneumonias. Cold agglutinin levels are helpful to the nurse in determining the stage of the disease, since the agglutinins reach their highest levels during the acute phase of the illness and decrease by 4–6 weeks after onset. Test results should be included in the data gathering when the nurse assesses the patient's condition, the response to treatment, and the possibility of complications.

10

Interventions. Nursing interventions are similar to those for patients with pneumonia. They include the following:

1. Provide adequate physical and mental rest;
2. Give frequent oral hygiene;
3. Promote good tracheobronchial hygiene;
4. Instruct the patient about the prevention of future respiratory infections.

COOMBS' ANTIGLOBULIN

Description
This is a nonspecific test used to detect antibodies that may attach to red cells. It may be used to differentiate between types of hemolytic anemia, detect immune bodies, or detect suspected erythroblastosis fetalis (hemolytic disease of the newborn). There are two forms of this test, the *direct* and the *indirect*. The direct form detects the presence of antibodies on the red cells; the indirect form detects the presence of free antibodies in the serum. The indirect form is valuable in detecting blood incompatibilities not found by other tests.

NORMAL RANGE

Normally, both the direct and indirect tests are negative.

Specimen Required
A 5–10-ml sample of venous blood is obtained in a plain collecting tube or syringe.

Preparation of the Patient
There are no food or fluid restrictions before venipuncture.

Causes of Deviation from Normal
The Coombs' test is positive when there are antibodies on red cells present in the serum. There are many causes of a positive Coombs' test, such as transfusion reaction, erythroblastosis fetalis, acute and chronic leukemia, malignant lymphomas, and autoimmune hemolytic anemia. There are also several drugs that can cause a false-positive Coombs' test (Table 10.4).

Nursing Implications of Abnormal Findings
Assessment and Interventions. When a transfusion reaction causes a positive Coombs' test, the patient should be observed for the same clinical manifestations discussed in the section on Crossmatches (Chapter 2). The patient with a hemolytic anemia should be assessed for the general manifestations of anemia, such as lassitude, fatigue, pallor, dyspnea, and palpitations, as well as jaundice, hepatosplenomegaly, and cholelithiasis. Nursing interventions include maintenance of fluid and electrolyte balance by keeping accurate records of intake and output, and slow, careful administration of blood transfusions. The latter is important because of the rapid destruction of transfused cells that occurs with an autoimmune hemolytic disease.

C-REACTIVE PROTEIN TEST

Description

C-reactive protein (CRP) is a glycoprotein thought to be synthesized in the liver. The CRP test is an antibody–antigen reaction test done to determine the presence of an inflammatory process or widespread tissue destruction which occurs in malignant disease, myocardial infarction, acute rheumatic fever, malaria, and bacterial infections. The C-reactive protein test is used less frequently than formerly, because it is nonspecific and similar to the sedimentation rate. Presence of C-reactive protein can occur in the blood serum 18–24 hours after tissue injury occurs. It peaks within 48–72 hours. The CRP may be used to monitor the acute phase of illnesses such as rheumatoid arthritis or the wound healing process in patients with burns or other conditions in which there is tissue damage.

NORMAL RANGE
Normally, either no C-reactive protein or a trace amount is present in the blood.

Specimen Required

A 10-ml sample of venous blood is collected in a plain collecting tube or syringe.

TABLE 10.4. Drugs that Cause a False-Positive Coombs' Test

Cephalexin (Keflex)	Isoniazid
Cephaloglycin	Levodopa
Cephaloridine (Loridine)	Mefenamic acid
Cephalothin (Keflin)	Melphalan
Methyldopa (effect lasts 6 months)	Oxyphenisatin
Penicillin	Procainamide
Rifampin	Quinidine
Chlorpromazine	Streptomycin
Diphenylhydantoin	Sulfonamides
Ethosuximide	Tetracyclines
Hydralazine	

10

Preparation of the Patient

Some laboratories require an 8–12-hour fast from food and fluids before venipuncture. There are no water restrictions.

Causes of Deviation from Normal

The CRP test is positive during certain acute inflammatory processes or during tissue destruction, such as in rheumatic fever, rheumatoid arthritis, and myocardial infarction; it also occurs in cases of malignant diseases that are acute and widespread. Although elevation indicates that inflammation is present, it does not give information about its cause. It is generally used to monitor the inflammatory process.

Nursing Implications of Abnormal Findings

Assessment and Interventions. An elevated CRP level is of limited value for a nursing assessment. It can be useful when assessing the long-term status of a patient with rheumatoid arthritis, particularly if the CRP level rises suddenly, indicating an exacerbation. In this instance, nursing interventions should shift from a focus on rehabilitation to a goal of reducing the inflammatory process and should remain so until the CRP levels begin to drop.

The nurse must remember that results of this test may be positive in women taking oral contraceptives or using an IUD.

HEMAGGLUTINATION INHIBITION TEST (HIA, RUBELLA ANTIBODY TEST, PASSIVE HEMAGGLUTINATION [RUBACELL], ENZYME LINKED IMMUNOSORBENT ASSAY [ELISA])

Description

The *Rubella antibody test* is done to determine the presence of antibodies in serum against the rubella virus. It is most often used to determine a person's level of immunity against rubella. The importance of this test is related to the dangers of rubella in a developing fetus. If a pregnant woman contracts this disease during the first trimester abortion, stillbirth, or congenital anomalies may occur in the baby. The *Hemagglutination Inhibition Test* is the classic test; however, it has been replaced in most instances by one of the other rubella antibody tests.

NORMAL RANGE

There is no specific normal range. An HIA titer of 1:10 indicates susceptibility to the virus. A titer of 1:20 indicates previous rubella infection or vaccination as does a positive result on a Rubacell or ELISA test.

Specimen Required

A 5-ml sample of venous blood is collected in a plain collecting tube or syringe.

Preparation of the Patient

Food and fluid restrictions are not required before collection of the specimen.

Causes of Deviation from Normal

Although there is no specific normal range, people who have an HIA titer of 1:10 are considered to be susceptible to the virus. If the test shows a titer of 1:20 or more, the person has enough antibodies for protection against rubella.

Nursing Implications of Abnormal Findings

Assessment and Interventions. When individuals have low antibody titers, the nurse should recommend they be immunized with rubella vaccine if they are women of childbearing age, men who plan to father children, hospital personnel working with children, day-care workers, or teachers. Patient education should include information about the effects on the fetus when a pregnant woman is infected. Potential carriers who work with or around women who are or may be pregnant should also understand the possible consequences if they become the source of a rubella infection. Pregnant women should be screened for rubella during their first prenatal visit. If their titer is low, they should be advised to limit their exposure to young children, particularly those who have an upper respiratory infection. Any pregnant woman who is exposed to rubella regardless of previous test results, should have another rubella antibody test. A rise in the titer indicates that both mother and fetus have been infected. If this occurs during the first trimester, the nurse should explain the consequences to the fetus and support the mother's decision to either continue with the pregnancy or have a therapeutic abortion.

CYTOMEGALOVIRUS ANTIBODY

Description

The *cytomegalovirus antibody test* is done to detect the titers of specific antibodies to cytomegalovirus. This virus belongs to the herpes family and is quite common. Antibodies can be detected by several methods including passive hemagglutination, latex agglutination, enzyme immunoassay, and indirect immunofluorescence. It is generally viewed as a qualitative test, detecting the presence of antibody at a single low dilution (for example, 1:5). Blood banks routinely screen for the CMV antibody.

10

N O R M A L   R A N G E
Titer $<$1:5

Preparation of the Patient

There are no food or fluid restrictions before venipuncture.

Causes of Deviation from Normal

Patients who have never had cytomegalovirus infection have no antibodies in their blood and should receive blood products or organ transplants that are from donors who are also seronegative. Infection with cytomegalovirus is usually asymptomatic and the virus persists in a latent stage in the host. Infants who acquire the virus during a maternal primary infection may develop severe cytomegalic inclusion disease (CID) which may be fatal or cause neurologic changes including mental retardation and deafness. CMV infection in immuno-compromised patients (post bone marrow transplant or AIDS) may develop interstitial pneumonitis which can be fatal.

Nursing Implications of Abnormal Findings

Patients who have titers >1:5 of cytomegalovirus antibody should be assessed for signs and symptoms of pneumonitis, especially if they are immunocompromised. Since this infection may be fatal, patients should be monitored carefully and watched for respiratory compromise. Medical-surgical and cancer-nursing textbooks should be consulted for further details on the nursing care of these patients.

HETEROPHILE ANTIBODY TEST (MONO-SPOT, MONO-SCREEN, EPSTEIN BARR VIRUS TEST)

Description

The *heterophile antibodies* produced by humans react with the red cells of another species. This test is used to detect the presence of infectious mononucleosis, which is caused by the Epstein-Barr virus. The diagnosis is made when it is demonstrated in the laboratory that the heterophile antibody agglutinates sheep or horse red cells, retains most of its activity after exposure to Forssman antigen, and is completely removed by absorption with bovine red cells.

NORMAL RANGE

Adults and Children
Normally, heterophile antibodies are present in small amounts in the serum. Some specimens have titers between 1:56 and 1:28. Generally, a titer of 1:56 indicates that infectious mononucleosis may be present. A titer of 1:2224 or higher is diagnostic of the disease. If the mono-spot is used for testing, positive results occur when the heterophile is greater than 1:28.

Specimen Required

A 5–10-ml sample of venous blood is collected in a plain collecting tube or syringe.

Preparation of the Patient

There are no food or fluid restrictions before venipuncture.

Causes of Deviation from Normal

Infectious mononucleosis is the most common cause of a rise in the antibody titer. The antibody titer peaks during the second to third weeks of the illness and usually disappears at 4–8 weeks.

Nursing Implications of Abnormal Findings

Assessment and Interventions. The heterophile test is helpful in the assessment of a patient with a sore throat, and lymphadenopathy, since these clinical data can be found in several diseases besides mononucleosis. If liver function tests have also been done, these data should be included in the patient evaluation, since liver function tests can also be elevated when infectious mononucleosis is present.

Because most patients with infectious mononucleosis are not hospitalized, they should be taught important aspects of self-care. These include (1) rest in bed during the febrile period, (2) analgesia such as aspirin for general discomfort and fever, and (3) warm saline gargles and throat lozenges to relieve sore throat. Patients should be told that they can still spread the disease to others while they are convalescing.

LEGIONNAIRE'S ANTIBODY TEST

Description

This test is performed to determine the presence of *Legionella pneumophila* in the serum. A four-fold increase in the titer is evidence of infection.

10

N O R M A L   R A N G E
Negative

Specimen Required

A 7-ml specimen of venous blood is collected in a plain collecting tube or syringe.

Preparation of the Patient
There are no food or fluid restrictions before venipuncture.

Causes of Deviation from Normal
Legionnaire's disease is caused by the inhalation of *Legionella pneumophila*. This organism is thought to be present in air conditioning and plumbing systems.

Nursing Implications of Abnormal Findings
Assessment and Interventions. Patients who have a positive Legionnaire's antibody test should be assessed for the signs and symptoms of Legionnaire's Disease such as malaise, high fever, chills, cough, chest pain, and tachypnea. Nursing interventions include activities that will help the patient mobilize and remove secretions such as breathing exercises, frequent position changes, and humidified air. The temperature should be monitored closely as fever may rise quickly to 102° F–105° F (39° C–41° C). Antipyretics and analgesics should be administered as needed.

LYME DISEASE ANTIBODY TEST

Description
The *Lyme Disease test* is done to detect the titers of specific antibodies to the *Borrelia burgdoferi* spirochete. The antibodies produced vary with the stage of infection. Titers are generally low during the first several weeks of the illness and increase several months later, often remaining elevated for years.

N O R M A L   R A N G E
Titer <1:256

Specimen Required
A 5-ml sample of venous blood is collected in a plain collecting tube or syringe.

Preparation of the Patient
There are no food or fluid restrictions before venipuncture.

Causes of Deviation from Normal
Lyme disease is an infection that occurs as a result of a deer tick bite. It is specifically caused by the spirochete *Borrelia burgdorferi*. Weeks to months following the tick bite, some people develop peripheral neuropathies, aseptic meningitis, cardiovascular abnormalities, or arthritis in one or

more joints. Patients with high rheumatoid factors may have false-positive results.

Nursing Implications of Abnormal Findings

Assessment and Interventions. When a patient has a positive Lyme disease test, the nursing assessment should include questions about the occurrence or evidence of a tick bite, asking the patient about the presence of a reddish, macular lesion. Patient education should include a discussion about the importance of wearing clothing that covers the arms and legs when in a tick infested area. Patients should also be told to report any tick bites to a physician as soon as possible. If the patient has any of the complications associated with Lyme disease, a medical-surgical textbook should be consulted for related nursing care.

LUPUS ERYTHEMATOSUS CELL TEST

Description

Lupus erythematosus (LE) cells are produced in the serum of approximately 75% of patients with lupus erythematosus. However, they are also found in patients with other conditions such as rheumatoid arthritis and scleroderma. LE cells result from immunological activity directed against nucleoproteins.

N O R M A L   R A N G E

Normally there are no LE cells present in the blood.

Specimen Required

A 5–10-ml sample of venous blood is collected. The laboratory should be consulted to determine if clotted or unclotted blood is required.

10

Preparation of the Patient

There are no food or fluid restrictions before venipuncture.

Note. There are several medications that may cause a false-positive test for LE cells (Table 10.5). If the patient is receiving any of these medications, a note should be made on the laboratory slip.

Causes of Deviation from Normal

LE cells are present in patients who have lupus erythematosus. However, they are not present in all cases. Since positive results may be seen in patients with rheumatoid arthritis, scleroderma, and some types of hepatitis, the LE

TABLE 10.5. Drugs that Affect the LE Cell Test

Clofibrate	Phenytoin
Hydralazine	Procainamide
Isoniazide	Quinidine
Mesantoin	Reserpine
Methyldopa	Streptomycin
Methysergide	Sulfonamides
Oral contraceptives	Tetracycline
Penicillin	Tridione
Phenylbutazone	

test is not considered to be primary in the diagnosis of systemic lupus erythematosus.

Nursing Implications of Abnormal Findings

Assessment and Interventions. Since the LE test is positive in only 50–75% of patients with systemic lupus erythematosus, results of this test should not be considered definitive when the diagnosis has not been confirmed. Nursing interventions should relate to the specific problems that have been identified in the assessment. See the section on antinuclear antibody tests (page 288) for a detailed discussion of nursing implications.

RHEUMATOID FACTORS

Description

Rheumatoid factors are antiglobulin antibodies that react specifically with the IgG human immunoglobulins. These are abnormal antibodies that develop against the host's own tissues, and are generally associated with rheumatoid arthritis and other autoimmune diseases. Elevated titers of these antibodies are used in diagnosing the presence and persistence of these diseases.

NORMAL RANGE

Adults	<1:20
Children	Consult laboratory for reference values.

Specimen Required

A 5–10-ml sample of venous blood is collected in a plain collecting tube or syringe.

Preparation of the Patient

Food and fluids are not restricted before venipuncture.

Causes of Deviation from Normal

Elevated titers of rheumatoid factors (>1:80) occur in 75–80% of patients with rheumatoid arthritis. These high titers are usually associated with acute episodes of the disease. Elevations also occur in patients with systemic lupus erythematosus, scleroderma, and, less frequently, tuberculosis, syphilis, infectious mononucleosis, and leprosy.

Nursing Implications of Abnormal Findings

Assessment. When a patient has an elevation of rheumatoid factors, repeat tests and other tests for autoimmune diseases are likely to be done to determine a specific diagnosis. For the patient with established rheumatoid arthritis, the titer is likely to remain high. For these patients, nursing assessment should include determining the joints that are involved and the symptoms of inflammation occurring in each joint. The extent and duration of symptoms after a night's sleep should be noted so that nursing care can be planned accordingly. Assessment should include the patient's personality and emotional response to the disease. The patient's ability to do self-care should be evaluated regularly.

Interventions. If the patient with elevated rheumatoid factors does not have a specific diagnosis, nursing interventions should focus on the patient's general needs. If rheumatoid arthritis is present, nursing interventions should emphasize rest, a well-balanced diet, and reduction of pain. A teaching plan will be needed to assist the patient in understanding what medications are being used and any side effects that should be reported, such as signs of salicylism (when salicylates are being taken). The plan should also include information about medications. For example, salicylates should be taken with milk, food, or antacids. Pain interventions should include positioning, application of heat, administration of medications, and either rest of the involved joint or passive to active exercise, depending upon the stage of illness present. Rheumatoid arthritis is a long-term, episodic illness, and the patient needs emotional support while adapting to the illness and the life changes that may result. Additional nursing interventions may be found in general medical-surgical nursing textbooks.

10

SYPHILIS SEROLOGY TESTS

Description

Syphilis is an infectious communicable disease caused by a thin, spiral-shaped anaerobe (spirochete) called *Treponema pallidum*. The disease is usually transmitted by sexual contact. The spirochete is so narrow that it cannot be visualized by conventional microscopy nor can it be cultured on artificial media.

There are two types of tests used to detect the presence of infection with *Treponema pallidum*. The first type is designed to detect the presence of reagin, a non-treponemal antibody, that is produced in response to infection with *Treponema pallidum*. The *Venereal Disease Research Laboratories* (VDRL), and the *Rapid Plasma Reagin* (RPR) are the most common and reliable tests used to detect reagin. These tests may show false non-reactive (negative) results in the early stages of infection; they are more accurate during the secondary and tertiary stages of disease. The second type of test is done to detect the presence of the treponemal antibody. The *fluorescent treponemal antibody absorption test* (FTA-ABS) is the most sensitive and reliable treponemal antibody test. It can be used to detect syphilis in any of its stages and is also used to confirm the diagnosis of syphilis when reagin tests may be showing false-positive results.

N O R M A L   R A N G E

VDRL, RPR, FTA-ABS   non-reactive (negative)

Test results are reported as non-reactive (negative), weakly reactive (borderline or doubtful), and reactive (positive).

Note: Table 10.6 shows conditions that may cause false-positive VDRL, RPR, and FTA-ABS reactions.

Specimen Required

A 5-ml sample of venous blood is obtained in a plain collecting tube or syringe.

Preparation of the Patient

Food and fluids are usually not restricted before venipuncture. The patient should not drink alcohol for 24 hours before venipuncture as this can cause a false-negative VDRL reaction. It should be noted if the FTA-ABS test is being performed on a person who has had syphilis before, because once this test becomes positive it remains so.

Causes of Deviation from Normal

Almost all cases of syphilis are acquired by sexual contact with a person infected with the organism. Other modes of transmission include non-sexual personal contact, contact with contaminated fomites, or transmission to the fetus *in utero*. Blood transfusions are also potential causes of transmission. The organism penetrates intact mucous membranes or abraded skin and rapidly enters the bloodstream, producing systemic infection. The primary lesion, or chancre, appears at the site of inoculation 10–90 days after contact. It heals spontaneously with or without treatment within 2–6 weeks. If the disease is

TABLE 10.6. Conditions that May Cause False-Positive Syphyllis Serology Tests

Conditions that May Cause False-Positive VDRL and RPR Reactions

Atypical pneumonia	Malaria
Chancroid	Measles
Chicken pox	Periarteritis nodosa
Collagen vascular diseases	Pneumococcal pneumonia
Common cold	Pregnancy
Hyperglobulinemia	Rheumatoid arthritis
Immunizations (DPT)	Rheumatic fever
Infectious hepatitis	Scarlet fever
Infectious mononucleosis	Subacute bacterial endocarditis
Leprosy	Tuberculosis
Leptospirosis	Thyroiditis
Lupus erythematosis	Typhus
Lymphogranuloma venerium	

Conditions that May Cause False-Positive FTA-ABS Reactions

Antinuclear antibodies	Lupus erythematosis
Chronic infection	Lymphoma
Cirrhosis of the liver	Pregnancy
Diabetes mellitus	Rheumatoid arthritis
Hypergammaglobulinemia	Scleroderma

untreated, a generalized secondary rash will appear, which also heals spontaneously within weeks or months. The untreated patient then enters the latent stage.

Nursing Implications of Abnormal Findings

Assessment. When a patient has a positive serology test for syphilis, the nursing assessment should include the following areas: (1) physical manifestations of the disease; (2) anxiety about the implications of the diagnosis; and (3) willingness of the patient to disclose recent sexual partners.

Interventions. When the patient with syphilis is symptomatic, nursing interventions should be related to the specific disease manifestations that are present. All lesions are assumed to be sources of contagion. When caring for a person with untreated syphilis, a gown and gloves should be used when direct contact with the lesions is made. Lesions are no longer sources of contagion 24 hours after antibiotic therapy has begun. Patients should be instructed to refrain from sexual activity for at least 4 hours after treatment and preferably until treatment has been completed.

10

When a person has latent syphilis, almost any body system may be involved. The two most common problem are disruptions in the functioning of the nervous and cardiovascular systems. Nursing-care plans should focus on problems related to cognitive, motor, and sensory impairment when neurosyphilis is present and on cardiac insufficiency when cardiovascular syphilis is present.

When the patient demonstrates anxiety about the diagnosis of syphilis, the nurse should reassure the person with primary or secondary syphilis that the manifestations are temporary and the disease can be completely cured. If the patient is anxious about informing a spouse or partner about the diagnosis, the nurse must provide nonjudgmental support and be available to the patient for further discussion.

The problem of infection control cannot be dealt with adequately unless the infected person is willing to reveal sexual contacts. If the patient is reluctant to provide the names of contacts, the nurse must help the patient understand the importance of sharing this information. A teaching plan can be developed for this purpose. It should include information about the way syphilis spreads, the difficulty in self-diagnosis for the female, the course of the disease if left untreated, and the importance of keeping follow-up appointments for evaluation of treatment. All patients should be taught about prevention; some measures that can be taken are the use of condoms and cleansing the genitals with warm water and soap before and after sexual intercourse. Men can help prevent organisms from invading the genitourinary tract by urinating immediately after intercourse. The use of intravaginal contraceptive preparations may provide some protection from venereal disease for women. Patients should also be told that although antibiotic therapy is effective it should not be considered a means of easy control. The possible development of resistant organisms due to overuse of antibiotics should be explained, as well as the possibility that patients can develop a latent allergic reaction to the drug.

TORCH TEST

Description

The term TORCH is an acronym which represents Toxoplasmosis, Other, Rubella, Cytomegalovirus, and Herpes Simplex. It is a screening test to determine the presence of organisms which can cross the placental barrier during pregnancy and have serious congenital effects on the fetus including congenital abnormalities, abortion, or premature labor.

NORMAL RANGE
Negative

Specimen Required

A 5-ml sample of venous blood is collected in a plain collecting tube or syringe.

Preparation of the Patient

Food and fluids are not restricted before venipuncture.

Causes of Deviation from Normal

A positive test for one of the organisms indicates exposure to one of the agents that can cause infection of the fetus. Toxoplasmosis is a parasitic infection caused by toxoplasma gondii, found in raw meat and cat feces. If infection occurs in the mother following conception, fetal infection will occur with resultant congenital anomalies such as hydrocephalis, microcephalis, chronic retinitis, and psychomotor retardation. The other category encompasses a variety of infections including syphilis-See Syphilis Serology Tests. Rubella is discussed in the section on Rubella Antibody Test. Cytomegalovirus is a latent virus present in many adults. Pregnant women may transmit the virus to the fetus either *in utero* or during delivery, through an infected cervix. The cytomegalovirus can cause congenital infections resulting in microcephaly, mental retardation, deafness, growth retardation and other anomalies. Herpes simplex virus is a common virus classified as type I or type II. *Type I* may be present in the eyes, mouth, or upper respiratory tract; *type II* may be present on the genitalia. Neonatal infection can occur during vaginal delivery by exposure to genital lesions.

Nursing Implications of Abnormal Findings

Assessment and Interventions. If the TORCH test is positive, a history of previous infections should be obtained. The nurse should also assess the patient's response to a positive test and be prepared to answer questions about the need for further testing. When final test results are shared with the patient, the nurse should answer questions regarding the possibility of congenital anomalies to her child and support her in decisions regarding abortion, if it is suggested as an option.

10

HIV ANTIBODY TO HUMAN IMMUNODEFICIENCY VIRUS

Description

The *HIV Antibody test* is used to detect the antibody to human immunodeficiency virus (HIV). The virus is the cause of acquired immune deficiency syndrome (AIDS). The most common approach to identifying the virus is the *ELISA* (enzyme-linked immunosorbent assay). A positive test is only reported when positive findings are also found on a repeat testing of the same sample, and a confirmatory positive test, usually the Western blot procedure, has been performed.

N O R M A L   R A N G E

Negative

Specimen Required

A 5–10-ml sample of venous blood is collected in a red-top tube.

Preparation of the Patient

No food or fluids are restricted prior to collection of the specimen. Written, informed consent is generally required. In some states, a positive result has to be reported to the state health authorities, so that epidemiologic studies can be conducted, and potential contacts can be notified and counseled.

Causes of Deviation from Normal

While the presence of HIV does not always lead to AIDS, the virus is present in patients with AIDS. Following initial infection, progression to AIDS may take up to ten years. The virus may be absent in late-stage AIDS. The test is used to detect the virus in patients, to screen blood and blood products, and to track reactions of health-care personnel exposed to potential contamination by the virus in the work setting. HIV appears in the plasma and circulating mononuclear cells 1 to several weeks after infection. The HIV antibodies usually appear within 1–3 months, with occasional individuals not exhibiting them for up to 12 months. Presence of antibody does not cause immunity; thus, antibody-positive individuals may transmit the virus to others.

Those at risk for the infection include sexually active homosexual and bisexual men with multiple partners, IV drug abusers, persons receiving blood transfusions before 1985, and infants exposed to the virus during gestation. Since March, 1985, blood in blood banks has been tested for HIV and donations that test positive are discarded.

Nursing Implications for Abnormal Findings

Assessment. Assess the patient with positive findings for symptoms of AIDS, including fatigue, fever, anorexia, weight loss, diarrhea, night sweats, and swollen lymph glands in the axilla or groin. Because of the lethal potential and the social stigma associated with AIDS, the patient's emotional responses should be evaluated carefully, and supportive care provided.

Interventions. For patients who are HIV+ and have no other signs of AIDS, counseling for healthy living is needed. Patients should be encouraged to maintain their general health, nutritional status, abstain from sexual activities that may provide for transmission of the virus, and avoid sharing needles. For patients who have progressed to AIDS, protection from infection and injury is needed. Patients need to be instructed in ways to prevent spread of the virus to others. They should not donate blood, plasma, body organs, other tissue, or sperm. They should be instructed that there is risk of passing the infection to others through sexual contact, sharing of needles, and possibly through saliva in oral-genital contact or intimate kissing. Tooth brushes, razors and other implements contaminated with blood should not be shared. Women who are infected with the virus who become pregnant risk passing the virus and the disease to their offspring.

Frequently, health-care personnel and the patient's family and friends are concerned about being contaminated with the virus and contracting the disease. Explanation that casual contact does not put persons at high risk for contracting AIDS should be included. Intimate sexual contact (oral, genital, rectal) with a person with AIDS put the individual at high risk to contract AIDS.

HIV seropositive women should be counseled on the possibility of infecting their infant. Men and women should be encouraged to avoid casual, unprotected sexual activities. The public should be taught that blood donation does not put the blood donor at risk (a common misperception).

Precautions essential to those caring for the patient include protection from the patient's body fluids, especially blood and semen. Table 10.7 lists the precautions that are needed when providing direct care. Current references should be sought to identify further nursing interventions in caring for these patients.

VAGINAL SMEAR

Description

A *vaginal smear* involves preparation of microscopic slides with vaginal secretions and wet-mount or immediate microscopic examination. Vaginal secretions collected during a vaginal examination are used and examined for characteristics specific to microorganisms associated with vaginitis.

10

NORMAL RANGE

A normal vaginal smear reveals no evidence of the various characteristics of pathogenic vaginal microorganisms. Positive or abnormal results differ depending on the specific organism present.

Specimen Required

Exudate from the vaginal walls or the cervix when cervicitis is present, is used to prepare two slides, one with potassium hydroxide solution and one with saline. The solutions must be fresh. A typical procedure involves both a smear

TABLE 10.7. Guidelines for Nursing Care of the Patient with AIDS

The plan for nursing care of the patient with AIDS is based on the following anticipated needs:

1. The need for a *safe environment.*
2. The patient's need for *information* on self-care and management of disease complications.
3. The patient's need for *psychological support.*

The approach to providing a *safe environment* is based on:

1. Preventing the occurrence of potentially fatal infections.
2. Preventing the spread of the AIDS virus to health personnel and other patients by observing appropriate precautions for anything containing or contaminated with body fluids or blood.

The *safe environment* for the AIDS patient is similar to that for the patient with hepatitis and includes:

1. Carrying out usual hand-washing procedures before and after contact with the patient.
2. Assigning the patient to a private room.
3. Use of gowns and gloves when giving care that involves handling specimens or performing nursing interventions during which body fluids or blood may be involved, such as caring for an incontinent patient or collecting blood specimens.
4. Use of masks and goggles or other protective eye coverings to prevent contamination during procedures that generate sprays from body fluids such as oral suctioning procedures and wound care.
5. Disposal of all equipment with potentially or actually contaminated materials, using containers and procedures for blood and secretion precautions.
6. Provision of a two-way airway in the patient's room to be used during implementation of cardiac arrest procedures.

The *information* necessary for the AIDS patient to maintain appropriate self-care and management of disease complications includes:

1. Precautions needed to protect the patient from opportunistic infections.
2. Safe sex guidelines.
3. Reportable signs and symptoms.

TABLE 10.7. (*Continued*)

Psychological support for the AIDS patient includes:

1. Assessing the patient's emotional state and providing interventions appropriate to the mood state identified (depression, anxiety, anger, etc.)
2. Checking the patient at regular intervals to avoid having the patient feel abandoned.
3. Providing opportunities for family and friends to visit and assist with care as appropriate.
4. Referring to a psychologist or psychiatric social worker to assist the patient as needed.

and a culture taken during a vaginal exam. It is performed by a physician, nurse practitioner, or a registered nurse with specific training in vaginal examinations.

Preparation of the Patient

The patient should be prepared for a vaginal examination. Instructions should include what the patient can expect to experience during the procedure and methods to relax during the examination and specimen collection. No food or fluid restrictions are needed. Patients should be instructed not to douche prior to vaginal examination, since such a procedure may temporarily wash away organisms causing disease and lead to false-negative results.

Causes of Deviation from Normal

The presence of a fishy amine-like odor on the slide with potassium hydroxide indicates that *Gardnerella* is present. This is generally called the "whiff" test. Yeasts such as *Candida albicans* are identified by the presence of budding cells, pseudohyphae, and spores during microscopic examination of the potassium hydroxide slide. These characteristics of the yeast are seen most easily on the potassium hydroxide slide since the medium destroys leukocytes, epithelial cells, and bacteria. On the normal saline slide, *Gardnerella* is identified by the presence of clue cells, which have a typical stippled or granulated appearance. *Trichomonas* is identified by its flagella, a typical pear or corkscrew shape.

10

Nursing Implications of Abnormal Findings

Assessment. Assessment of the patient with vaginitis includes information gained from the vaginal smear and culture, as well as other objective signs and patient subjective symptoms (Fig. 10.1). A thorough assessment is needed for

---

Interview

A. **Menstrual Cycle:**
  1. LMP's _____ _____
  2. Length
  3. Due Date
B. **Self-Care Practices:**
  1. Douching:
    a. Number of
       times/week _____
    b. Solution
  2. Lingerie
  3. Clothing
  4. Urination/Defecation
     Practices
C. **Sexual Activity:**
  1. Frequency
  2. Types:
    a. Heterosexual
    b. Homosexual
    c. Bisexual
  3. Partner(s)
  4. Dyspareunia
  5. Other:
    a. Masturbation
D. **Contraception Practices:**
  1. IUD
  2. Condom
  3. Diaphragm
  4. The "Pill"–Name _____
  5. Jelly/Foam
  6. Vasectomy/tubal
     ligation
  7. Other: _____

E. **Drugs**
  1. Birth Control Pills
  2. Antibiotics
  3. Steroids
  4. Tranquilizers
  5. Barbiturates
  6. Alcohol
  7. Antihypertensives
F. **Vaginitis History:**
  1. Pruritus:
    a. Labia
    b. Ant. Perineum
    c. Peri-Anal
  2. Discharge:
    a. Amount
    b. Color
  3. Odor
  4. Vaginal Burning
  5. Vaginal Pressure
  6. Vaginal Soreness
  7. Dysuria
  8. Fever
  9. Lesions
  10. Other_____
G. **Psychosocial Responses:**
  1. Depression
  2. Anxiety
  3. Anger
  4. Sadness
  5. Fear
  6. Other:_____
  _____

FIGURE 10.1. Vaginitis Assessment Form

accurate identification of the specific causative organism, since these signs and symptoms differ across infections (Table 10.8). Assessment should continue during treatment in order to monitor responses. Assessment and treatment of the sexual partner are frequently needed as well.

Interventions. When the patient has a positive smear for a specific vaginal pathogen, treatment may involve a medication specific to the organism, as in

			Physical Exam		
External Exam	**Yes**	**No**	**Internal Exam**	**Yes**	**No**
Erythema:			**Color:**		
Labia			Abnormal		
Ant. Perineum			Erythema		
Peri-Anal			Beefy-Red		
Pustules:			Cyanotic, Pale		
Labia Majora			**Edema** (Congested)		
Labia Minor			**Secretions:**		
Ant. Perineum			Small		
Peri-Anal			Moderate		
Edema:			Profuse		
Labia			**Odor**		
Ant. Perineum			**Discharge:**		
Peri-Anal			Clear		
Odor			White		
Discharge:			Yellow/Green		
White			Gray		
Yellow-Green			Other: _____		
Gray			**Placques**		
Bloody (Menses)			**Cervical Os:**		
Groin, Abdominal Folds:			Round		
Erythema			Transverse		
Odor			Excoriated		
Vesicles			Lesions		
Discharge					

	Laboratory Tests	
	+ —	
Wet Mount:		**Additional Information**
Hyphae		
Flagella		
Other: _____		
pH		**Problems/Diagnosis**
Vaginal Glucose		
Culture		

10

FIGURE 10.1. (*Continued*)

infections with *Trichomonas*, or multiple antibiotic therapy for infections where therapy specifically sensitive to the organism has not yet been developed (Table 10.9). Patient teaching should include how to take whatever medical

TABLE 10.8. Symptom Patterns in Specific Vulvovaginal Infection

	Candida	Trichomonas	Gardnerella	Herpes	Gonorrhea	Chlamydia	Condylomata
Pruritus	Intense, painful	Sometimes	Seldom	Sometimes			Sometimes
Lesions		Petechial spots on cervix and fornix; "Strawberry spots"		Stinging sensations Vesicles on vulva, vagina and cervix	Abscess of Bartholin glands		Pink, elongated, soft
Pain				Tender groin nodes	Right upper quadrant pain		Vulva and vagina pain sometimes
Discharge	White, curd-like	Yellowish-green, frothy	Grayish-yellow		Mucopurulent from cervix	Mucopurulent from cervix	
Odor		Foul	Fish-like				
Dyspareunia	Present						
Dysuria	Present			Present	Present	Present	
Fever				Moderate			
Asymptomatic		25%	50%		70–80%	50%	
Inflammation	Present	Present					
Other					Urethritis with edema and inflammation of urethral orifice		Present

treatment is prescribed, and changes needed in sexual activity. Instruction to the patient should include the usual ways the infection is spread, the needed medical treatment, the complications that can occur if treatment is not completed, and the importance of keeping follow-up appointments. Instruction in general hygiene measures should be given. Discussion of the need for treatment of the patient's sexual partner is necessary so that reinfection does not occur. Since the treatment of each of these diseases is different, gynecological textbooks should be consulted in planning nursing care.

VAGINAL CULTURE

Description

A *vaginal culture* is used to identify microorganisms causing vaginitis and cervicitis. It is used along with a vaginal smear to identify the specific organisms present when patients have signs and symptoms of vaginal disease. Treatment is prescribed depending upon the results of the culture.

N O R M A L   R A N G E

Normally, there are no pathogenic organisms cultured from vaginal secretions. However, many skin organisms are present and grow when cultured.

Specimen Required

Exudate from the vaginal walls or cervix for cervicitis is obtained on cotton swabs and transported to the laboratory for preparation of cultures. Rapid transportation for fragile organisms such as *Neisseria gonorrhoeae* is critical. Different kinds of media are used to foster the growth of specific organisms (Table 10.10). Following incubation of the cultures, the presence of specific organisms is determined by the characteristics of the colonies and by carrying out various tests such as a Gram stain of the organisms that have grown.

Preparation of the Patient

The patient should be prepared for a vaginal examination. Instructions should include what the patient can expect to experience during the procedure and methods to be used to relax during the examination and specimen collection. No food or fluid restrictions are needed. Patients should be instructed not to douche prior to vaginal examination, since such a procedure may temporarily wash away organisms causing disease and lead to false-negative results.

10

TABLE 10.9. Usual Medical Treatment for Common Sexually Transmitted Diseases

Organism	Usual Treatment
Candida albicans	Nystatin or imidazole antifungals such as clotrimazole, miconazole nitrate, and ketoconazole
Chlamydia trachomatis	Multiple antibiotic therapy with tetracycline, doxycycline, minocycline, erythromycin, trimethoprimsulfamethoxazole
Condylomata	Local topical acidic agents (bichloroacetic acid, trichloroacetic acid), laser vaporization, cryotherapy cautery
Bacterial Vaginosis	Metronidazole, ampicillin, or tetracycline
Herpes simplex virus type 2, sometimes type 1	Acyclovir
Neisseria gonorrhoeae	Penicillin for nonresistant strains; spectinomycin for resistant strains
Trichomonas vaginalis	Metronidazole
Treponema pallidum	Penicillin, erythromycin, and tetracycline

TABLE 10.10. Culture Media Used for Detection of Vaginal Pathogens

Organism	Media
Candida albicans	Nickerson's medium Sabouraud's medium
Chlamydia trachomatis	Tissue culture McCoy cells
Bacterial vaginosis	Casman blood agar
Herpes simplex virus	Viral culture
Neisseria gonorrhoeae	Thayer-Martin Transgrow Martin-Lewis New York City medium
Trichomonas vaginalis	Feinberg-Whittington medium Trichosal broth

Causes of Deviation from Normal

Two organisms commonly associated with vaginitis are *Candida albicans*, which is a fungus previously referred to as *Monilia*, and *Trichomonas vaginalis*, which is a flagellated protozoa. In the past, cases in which neither of these pathogens has been identified have been referred to as nonspecific vaginitis and associated with *Hemophilus vaginalis*, also called *Corynebacterium vaginale* and *Gardnerella*. It has recently been renamed *bacterial vaginosis*, which is a more descriptive term for this infection which is caused by various aerobic and anaerobic organisms. Infections with the herpes virus are less frequent and generally involve the vulvar tissues, causing blisters that become shallow, painful ulcerations. Herpes occasionally infects both the vagina and cervix.

Vaginitis may also be associated with other sexually transmitted diseases. It is estimated that only one in 5 actual cases of gonorrhea is reported. However, 70–80% of these infections in women are asymptomatic. Another very common sexually transmitted pathogen that causes cervicitis is *Chlamydia trachomatis*; an estimated 3–4 million cases occur in the United States each year. In women, *Chlamydia* may cause cervicitis, salpingitis, and acute urethral syndrome, but it is common for symptoms to be nonspecific, mild, or nonexistent. Venereal warts, *condyloma acuminatum*, may occur on the vulva, vagina, or cervix of infected patients. Condylomata is caused by the human papillomavirus (HPV), and is the most prevalent sexually transmitted disease, with 20 million cases identified per year. It infects both men and women. A link between HPV infection, cervical intraepithelial neoplasia, and invasive cancer has been established, but to date lacks clear epidemiologic support. The course of infection with HPV is characterized by regression, persistence, and progression. Carefully designed studies are needed to demonstrate the exact role of HPV in carcinogenesis.

Nursing Implications of Abnormal Findings

Assessment. Assessment of the patient with vaginitis includes information gained from the vaginal smear and culture, as well as other objective signs and patient subjective symptoms (Fig. 10.1). A thorough assessment is needed for accurate identification of the specific causative organism, since these signs and symptoms differ across infections (Table 10.8). Assessment should continue during treatment in order to monitor responses. Assessment and treatment of the sexual partner are frequently needed as well.

Interventions. When the patient has a positive smear for a specific vaginal pathogen, treatment may involve a medication specific to the organism or multiple antibiotic therapy for infections where therapy specifically sensitive to the organism has not yet been developed (Table 10.9). Patients should be instructed how to take whatever medical treatment is prescribed and what changes are needed in sexual activity. Instructions to the patient should include the usual ways the infection is spread, the needed medical treatment,

10

the complications that can occur if treatment is not completed, and the importance of keeping follow-up appointments. Instruction in general hygiene measures should be given. Discussion of the need for treatment of the patient's sexual partner is necessary so that reinfection does not occur. Since the treatment of each of these diseases is different, gynecological textbooks should be consulted in planning nursing care.

PAPANICOLAOU SMEAR (PAP SMEAR)

Description

The *pap smear* is a screening test used to identify cervical cancer. It consists of an evaluation of cells obtained from scraping of the cervix. By identification of cellular characteristics, the pap smear can be used to detect early precancerous conditions or the presence of malignant cells.

NORMAL RANGE

Results of a pap smear are reported on a five-point scale.

Grade or Class I	Negative, absence of atypical or abnormal cells.
Grade or Class II	Atypical cytology, dysplasia, borderline but not neoplastic.
Grade or Class III	Suspicious cytology suggestive of malignancy.
Grade or Class IV	Probably positive, strongly suggestive of malignancy.
Grade or Class V	Positive, conclusive for malignancy, cancer cells present.

Specimen Required

A pap stick (small wooden spatula) is used to obtain scrapings from the cervix during a vaginal examination. Because of high false-negative results ranging from 15–50%, careful and accurate collection of the cervical smears are essential. Two samples are needed. The first is taken where the stratified squamous epithelium of the exocervix meets the columar epithelium. The second sample should be from the endocervical canal. The specimens should be obtained from the correct sites, spread quickly but gently as a thin film onto a clean glass slide, and fixed immediately. If a spray fixative is used, the nozzle needs to be about 6 inches from the slide. Because of the critical value of the Pap smear, procedures should ensure obtaining the best possible specimen. Current gynecologic textbooks should be consulted.

Preparation of the Patient

No food or fluid restrictions are needed prior to the test. The patient should be instructed about the vaginal examination and the potential associated discomforts. Instructions about how to relax and minimize discomfort during the examination should be included. The patient needs to be instructed not to douche or insert vaginal medication 24–48 hours prior to the examination.

Causes of Deviation from Normal

Several factors can interfere with test results, such as menstruation, douching prior to the examination, lubricating jelly used on the vaginal speculum, and some drugs, namely digitalis preparations and tetracycline. Atypical cells can occur with long-term oral contraceptive therapy or prolonged use of hormones. Malignant changes occur over a long period of time. Therefore, yearly pap smears are recommended. Gradual changes can be identified and appropriate preventive measures and early treatment of cervical cancer can be implemented.

Nursing Implications of Abnormal Findings

Assessment. A number of factors should be included in the assessment of the patient undergoing a pap smear. The history should include information on menstruation, menstrual problems, use of contraceptives or hormone therapy, and vaginal infections. It should be noted whether the patient is taking digitalis products or tetracycline. When results indicate a precancerous condition or the presence of malignancy, the patient's emotional response and the need for emotional support should be addressed.

Interventions. The patient should be instructed as to the meaning of a positive pap smear and reassured when the results indicate changes that are not malignant. Counseling women on the need for follow-up testing on an annual basis is critical. Education should include the need to protect the cervix from re-exposure to those elements that may contribute to abnormal transformation of the cervix. This may mean incorporating barrier methods such as condoms into sexual practice. Promotion of a healthy lifestyle with proper nutrition and adequate sleep and exercise should be encouraged in order to maintain an immune system that is functioning at its optimum. If the patient smokes, she needs to be advised that beginning data have illustrated women who smoke are more vulnerable to carcinoma of the cervix. If repeat tests indicate the presence of cervical malignancy, additional tests and biopsy will be performed. Supporting the patient during this time is essential. If additional tests confirm the diagnosis of cancer, hospitalization may be required, and the patient prepared for surgical or radiation procedures.

10

URINE CULTURE

Description

A *urine culture* is used to identify microorganisms associated with the occurrence of a urinary-tract infection. The culture is frequently accompanied by a sensitivity test to determine what antibiotics are effective against the pathogenic organisms cultured.

NORMAL RANGE

While the urinary tract is sterile at birth, small amounts of a number of microorganisms may be found in noninfected urine (Table 10.11). These organisms come from the surrounding tissues; however, they can cause urinary tract infections if in sufficient quantities. Other organisms are pathogenic as well (Table 10.11). Cultures of less than 1,000 bacterial colonies/ml usually represent contamination during specimen collection. Cultures of between 10,000 and 100,000/ml represent significant numbers, but are frequently repeated to confirm results. Cultures of more than 100,000/ml represent significant bacteriuria and are considered sufficient evidence for the diagnosis of a urinary-tract infection. Contamination is less common in the male because it is fairly easy to obtain a midstream specimen. In women, contamination is common because of the close proximity of the urethra to the vagina and rectum.

TABLE 10.11. Normal Urinary-Tract Flora When Found in Sufficiently Low Quantities

Fungus	Bacteria
Candida albicans	*Bacillus* species
Pityrosporon species	*Corynebacterium diphtheriae*
	Enterobacter species
	Escherichia coli
	Lactobacillus species
	Proteus species
	Staphylococcus albus
	Staphylococcus aureus
	Streptococcus faecalis
	Streptococcus species

Specimen Required

A clean-voided midstream specimen is needed for patients who do not have an indwelling catheter. If an indwelling catheter system is in place, the specimen is collected via a needle through the catheter or a side port following cleansing.

Patient Preparation

The patient needs specific instructions as to the method needed to collect the specimen when a midstream specimen is required. For patients with indwelling catheters, the nurse should collect the specimen. See Chapter 1 for the process of collection of each of these specimens.

Causes of Deviation from Normal

A number of organisms are associated with urinary-tract infections (Table 10.12). Sources of infection with microorganisms such as *Escherichia coli* and *Candida albicans* are the rectum, the vagina, and urinary catheters. In these infections the source of infection has ascended into the urinary tract. The frequency of ascending urinary-tract infections associated with catheterization is very high. The source of infection with organisms such as *Staphylococcus* and *Streptococcus* is generally the blood, and the infection has descended into the urinary tract.

Nursing Implications of Abnormal Findings

Assessment. When the patient has a positive urine culture, the nurse should assess the patient for other clinical manifestations of infection. The temperature should be monitored, urine inspected for indications of cloudiness, and the patient should be interviewed for evidence of dysuria. Several urine cultures

TABLE 10.12. Common Urinary-Tract Infection Pathogens

10

Candida albicans	*Proteus* species
Corynebacterium vaginalis	*Providencia* species
Enterococcus species	*Pseudomonas aeruginosa*
Escherichia coli	*Salmonella* species
Hemophilus species	*Serratia* species
Enterobacter species	*Shigella* species
Klebsiella pneumoniae	*Staphylococcus* species
Mycobacterium species	*Streptococcus faecalis*
Neisseria gonorrhoeae	*Streptococcus pyrogens*
Proteus mirabilis	*Trichomonas vaginalis*

may be obtained. Continued assessment is needed to evaluate the effectiveness of treatment.

Interventions. Patients with positive urinary-tract infections will be placed on antibiotic therapy specific to the organisms identified. If therapy has begun before the results of the sensitivity have been received, the report should be reviewed as soon as possible, and the antibiotics evaluated as to their appropriateness. Patients should be instructed to maintain adequate fluid intake, and intake and output should be evaluated.

BIBLIOGRAPHY

Baltimore, D., and S. Wolff. *Confronting AIDS—Update 1988*. Washington DC: Institute of Medicine, National Academy of Sciences, 1988.

Bloch, K.J., and J.E. Salvaggio. "Use and Interpretation of Diagnostic Immunologic Laboratory Tests." *Journal of the American Medical Association*, 248:2734–2758 (November 26, 1982).

Breslin, E. "Genital Herpes Simplex." *Nursing Clinics of North America*, 23:907–915 (December 1988).

Byrne, C.J., D.F. Saxton, P.K. Pelikan, and P.M. Nugent. *Laboratory Tests: Implications for Nursing Care*. Menlo Park: Addison-Wesley, 1986.

Centers for Disease Control. "Recommendations for Preventing Transmission of Infection with Human T-Lymphotropic Virus Type III/Lymphadenopathy-Associated Virus in the Workplace." *Morbidity and Mortality Weekly Report*, 34:681–686, 691–695 (November 15, 1985).

Centers for Disease Control. "Recommendations for Prevention of HIV Transmission in Health-Care Settings." *Morbidity and Mortality Weekly Report*, 36:1–17 (Supplement No. 2S) (August 21, 1987).

Centers for Disease Control. "Update: Universal Precautions for Prevention of Transmission of Human Immunodeficiency Virus, Hepatitis B Virus, and Other Bloodborne Pathogens in Health-Care Settings." *Morbidity and Mortality Weekly Report*, 37:377–382, 387–388 (June 24, 1988).

Centers for Disease Control. "Guidelines for Prevention of Transmission of Human Immunodeficiency Virus and Hepatitis B Virus to Health-Care and Public-Safety Workers." *Morbidity and Mortality Weekly Report*, 38:1–37 (Supplement No. S-6) (February 1989).

Centers for Disease Control. "Recommendations for Preventing Transmission of Human Immunodeficiency Virus and Hepatitis-B Virus to Patients During Exposure-Prone Invasive Procedures." *Morbidity and Mortality Weekly Report*, 40:1–9 (Recommendations and Reports) (July 12, 1991).

Corbett, J.V. *Laboratory Tests and Diagnostic Procedures with Nursing Diagnoses*. Norwalk, CT: Appleton and Lange, 1992.

Crummy, V. "Hospital Acquired Urinary Tract Infection." *Nursing Times,* 81:6–11 (June 1985).

Davies, K. "Genital Herpes: An Overview." *Journal of Obstetrics, Gynecology and Neonatal Nursing,* 19:401–406 (October 1990).

Dawkins, B.J. "Genital Herpes Simplex Infections." *Primary Care,* 17:95–111 (March 1990).

Ferenczy, A. "Human Papillomavirus." *Obstetrics and Gynecology Reports,* 1:167–191 (1991).

Fischbach, R.T. *A Manual of Laboratory and Diagnostic Tests.* Philadelphia: J.B. Lippincott Company, 1992.

Fiumara, J.J. "Lymphogranuloma Venereum." *Medical Aspects of Human Sexuality,* 20:82, 87–88 (October 1986).

Fiumara, N.J. "Trichomoniasis." *Medical Aspects of Human Sexuality,* 20:33–34 (February 1986).

Fogal, C. "Gonorrhea: Not a New Problem but a Serious One." *Nursing Clinics of North America,* 23:885–897 (December 1988).

Guinan, M.E. "Oral Acyclovar for Treatment and Suppression of Genital Herpes Simplex Virus Infection." *Journal of the American Medical Association,* 255:1747–1749 (April 4, 1986).

Heller, M.B. "Generally Unrecognized Effects of Sexually Transmitted Diseases." *Medical Aspects of Human Sexuality,* 19:186–188, 193 (January 1985).

Hubbard, S.B., P.E. Greene, and M.T. Knobf. "Cervical Cancer: the Role of Human Papillomavirus." *Current Issues in Cancer Nursing Practice Updates,* 1(2): 1–9 (1992).

Ignatavicius, D.D., and M.V. Bayne. *Medical-Surgical Nursing: A Nursing Process Approach.* Philadelphia: W.B. Saunders, 1991.

Lewis, S.M., and I.C. Collier. *Medical-Surgical Nursing: Assessment and Management of Clinical Problems.* St. Louis: Mosby Yearbook, 1992.

Luckman, J., and K.C. Sorensen. *Medical-Surgical Nursing: A Psychophysiological Approach.* Philadelphia: Saunders, 1987.

Martin, L.D., and P.S. Braly. "Gynecologic Cancers." In S. Baird, R. McCorkle, and M. Grant. *Cancer Nursing: A Comprehensive Textbook.* Philadelphia: W.B. Saunders, 1991.

McElhose, P. "The Other STDs." *RN,* 51:52–57 (June 1988).

NCI Workshop. "The 1988 Bethesda Report on Cervical/Vaginal Cytologic Diagnoses." *Journal of the American Medical Association,* 262:931–934 (August 18, 1989).

Paavonen, J. "Mucopurulent Cervicitis: An Often Ignored STD." *Medical Aspects of Human Sexuality,* 6:132, 134, 138–140 (June 1985).

10

Phipps, W.S., B.C. Long, N.F. Woods, and V. Cossmeyer. *Medical-Surgical Nursing*. St. Louis: Mosby Yearbook, 1991.

Ravel, R. *Clinical Laboratory Medicine*. Chicago: Year Book Medical Publishers, 1989.

Rein, M.F. "Evaluation of Women with Vulvovaginitis." *Medical Aspects of Human Sexuality*, 19:100, 102, 107–110, 113, 114 (December 1985).

Sacher, R.A., and R.A. McPherson, *Widmann's Clinical Interpretation of Laboratory Tests*. Philadelphia: F.A. Davis, 1991.

Secor, R. "Bacterial Vaginosis: A Comprehensive Review." *Nursing Clinics of North America*, 23:865–875 (December 1988).

Smetzer, S.C., and B.G. Ball. *Brunner and Sudarth's Medical-Surgical Nursing*. New York: J.B. Lippincott, 1992.

Swanson, J.M., and W.C. Chanitz. "Psychosocial Aspects of Genital Herpes: A Review of the Literature." *Public Health Nursing*, 7:96–104 (June 1990).

Wallach, J. *Interpretation of Diagnostic Tests*. Boston: Little, Brown, and Company, 1992.

Washington, A.E., S. Gove, J. Schachter, and R.L. Sweet. "Oral Contraceptives, *Chlamydia trachomatis* Infection and Pelvic Inflammatory Disease." *Journal of the American Medical Association*, 253:2246–2250 (April 19, 1985).

Wasley, G. "Detecting Sexually Transmitted Diseases." *Nursing Times*, 84:59–61 (September 28, 1988).

Wasley, G. "No Ordinary Microbes." *Nursing Times*, 84:50–51 (September 28, 1988).

Wilson, J.D., *et al. Harrison's Principles of Internal Medicine*. New York: McGraw-Hill, 1991.

11

Laboratory Tests of Reproductive System

Estrogens
  Estrone (E₁)
  Estradiol (E₂)
  Estriol (E₃)

Progesterone

Prolactin (Lactogenic Hormone, Lactogen, Luteotrophic)

Gonadotropins

Testosterone

Urine Pregnanediol

Urine Pregnanetriol

Urine Follicle-Stimulating Hormone and Luteinizing Hormone

Alpha₁-Fetoprotein (AFP)

Amniotic Fluid Analysis

Human Chorionic Gonadotropin

Human Placental Lactogen

Semen Examination and Analysis

ESTROGENS

Description

Estrogens are hormones secreted by the ovaries and placenta during pregnancy. Over thirty estrogens have been identified but only 3 are measured—*estrone* (E_1), *estradiol* (E_2), and *estriol* (E_3). In post menopausal women, all estrogen is produced from the conversion of androsenedione from the adrenal glands. In men, estradiol is secreted by the testes from extraglandular conversion of testosterone and estrone.

ESTRONE (E₁)

Estrone is derived from estradiol metabolism and is the principle precursor for the formation of other estrogens.

11

ESTRADIOL (E₂)

Estradiol is the most biologically active hormone and is secreted almost entirely by the ovaries.

ESTRIOL (E₃)

Estriol is derived partly from the placenta and partly from the fetal adrenal glands. Its production correlates with fetal growth rate and changes as pregnancy progresses. Urinary estriol levels vary, as they are influenced by the maternal excretory function and urine volume.

NORMAL RANGE

Estrone (E₁)	
Men	100–175 pg/mL
Women—non-pregnant	80–400 pg/mL
Estradiol (E₂)	
Men	10–50 pg/mL
Women—non-pregnant	10–340 pg/mL
Women—post-menopausal	10–50 pg/mL
Estriol (E₃)	
Pregnant women	
25–28 weeks	25–140 pg/mL
29–32	31–180 pg/mL
33–34	40–270 pg/mL
35–36	50–340 pg/mL
37–38	75–410 pg/mL
39–40	98–450 pg/mL
Urine	
Estrone (E₁)	
Men	3.4–8.2 μg/24 hours
Women—non-pregnant	4–32 μg/24 hours
Women—post-menopausal	0.8–7.1 μg/24 hours
Children	0.2–1.0 μg/24 hours
Estradiol (E₂)	
Men	0–0.4 μg/24 hours
Women—non-pregnant	0–14 μg/24 hours
Women—post-menopausal	0–2.3 μg/24 hours
Children	0–0.2 μg/24 hours
Estriol (E₃)	
Men	0.3–2.4 μg/24 hours
Women—non-pregnant	0–54 μg/24 hours
Women—post-menopausal	0.6–6.8 μg/24 hours
Women—pregnant	
<15 weeks	0.4–3.5 μg/24 hours

16–20 weeks	3.5–7 µg/24 hours
21–28 weeks	4–1.5 µg/24 hours
29–32 weeks	6–20 µg/24 hours
33–36 weeks	10–30 µg/24 hours
37–40 weeks	15–42 µg/24 hours
Children	generally not done

Note: Normal values may vary. The above are general reference values. Consult local laboratories for variation in values.

Specimen Required
BLOOD

A 10-ml sample of venous blood is collected in a plain collecting tube or syringe or a collecting tube or syringe containing EDTA or heparin. The specimen should be collected in the morning and delivered to the laboratory immediately. The phase of the menstrual cycle in pre-menopausal women should be noted on the laboratory slip.

URINE

A 24-hour urine specimen is collected in a bottle containing 15 ml of concentrated hydrochloric acid.

Preparation of the Patient
BLOOD

There are no food or fluid restrictions before venipuncture.

URINE

There are no food or fluid restrictions before urine collection. If the patient collects the specimen at home, he or she should be told about the importance of obtaining a complete specimen.

Causes of Deviation from Normal
ESTRIOL

Serious fetal disease causes estriol levels to fall. A sharp downward trend indicates fetal difficulty. A drop of 30–40% below previous levels on 2 consecutive days, or a fall of 35% or more on a single day from the preceding 3 days' average is a serious drop.

Decreases can also be caused by maternal renal or liver dysfunction. Ovarian agenesis and ovarian dysfunction are also causes in a non-pregnant woman. Increased estriol levels can be seen in cases of adrenocortical hyperplasia, adrenocortical tumor, and some ovarian and testicular tumors.

11

TABLE 11.1.	Drugs that Cause an Increase in Estriol Levels

Ampicillin
Adrenocorticosteroids
Hydrochlorthiozide (Hydrodiuril)
Neomycin

ESTRADIOL

Increases may be seen with ovarian tumors, testicular tumors, and adrenal hyperplasia or tumors. Decreases are associated with primary amenorrhea, ovarian dysfunction, pituitary insufficiency and menopause. Estradiol is most often measured to evaluate gonadal dysfunction.

Nursing Implications of Abnormal Findings
ESTRIOL

Assessment and Interventions. When assessing a patient with a decrease in estriol values, the nurse should look for evidence of developing trends. Urine specimens collected for several days should be examined. In pregnant women, a drop that equals or exceeds 50% of the previous value is firm evidence that fetal distress is present. The physician should be notified and the patient closely monitored for further signs and symptoms of fetal distress. Uterine contour should be examined, fetal movement assessed, and the fetal heart rate auscultated.

The nurse should be aware of the fear and anxiety that will be experienced by most patients who are told about the possibility of fetal distress. The nurse should allow time for the patient to express concern and ask questions. The father should be included in teaching or information-giving sessions whenever possible. The parents should be told that fetal monitoring may be used during labor, and the procedure and equipment should be described. The possibility of delivery by caesarian section should also be discussed and the reasons explained.

The nurse must remember that estriol levels are not reliable indicators of fetal well-being in Rh-sensitized women or in pregnancies complicated by eclampsia. The patient should also be asked if she is taking any drugs that depress estriol levels (Table 11.2).

ESTRADIOL

Assessment and Interventions. Since there are several causes of increases and decreases in estradiol levels, a medical-surgical or gynecological nursing textbook should be consulted when the cause of abnormal estradiol levels is diagnosed.

TABLE 11.2. Drugs that Can Depress Estriol Levels

Ampicillin	Methenamine mandelate
Cascara	Phenazopyridine
Corticosteroids	Phenolphthalein
Diethylstilbestrol	Senna
Hydrochlorothiazide	Tetracyclines
Meprobamate	

PROGESTERONE

Description

The steroid hormone *progesterone* is secreted by the corpus luteum in non-pregnant women during child-bearing years. Progesterone causes preparation of the endometrium for implantation of the fertilized ovum. A pregnancy is maintained by placental secretion of progesterone. Along with estrogen, progesterone prepares the breasts for lactation. If implantation of a fertilized ovum does not occur, progesterone levels drop and menstruation begins. Small amounts of progesterone are also secreted by the adrenal glands in both men and women.

NORMAL RANGE

Female	
Follicular Phase	0.1–1.5 ng/mL
Luteal Phase	1.2–28 ng/mL
Pregnancy	
First Trimester	9–50 ng/mL
Second Trimester	17–146 ng/mL
Third Trimester	55–260 ng/ml
Post-menopause	0–0.2 ng/mL
Male	0–1.0 ng/mL

Note: Consult laboratory as normal values vary among laboratories.

11

Specimen Required

A 7–10-ml sample of venous blood is collected in a plain collecting tube or syringe or in a tube or syringe containing heparin. If the patient is taking a progesterone preparation, such as birth control pills or ACTH, a note should be made on the laboratory slip.

Preparation of the Patient

All food and fluids except water should be withheld for 12 hours before the test.

Causes of Deviation from Normal

Increased levels of progesterone not associated with pregnancy may be caused by ovarian tumors or cysts, adrenocortical hypoplasia and adrenal tumors. Progesterone levels may also be elevated in patients who are on ACTH or progesterone therapy. Progesterone levels are decreased in panhypopituitarism, gonadal dysfunction, and Stein-Leventhal syndrome. In pregnant women, progesterone decreases when there is a threatened abortion, toxemia of pregnancy, fetal death, or placental failure.

Nursing Implications of Abnormal Findings

Assessment and Interventions. When the nurse has an opportunity to work with a patient with an abnormal menstrual cycle, assessment should include an evaluation of how the patient views herself, her concept of what an abnormal menstrual cycle means, and if she hopes to have children. If the patient hopes to have children, she should be referred to a clinic or physician who deals with problems of hormone imbalance. It is essential to provide emotional support without giving false hope or high expectations of successful treatment.

If the patient is pregnant and has a decrease in progesterone levels, the nurse should determine what the patient knows about the test and its relationship to the possibility of fetal distress due to placental dysfunction. Emotional support is the focus of nursing care when progesterone levels are falling before delivery of the infant.

PROLACTIN (LACTOGENIC HORMONE, LACTOGEN, LUTEOTROPHIC HORMONE)

Description

Prolactin is secreted by the acidophil cells of the anterior pituitary gland unless inhibited by prolactin-inhibiting factor from the hypothalamus. Prolactin is secreted in both men and women; levels in women during child-bearing years are elevated. In men and non-pregnant women, secretion rises in response to exercise, sleep, stress and hypoglycemia. Prolactin levels rise during pregnancy and increase during breast feeding. Prolactin levels fall after delivery in mothers who do not breast feed their infants.

NORMAL RANGE	
Men and children	1–20 ng/mL
Women	
Pre-menopausal	
Follicular Phase	1–23 ng/mL
Luteal Phase	5–40 ng/mL
Women	
Post-menopausal	1–20 ng/mL

Specimen Required

A 5-ml sample of venous blood is obtained in a plain collecting tube or syringe or in a tube or syringe containing EDTA. Venipuncture should be performed at least 2 hours after the patient awakens because of sleep-induced rises in prolactin. A note should be made on the laboratory slip if the patient is taking a drug that may cause an elevation in prolactin level. (Table 11.3).

Preparation of the Patient

All food and fluids except water should be withheld for 12 hours before the test.

Causes of Deviation from Normal

An increase in prolactin levels may be caused by disorders of the hypothalamus, diseases of the pituitary stock, a pituitary tumor that secretes prolactin, or hypothyroidism. Some tumors of the lungs and kidneys may also be associated with increased levels of prolactin.

Nursing Implications of Abnormal Findings

Assessment and Interventions. Women who have increased prolactin levels should be assessed for amenorrhea, anovulation, and galactorrhea. The nursing assessment of men with increased levels should include questions about

TABLE 11.3. Drugs that may Cause an Increase in Prolactin Levels

11

Aldomet (methyldopa)	Meprobamate
Amphetamines	Phenothiazines
Benzamides	Procainamide
Estrogens	Reserpine
Haloperidol	Tricyclic antidepressants

the presence of impotence. The chest should be observed for signs of gyneco-mastia. Since increased prolactin levels affect sexual function in both men and women, the nurse should assess the patient's psychological response to the changes and their effect on the patient's life. A teaching plan should include a discussion of why these changes have occurred and a discussion of the medical plan of care. Emotional support for the patient, family, and significant others is an important aspect of nursing care.

Additional areas of assessment and interventions are related to the patho-physiological cause of increased prolactin levels. A medical-surgical nursing textbook should be consulted for related nursing care.

GONADOTROPINS

Description

The *gonadotropins* include follicle-stimulating hormone (FSH), luteinizing hor-mone (LH), and luteotropic hormone (LTH). FSH and LH are largely protein hormones that regulate hormonal secretion from the ovaries and testes. Their secretion is regulated by the sex hormones and the hypothalamus. The hypo-thalamus secretes hormones that control the release of FSH, LH, and LTH from the pituitary gland (Fig. 11.1). FSH promotes maturation of the ovarian follicle in women. LH is produced when there is a rise in the amount of estro-gen produced by the maturing follicle. The activity of FSH and LH causes the ovum to mature and the follicle to rupture. In men, FSH stimulates spermato-genesis and LH stimulates the secretion of androgens.

NORMAL RANGE	
FSH	
Men	up to 15 mIU/ml
Women	
Menstruating	up to 10 mIU/ml
Midcycle peak	up to 20 mIU/ml
Post-menopausal	up to 200 mIU/ml
Children	up to 12 mIU/ml
LH	
Men	up to 15 mIU/ml
Women	
Menstruating	up to 10 mIU/ml
Midcycle peak	up to 80 mIU/ml
Children	up to 12 mIU/ml

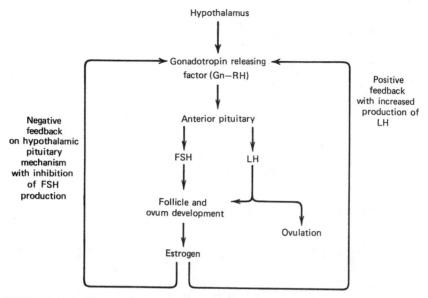

FIGURE 11.1. Hormonal control of FSH and LH and their effect on ovulation. FSH and LH secretions are stimulated by Gn-RH. When estrogen secretion begins with a low plasma concentration, there is a negative feedback inhibition of FSH. As estrogen plasma levels peak during the late follicular phase of ovulation, there is a positive feedback stimulation of LH.

During infancy, the serum values of both FSH and LH are low. Levels of both gonadotropins increase during puberty. FSH reaches a maximum at mid-puberty and LH at the end of puberty. The secretions of both FSH and LH are episodic in the adult man. FSH has a low oscillation level, whereas LH has 9–14 secretory surges every 24 hours. In about the sixth decade, decreasing testosterone and inhibin levels cause a gradual rise in LH and FSH with variations among individuals.

In adult women, all ovulatory menstrual cycles have similar patterns of FSH and LH secretions (Figs. 11.2, 11.3). After menopause, these hormones continue to have an episodic secretion pattern; levels of FSH are higher. This may be attributable to lack of inhibition of an ovarian substance. LH levels may also become slightly higher after menopause.

Specimen Required

A 5-ml specimen of venous blood is required for the test.

Preparation of the Patient

No food or fluid restrictions are required before collection of the specimen. The patient should be told if several specimens are to be collected over a period of time.

11

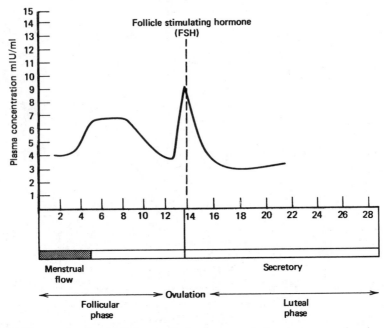

FIGURE 11.2. Levels of follicle-stimulating hormone during the menstrual cycle

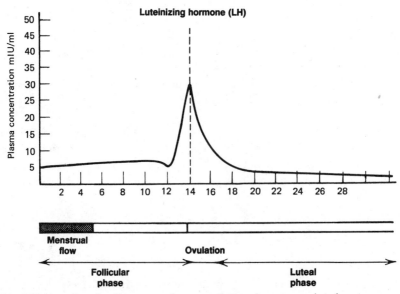

FIGURE 11.3. Levels of luteinizing hormone during the menstrual cycle

Causes of Deviation from Normal

The secretion of gonadotropins depends upon the activity of certain areas of the hypothalamus, normal functioning of the pituitary gland, and the activity of the sex hormones. The causes of abnormal gonadotropin secretion are many. Decreases can be caused by hypopituitarism, Kallman's syndrome, isolated gonadotropin deficiency, or delayed puberty. Increased levels occur with anorchidism, testicular failure, Klinefelter's syndrome, or menopause.

Nursing Implications of Abnormal Findings

Assessment and Interventions. Infertility, lack of development of secondary sex characteristics, and changes in sexual characteristics or sexual functioning are the most common reasons for measuring the gonadotropins. These are all sensitive problems for patients. The nursing assessment of patients with this problem should focus on psychological factors, such as denial, disappointment, and despair. Matter-of-fact responses to the nurse's questions or signs that the patient does not appear upset or disturbed may be clues to the patient's hidden emotional reaction.

The major focus of nursing interventions is to let the patient know that these feelings are normal. If the patient does not want to discuss them, the primary intervention may be to represent reality to the patient by giving permission to experience anger or depression rather than suppression.

The patient should also be encouraged to seek information about the nature of the physiological condition if infertility is present. The nurse should provide the information and the patient should be encouraged to join a support group for infertile couples or to consider alternate approaches to parenthood, such as adoption or foster parenthood.

TESTOSTERONE

Description

Testosterone is a sex hormone predominant in males, that is secreted by the adrenal glands and testes in men and by the adrenal glands and ovaries in women. It stimulates the seminiferous tubules in the testes, and, in conjunction with the pituitary follicle-stimulating hormone, stimulates spermatogenesis. Testosterone secretion initiates male secondary sexual characteristics.

11

N O R M A L R A N G E	
Men	406–950 mg/dl
Women	40–120 mg/dl
Children	>100 mg/dl

Specimen Required

Three 10-ml specimens of venous blood are collected from male patients and five specimens from female patients in plain collecting tubes or syringes. The name and sex of the patient should be specified on both the laboratory slip and the specimen.

Preparation of the Patient

Foods and fluids are not restricted before venipuncture.

Causes of Deviation from Normal

Decreased testosterone levels in men occur in hypogonadism, hypopituitarism, orchidectomy, and Klinefelter's syndrome. The deficiency may be associated with primary dysfunction of the testes or with inadequate pituitary stimulation. In women, increased levels of testosterone are associated with adrenogenital syndrome, Stein-Leventhal syndrome, and adrenal and ovarian neoplasms.

Nursing Implications of Abnormal Findings

Assessment and Interventions. Assessment of a man with decreased testosterone levels should include observation of changes in male secondary sexual characteristics. The pattern of hair growth, the pitch of the voice, the muscular development, and the external genitalia may all show signs of decreased male hormone levels. Increased levels of testosterone in a woman should be followed by assessment of female secondary sex characteristics. The pattern of hair growth, breast size, and muscular development may show signs of masculinization. The patient's emotional and mental state should also be included in the assessment. Interventions vary depending on the condition present, but they should include psychosocial support for the patient and family and protection of the patient from curious onlookers, including members of the nursing staff. Medications ordered should be administered and a teaching plan discussed if therapy is to continue after discharge.

Causes of Deviation from Normal

A positive result usually indicates pregnancy. However, the following conditions may also cause positive results: chorionepithelioma, hydatidiform mole, choriocarcinoma, chorioadenoma destruens, and conditions with an elevated erythrocyte sedimentation rate (ESR). Positive pregnancy tests occur in two-thirds of women with ectopic pregnancies.

Nursing Implications of Abnormal Findings

Assessment and Interventions. If a nurse is present when a patient receives the results of a pregnancy test, the nursing assessment should focus on determining whether the patient is pleased with the results. When the HCG test confirms a pregnancy desired by the patient, the nurse can use this opportunity to help the patient develop a plan for good prenatal care. If the pregnancy is not wanted, the nurse should help the patient seek the guidance and counseling necessary to help her make a decision about the outcome of the pregnancy.

When the results are negative in a women who was expecting positive results, the nurse should help the patient cope with her disappointment. See the section on gonadotropins for more detailed information.

If elevated levels of HCG are caused by a hydatidiform mole, the nurse should focus on the patient's response to learning that her pregnancy has not resulted in a fetus. Nursing interventions include: (1) psychological support for the patient based on her response to the diagnosis; (2) an explanation of the dilation and curettage (D&C) needed to remove the contents of conception; and (3) discussion of the importance of follow-up evaluation and testing to determine the continuing or recurring presence of HCG in the urine. The patient should understand the reason for follow-up. The mole can recur or choriocarcinoma can develop, thus early diagnosis is essential for successful therapy.

URINE PREGNANEDIOL

Description

Urine pregnanediol is a metabolite of progesterone. It provides a measurement of ovarian and placental functioning because of its relationship to circulating plasma progesterone. During a normal menstrual cycle, progesterone concentrations rise rapidly during the middle of the luteal phase and remain elevated until just before menses, when there is a rapid fall. Progesterone causes the secretory phase of the endometrium, preparing it for a fertilized ovum. If implantation does occur, the progesterone level remains elevated, since this hormone is necessary for placenta formation.

NORMAL RANGE	
Proliferative (preovulatory) phase	<1 mg/24 h
Luteal phase	2.5–6 mg/24 h
Post-menopausal	0.2–1 mg/24 h
Pregnancy	6–200 mg/24 h

11

Specimen Required

A 24-hour refrigerated urine specimen is required.

Preparation of the Patient

There are no food or fluid restrictions. The patient should be informed of the purpose and method of collection of a 24-hour urine specimen. Specific instructions are provided in Chapter 1.

Causes of Deviation from Normal

Decreased progesterone levels can occur with an abnormal menstrual cycle and may be accompanied by amenorrhea. During pregnancy, urinary pregnanediol levels drop with severe placental dysfunction, but not in time to detect impending problems. Pregnanediol assays are not useful in the diagnosis of problem pregnancies and fetal death because progesterone does not have fetal precursors.

Nursing Implications of Abnormal Findings

Assessment and Interventions. When the nurse has an opportunity to work with a patient who has an abnormal menstrual cycle, assessment should include an evaluation of how the patient views herself, her concept of what an abnormal menstrual cycle means, and if she hopes to have children. If the patient hopes to have children, she should be referred to a clinic or physician who deals with problems of hormone imbalance. It is essential to provide emotional support without giving false hope or high expectations of successful treatment.

If the patient is pregnant and has a decrease in pregnanediol levels, the nurse should determine what the patient knows about the test and its relationship to the possibility of fetal distress due to placental dysfunction. Emotional support is the focus of nursing care when progesterone levels are falling before delivery of the infant.

URINE PREGNANETRIOL

Description

Pregnanetriol is a precursor of the synthesis of adrenal corticoid hormones. It is used in hormone synthesis.

N O R M A L R A N G E	
Adults	up to 2 mg/24 h
Children	up to 1.5 mg/24 h
Newborns	up to 0.2 mg/24 h

Specimen Required

A 24-hour urine specimen is required for the test. The specimen container should contain a preservative.

Preparation of the Patient

Restriction of bananas, pineapples, and avocados is required for at least 24 hours before the test. The procedure for collection of a 24-hour urine specimen is described in Chapter 1.

Causes of Deviation from Normal

Elevations of pregnanetriol are rare and occur in *adrenogenital syndrome* (congenital adrenocortical hyperplasia) and in *Stein-Leventhal syndrome*.

Nursing Implications of Abnormal Findings

Assessment and Interventions. Assessment of patients with elevations in pregnanetriol includes observation for changes in external genitalia, virulism in women, and early puberty in boys. Treatment involves injection of cortisone or cortisone products. Nursing interventions include teaching the patient and family about the need for prescribed administration of medication and the need for follow-up medical care.

URINE FOLLICLE-STIMULATING HORMONE AND LUTEINIZING HORMONE

Description

Follicle-stimulating hormone (FSH) and *luteinizing hormone* (LH) are gonadotropins secreted by the pituitary gland. In women, FSH stimulates the maturation of the ovarian follicle in which the ovum is located. Both hormones together induce ovulation. In men, FSH stimulates spermatogenesis and LH stimulates secretion of androgens.

NORMAL RANGE	
Follicle-Stimulating Hormone (FSH)	
Adult men	1–20 IU/24 h
Adult women	5–20 IU/24 h
Post-menopausal women	30–440 IU/24 h
Children	Consult Laboratory
Newborns	Consult Laboratory
Luteinizing Hormone (LH)	
Adult men	5–20 IU/24 h
Adult women	5–15 IU/24 h
Post-menopausal women	50–100 IU/24 h
Children	Consult Laboratory
Newborns	Consult Laboratory

11

Specimen Required

A 24-hour urine specimen is required.

Preparation of the Patient

Food and fluid restrictions are not necessary before or during collection period. See general rules for 24-hour collection in Chapter 1.

Causes of Deviation from Normal

The most usual causes of decreases in FSH and LH are ovarian tumors. Increases in FSH and LH levels occur in Turner's syndrome and hypogonadism.

Nursing Implications of Abnormal Findings

Assessment and Interventions. The nurse should evaluate the results of other laboratory tests when assessing the patient with increases or decreases in urine FSH and LH. Observation of sexually related symptoms should be carried out. Interventions depend on the kind of problems presented and are likely to include psychosocial support.

ALPHA$_1$-FETOPROTEIN (AFP)

Description

The glycoprotein *alpha$_1$-fetoprotein* (AFP) is produced by the fetal liver and is the major serum protein in the fetus. It is produced from the second to the thirty-second weeks of gestation. Normally, serum alpha$_1$-fetoprotein levels are present in small amounts in maternal serum and in larger amounts in amniotic fluid as a result of fetal urination. The peak level of AFP in amniotic fluid is reached by 13–15 weeks. In normal pregnancies, the maternal serum level of alpha$_1$-fetoprotein increases as the pregnancy progresses, but the amniotic fluid level begins to decrease after the sixteenth week.

NORMAL RANGE	
Maternal Serum	
Non-pregnant women	<15 ng/ml
Pregnant women	
12 weeks	<130 ng/ml
24 weeks	<400 ng/ml
32 weeks	<450 ng/ml
40 weeks	<375 ng/ml
Amniotic Fluid	
14 weeks	<36 μg/ml
22 weeks	<15 μg/ml
35 weeks	2 μg/ml
40 weeks	0.8 μg/ml

Specimen Required

SERUM

A 7-ml sample of venous blood is collected in a plain collecting tube or syringe.

AMNIOTIC FLUID

An amniocentesis is performed and amniotic fluid aspirated. A sample of clear amniotic fluid is transferred from the collecting syringe to a specified container and immediately sent to the laboratory.

Note. A specimen contaminated with blood will result in falsely elevated levels of AFP.

Preparation of the Patient

An informed consent should be signed and the patient told that results of the test will probably not be available for 3 weeks. The patient is asked to void immediately before the test. Food and fluids are not restricted prior to amniocentesis. Specific details of this procedure are discussed in Chapter 1.

Causes of Deviation from Normal

In non-pregnant individuals, elevated AFP levels occur with some malignancies such as primary cancer of the liver. Alpha$_1$-fetoprotein concentrations are elevated in amniotic fluid and maternal serum when there are open neural-tube defects. Levels are also elevated in multiple pregnancies, missed or threatened abortions, fetal death, congenital nephrosis, omphalocele, esophageal and duodenal atresia, and Turner's syndrome.

Nursing Implications of Abnormal Findings

Assessment and Interventions. Alpha$_1$-fetoprotein studies are done on women who are at risk for having a child with an open neural-tube defect. A pre-procedure nursing assessment should be done to determine the amount of knowledge the patient has about open neural-tube defects and the amount of anxiety she has about the test results. Since there are biological factors that affect serum alpha$_1$-fetoprotein levels, decisions about termination of the pregnancy should not be made on AFP levels alone. Exact gestational age must be determined and other causes of elevated AFP levels ruled out. Once the screening process is complete and the presence of an open neural-tube defect confirmed, the nurse should be prepared to give as much information to the parents as possible so then they can make an informed decision regarding termination of the pregnancy. If they choose not to do so, the nurse should assist them in planning for the child's birth. Pediatric and obstetric textbooks should be consulted for specific nursing care related to open neural-tube defects, as well as other congenital defects associated with elevations of alpha$_1$-fetoprotein.

11

AMNIOTIC FLUID ANALYSIS

Description

Amniotic fluid consists of the products of fetal pulmonary secretions and fetal metabolism. As the fetus matures, it also contains fetal urine. Amniotic fluid is produced by the cells of the amniotic sac's membrane; as the pregnancy progresses it is produced from the mother's blood. The volume of amniotic fluid varies with each individual. It increases from 50–350 ml after 20-weeks gestation to approximately 1,000 ml of fluid at term. Amniotic fluid analysis is done for the following reasons:

1. Maternal age of 35.
2. History of genetic disorders or chromosomal aberrations.
3. Mother is a probable carrier of X-linked inheritable disorders.
4. Potential risk of neural-tube defect.
5. Elevated maternal alpha$_1$-fetoprotein.
6. Assessment of fetal maturity.
7. Suspected hemolytic diseases of newborn.
8. Parental history of metabolic autosomal recessive disorder (e.g., cystic fibrosis).

NORMAL RANGE

Color	Clear—may be flecks of vernix caseosa in the mature fetus
Alpha$_1$-fetoprotein	Varies with length of gestation 15–4 µg/ml at 13–14 weeks 0.2–3.0 µg/ml at term
Bilirubin	Highest early in pregnancy Minimal amounts at term <0.075 mg/dl at 14–24 weeks <0.02 mg/dl at term
Creatinine	2–4 mg/dl at term
Lecithin/sphyngomyelin (L/S Ratio)	1.5:1–2:1 = 40% risk of Respiratory Distress Syndrome (RDS) 2:1 = 1–2% risk of RDS 3:1 = fetal pulmonary maturity
Phosphatidylglycerol	Present at 36 weeks. Absent in pulmonary immaturity

Specimen Required

An amniocentesis is performed and amniotic fluid aspirated. A 10–15-ml sample of amniotic fluid is transferred from the collecting syringe to a specified container and immediately sent to the laboratory.

Preparation of the Patient

An informed consent should be signed and the patient told that results of the test will probably not be available for 3 weeks. The patient is asked to void immediately prior to the test. Food and fluids are not restricted prior to amniocentesis. Specific details of this procedure are discussed in Chapter 1.

Causes of Deviation from Normal

The following abnormalities can be detected by examination of amniotic fluid: Downs syndrome, Turners syndrome, Trisomy 13, Trisomy 18, Tay-Sachs disease, neural-tube defects such as anancephaly, spina bifida, meningocele, myelomeningocele, encephalocele, sickle cell anemia, thalassemia, hemoglobinopathies, hemolytic disease of the newborn, fetal maturity, and maturity of pulmonary function.

Nursing Implications of Abnormal Findings

Assessment. The nursing assessment of the patient who has had an amniocentesis should begin prior to the procedure so the nurse will know the amount of information the patient has been given about the disorder and/or defect that has been diagnosed. A pre-procedure assessment will also help the nurse with the level of grieving the patient might be experiencing. Determining the patient's beliefs on abortion is also an important part of the nursing assessment.

Interventions. Nursing interventions must be planned depending on the specific diagnosis as a result of the amniocentesis and the patient's beliefs on abortion. When the test results indicate that there is a chromosomal aberration or genetic disorder, the parents should be given enough information about the disease and its potential problems to make an informed decision about abortion. Patients who choose not to terminate a pregnancy when informed of a fetal anomaly should be given support for their decision. The nurse can assist the parents with plans for caring for the infant by giving them information about the birth defect and the names of support groups in the area. The parents can also take an active role in decision-making regarding the place of delivery and postnatal care, particularly if surgery will be needed following delivery. If the amniocentesis is done to determine fetal maturity when fetal distress has been observed, the nurse should encourage parents to verbalize their concerns. Questions should be answered accurately and data given so that the family understands the status of the fetus and the risks involved.

Note: Parents should be told that the results of amniocentesis are not 100% accurate and that negative results do not guarantee that the child will be free of congenital defects.

11

HUMAN CHORIONIC GONADOTROPIN

Description

Human chorionic gonadotropin (HCG) is a glycoprotein produced by placental trophoblastic tissue. It may be detected in the blood and urine shortly after implantation of a fertilized ovum. Animal pregnancy tests for HCG have been replaced by immunoassay tests, which are easier to perform.

NORMAL RANGE

Negative blood and urine tests are normal for non-pregnant women. When concentrations of HCG are present, they are expressed as IU/ml urine or serum or ng/ml urine or serum. The relationship between IU/ml and ng/ml is:

$$1 \text{ IU/ml} = 83.3 \text{ ng/ml}$$
$$1 \text{ mIU/ml} = 0.08 \text{ ng/ml}$$
$$1 \text{ ng/ml} = 12 \text{ MIU/ml}$$

Blood
Men	<0.01 IU/ml
Women (non-pregnant)	<0.01 IU/ml
Women (pregnant)	
1 week	0.010–0.04 IU/ml
4 weeks	1–10 IU/ml
5–12 weeks	10–100 IU/ml
13–24 weeks	10–30 IU/ml
25 weeks	5–15 IU/ml

Urine
Men	negative
Women (non-pregnant)	negative
Women (pregnant)	
1–12 weeks	6000–500,000 IU/24 hours
13–24 weeks	5000–350,000 IU/24 hours
25 weeks	2500–150,000 IU/24 hours

Note: False-positive test results may be caused by proteinuria, hematuria, the presence of excessive gonadotropin, or by several drugs, such as tranquilizers and oral contraceptives. False-negative test results may be caused by use of very dilute urine as a sample, proteinuria, or hematuria.

Specimen Required
URINE
Collecting an early-morning urine specimen is most desirable, since the greatest concentration of HCG is present at that time. However, a specimen collected at any time of day may be used provided it is not grossly contaminated and does not contain blood.

BLOOD
A 10-ml sample of venous blood is collected in a plain collecting tube or syringe.

Preparation of the Patient

Food and fluids are not usually restricted before venipuncture. A note should be made on the laboratory slip if the patient is taking any medications that can interfere with test results.

HUMAN PLACENTAL LACTOGEN

Description

The hormone *human placental lactogen* (hPL) is secreted by the placental trophophoblasts. Production begins about the fifth week of gestation and increases gradually throughout pregnancy, with a rapid decline following delivery. hPL exerts its effect on the mother causing insulin resistance and the circulation of few fatty acids, making glucose and free fatty acids available for utilization by the growing fetus. This test is performed on women who have high-risk or difficult pregnancies or when fetal distress is present. It is often used with tests for estriol levels. Together, they are reliable indicators of placental function.

NORMAL RANGE	
Men	$<.5$ µg/ml
Women	
Non-pregnant	$<.5$ µg/ml
Pregnant	
5–27 weeks	<4.6 µg/ml
28–31 weeks	2.4–6.1 µg/ml
32–35 weeks	3.7–7.7 µg/ml
36 weeks—term	5.0–8.6 µg/ml
Diabetic—term	9–11 µg/ml

Specimen Required

A 5-ml sample of venous blood is collected in a plain collecting tube or syringe or in a tube or syringe with heparin.

Preparation of the Patient

There are no food or fluid restrictions before venipuncture.

Causes of Deviation from Normal

During the first trimester, hPL levels fall when there is an impending spontaneous abortion. In general, hPL levels will fall during the third trimester if there is fetal distress; however, falsely elevated levels may occur. Serial determinations will give the best indication of this.

11

Nursing Implications of Abnormal Findings

Assessment and Interventions. When serial determinations show a decrease in hPL levels, the nurse should assess the woman for signs and symptoms of fetal distress. Included are examination of uterine contour, assessment of fetal movements and auscultation of fetal heart tones.

The nurse should be aware of the fear and anxiety that will be experienced by most patients who are told about the possibility of fetal distress. The nurse should allow time for the patient to express concern and ask questions. The father should be included in teaching or information-giving sessions whenever possible. The parents should be told that fetal monitoring may be used during labor and the procedure and equipment should be described. The possibility of delivery by caesarian section should also be discussed and the reasons explained. If fetal death has occurred, the nurse should assess the stage of the parents' grieving process and plan appropriate nursing care. The nurse can also offer information about available counseling and local support groups for parents who have experienced fetal death.

SEMEN EXAMINATION AND ANALYSIS

Description

Semen examination and analysis is performed to:

1. evaluate male fertility;
2. determine the effectiveness of vasectomy as indicated by two sperm-free samples, one month apart;
3. detect semen on or in the body or clothing of an alleged rape victim;
4. determine the presence of sterility in a paternity suit.

NORMAL RANGE	
Volume	0.7–6.5 ml/ejaculate
Sperm Count	60–150 million/ml
Sperm Motility	60% or more show good movement
Sperm Morphology	Less than 30% abnormal forms
Fructose	Present
pH	7.3–7.7

Specimen Required

A semen sample is collected at home or in the doctor's office. It may be obtained by masturbation (the most common method of collection), coitus interruptus, or intercourse using a condom. When the patient uses masturbation or coitus interruptus, the specimen should be collected in a clean, plastic specimen container. If a condom is used, it should be washed and dried to remove spermatacidal material. The specimen should be taken to the laboratory within one hour and should *not* be allowed to become chilled.

When a semen specimen is collected from a rape victim, a post-coital pelvic examination is done and the specimen collected from vaginal secretions. When a specimen is to be obtained from a rape victim's wet or moist clothing, the clothing should be handled as little as possible and placed in a *paper* bag. A plastic bag may cause semen on clothing to mold. Dried semen may be collected from the skin by washing it with a small piece of gauze moistened with saline.

Preparation of the Patient

The ingestion of alcohol should be restricted for at least 24 hours before specimen collection. The patient should also abstain from intercourse for 3 days before semen collection.

Causes of Deviation from Normal

Male infertility may be caused by a decrease in the number of sperm, impaired sperm motility, or abnormal sperm forms. In many men the cause of these abnormalities may not be known. Others may have hypothyroidism, liver disease, hypoglycemia, alcoholism, or severe liver disease.

Nursing Implications of Abnormal Findings

The nursing care of patients with infertility should focus on psychological factors such as denial, disappointment, and despair. Matter-of-fact responses to the nurse's questions or signs that the patient does not appear upset or disturbed may be clues to the patient's hidden emotional reaction.

The major focus of nursing interventions is to let the patient know that these feelings are normal. If the patient does not want to discuss them, the primary intervention may be to represent reality to the patient by giving permission to experience anger or depression rather than suppression. The patient should be told that the nurse understands that the diagnosis of infertility is a severe disappointment. The patient should also be encouraged to seek information about the nature of the physiological condition responsible for the infertility. The nurse should provide information, if possible. The patient can be encouraged to join a support group for infertile couples or to consider alternate approaches to parenthood such as adoption or foster parenthood.

When a semen analysis is done on a rape victim, a psychological assessment and emotional support are important aspects of nursing care. A discussion of

11

the trauma associated with rape are not within the scope of this book. Nursing textbooks that include information about all aspects of rape should be consulted for appropriate nursing care of the rape victim.

BIBLIOGRAPHY

Byrne, C.J., D.F. Saxton, P.K. Pelikan, and P.M. Nugent. *Laboratory Tests: Implications for Nursing Care*. Menlo Park: Addison-Wesley, 1986.

Cohen, R. "Neural-Tube Defects: Epidemiology, Detection and Prevention." *Journal of Obstetrics and Gynecological Neonatal Nursing*, 16:105–114 (March–April 1987).

Davies, D. "Genital Herpes—An Overview." *Journal of Obstetrics, Gynecology and Neonatal Nursing* 19:401–406 (September–October 1990).

Hoegsberg, B. "Surveillance of High Risk Pregnancies." *Journal of Medical Technology*, 3:486–489 (September 1986).

Luckman, J., and K.C. Sorensen. *Medical-Surgical Nursing: A Psychophysiological Approach*. Philadelphia: Saunders, 1987.

Ravel, R. *Clinical Laboratory Medicine*. Chicago: Year Book Medical Publishers, 1989.

Sacher, R.A., and R.A. McPherson. *Widmann's Clinical Interpretation of Laboratory Tests*. Philadelphia: F.A. Davis, 1991.

Smetzer, S.C., and B.G. Ball. *Brunner and Sudarth's Medical-Surgical Nursing*. New York: J.B. Lippincott, 1992.

Whalen, M. "Nursing Management of the Patient with *Chlamidia Trachomitis* Infection." *Nursing Clinics of North America*, 23:877–883 (December 1988).

Zorn, E. "Amniocentesis: Its Uses and Abuses and How to Prepare Patients." *Consultant*, 25:69–72, 76, 78–9 (November 30, 1985).

Laboratory Tests: Miscellaneous

CEREBROSPINAL FLUID TESTS

Description

Cerebrospinal fluid (CSF) is formed in the choroid plexus of the third, fourth, and lateral ventricles and circulates over the brain and around the spinal cord. Its formation from the venous bed in the choroid plexus involves both secretion and diffusion. It is a clear, colorless, odorless fluid similar to water, has a specific gravity of 1.007, and contains an occasional lymphocyte plus traces of mineral and organic substances from the blood. After circulating, it is absorbed back into the venous circulation from the cranial subarachnoid space through the arachnoid villi. The primary purpose of CSF is mechanical protection of the brain and spinal cord from injury through its action as a shock absorber.

12

Description

PRESSURE

The *pressure* of CSF results from the amount of fluid contained within the cerebrospinal space. It varies directly with venous pressure and has no constant relationship with arterial pressure.

N O R M A L   R A N G E

Adults	100–200 mm H_2O
Children	50–100 mm H_2O

If the Queckenstedt sign is used, the jugular veins are compressed; this normally causes an increase in CSF pressure in the lumbar region.

Specimen Required

A lumbar puncture is performed to measure the pressure of CSF. A water manometer is attached to a needle which has been introduced into the cerebrospinal space. Both opening and closing pressures are generally made; these correspond to pressures before and after withdrawal of CSF for laboratory analysis.

Preparation of the Patient

There are no food or fluid restrictions before the procedure.

Causes of Deviation from Normal

Increases in the CSF pressure occur with brain tumors, cerebral edema, congestive heart failure, encephalitis, neurosyphilis, low-grade inflammations, purulent or bacterial meningitis, subarachnoid hemorrhage, and extradural hemorrhage. Decreases may occur in tumors of the spinal cord, diabetic coma, when the cerebrospinal fluid is bloody, circulatory collapse, leakage of spinal fluid, and hyperosmolality.

Nursing Implications of Abnormal Findings

Assessment. When patients have increases in CSF pressure, an acute neurological problem is occurring and vigilant continuous neurological assessment is in order (Table 12.1). Any deterioration in these parameters should be reported to the physician. Further assessment is needed, depending on the suspected or identified pathology.

Interventions. If the patient is acutely ill and has an elevated CSF pressure, the nurse should be concerned about maintaining a patent airway, respirations,

TABLE 12.1. Neurological Assessment Parameters

Vital Signs	Blood pressure
	Central venous pressure
	Pulse
	Respirations
	Temperature
	Intracranial pressure
Pupillary response	Size
	Response to light
Arousal state	Arouses when called
	Arouses when shaken
	Arouses with light pain
	Arouses with deep pain
Consciousness status	Awake, alert
	Alert, memory lapses
	Drowsy
	Confused
	Stuporous
	Comatose
Movement	Moves arms
	Moves legs
	Involuntary movements
	Seizures
Pain response	Normal
	Withdrawal
	Decorticate
	Decerebrate

and circulation. Additional nursing interventions depend on the problems identified and the underlying pathology. A brief summary of some of the problem areas common to neurological patients and their associated nursing interventions is found in Table 12.2.

12

Description
BLOOD

The presence of *red cells* in the CSF is abnormal. It is an indication of bleeding into the cerebrospinal space.

Normally, there are no red cells in the CSF. Changes that occur in the color of CSF when red cells are present range from a yellowish discoloration to frank blood. The exact color depends upon the amount of bleeding and when it occurred.

Specimen Required

A small tube of 5–10 ml of CSF is required to examine the color and carry out a microscopic examination.

Preparation of the Patient

There are no food or fluid restrictions before the lumbar puncture. The nurse should note whether any trauma occurs with the insertion of the spinal needle, since this can be the cause of blood in the CSF.

Causes of Deviation from Normal

Blood is present in the CSF in cases of subarachnoid hemorrhage and ruptured cerebral aneurysm.

TABLE 12.2. Problems Common to Neurological Patients

Problem	Intervention
Hyperpyrexia	Sponge the patient with tepid water and provide for evaporation of body heat without shivering. A hypothermia blanket may be ordered.
Drainage of CSF from nose or ears	The drainage should be allowed to flow freely. The nurse should follow medical aseptic technique in handling the drainage.
Seizures	Protect the patient from injury during seizures by means of proper padding and positioning. Rapid administration of antiseizure medications can be facilitated by having the medication ready for prompt administration.
Immobility	Measures to prevent pneumonia, thrombus formation, and contractions should be implemented when danger of potentially fatal hemorrhage has passed. Skin breakdown may be prevented by positioning and the use of special mattresses.

Nursing Implications of Abnormal Findings

Assessment and Interventions. The nurse should do a neurological assessment when the patient returns from an acute-care setting to the regular unit. Interventions needed depend on the symptoms present and underlying pathology.

Description

CELLS

The presence of *cells* other than an occasional lymphocyte in the CSF is abnormal. Presence of red cells is discussed in the preceding section. Other cells that can be present in CSF in pathological conditions include neutrophils, monocytes, lymphocytes, malignant cells, lymphocytoid and plasmacytoid cells, macrophages, and various neurological cells, including glial, ependymal, and plexus cells.

N O R M A L   R A N G E

Normally there are no cells, except for an occasional lymphocyte, in CSF.

Specimen Required

A small tube of 5–10 ml of CSF is required. The specimen may be examined directly under the microscope or centrifuged and then examined.

Preparation of the Patient

There are no food or fluid restrictions before the lumbar puncture.

Causes of Deviation from Normal

Presence of different cells in the CSF is associated with different disease processes. In general, the presence of white cells indicates an inflammatory condition, usually an infection. The higher the white cell count, the more severe the infection. Repeat lumbar punctures may be done during an acute period to determine whether the white cell count is rising, stabilizing, or falling. Table 12.3 lists cells found in CSF during specific neurological conditions.

Nursing Implications of Abnormal Findings

Assessment and Interventions. The nursing assessment and interventions for patients with abnormal cells in the CSF depend on the pathology present and the problems identified. The nurse can generally prepare the patient for the possibility of repeat lumbar punctures and can arrange to have the equipment needed for this procedure readily available. When the CSF examination

12

reveals white cells, an infectious condition is likely to be present, and the nurse should institute precautionary measures to prevent the spread of infection.

Description
GLUCOSE

Glucose is the predominant form of carbohydrate found in the body. It is normally present in CSF; amounts vary with the amount of glucose in the serum.

NORMAL RANGE

The glucose level in CSF is usually one-half to two-thirds the blood glucose level. Changes in CSF glucose levels lag 1–3 hours behind changes in the blood.

Adults	40–80 mg/dl
Children	35–75 mg/dl
Newborns	20–40 mg/dl

Specimen Required
A 5–10-ml sample of CSF is needed for analysis. The specimen should be taken to the laboratory immediately for analysis.

Preparation of the Patient
There are no food or fluid restrictions before the lumbar puncture.

Causes of Deviation from Normal
Although both increases and decreases in CSF glucose levels can occur, the decreases are more significant pathologically and are associated primarily with both bacterial and tuberculous meningitis. These decreases occur because pyrogenic bacteria, the tubercle bacillus, fungi, and protozoa consume glucose and can lower content in the CSF to zero. Other conditions that are associated with decreased glucose levels are metastatic carcinoma of the meninges, subarachnoid hemorrhage, and mumps meningo-encephalitis. If the patient has hypoglycemia, the CSF glucose levels will be decreased proportionately. Increased glucose levels are associated with hyperglycemia.

Nursing Implications of Abnormal Findings
Assessment and Interventions. In order to evaluate the significance of CSF glucose levels, a comparison with blood glucose level is necessary. The blood glucose specimen is drawn about 30 minutes before the lumbar puncture and a

TABLE 12.3. Cells Found in Abnormal CSF and Associated Diseases

Cells	Pathological Conditions
Polymorphonuclear cells plus low glucose	Acute bacterial meningitis.
Polymorphonuclear cells plus normal glucose	Brain abscess, early viral meningitis, amoebic meningitis in the early phase, leptospiral meningitis.
Lymphocytes plus low glucose	Tuberculous meningitis, mumps meningoencephalitis, meningeal carcinomatosis, meningeal sarcoidosis.
Lymphocytes plus normal glucose	Viral meningitis, viral encephalitis, postinfectious meningitis, lead encephalopathy, CNS syphilis, brain tumor.
Monocytes, some lymphocytes	Poliomyelitis, aseptic meningitis, multiple sclerosis, tumors, abscess.
Malignant cells	Primary and metastatic brain tumors.
Lymphocytoid and plasmacytoid cells	Multiple sclerosis, leukoencephalitis, delayed hypersensitivity reactions, subacute viral encephalitis, meningitis, some brain tumors.
Macrophages	Traumatic and ischemic cranial infarcts.
Neurological cells, glial, ependymal, and plexis cells	Postsurgical conditions and after trauma to the spinal cord.

cerebrospinal fluid specimen is obtained. This allows for the lag time for blood glucose to diffuse into the cerebrospinal fluid. If a decrease in the CSF glucose level occurs, the nurse should seek information about the underlying pathology. If an infectious process is suspected, precautions should be instituted to protect the staff and other patients until the diagnosis is confirmed and isolation procedures specified. If the patient is a diabetic, the nursing assessment should include those factors having to do with the diabetic status (urine and blood glucose levels, dietary intake, hypoglycemic medication, or insulin administration), as well as the CSF glucose level. Other assessments and interventions for patients with increases and decreases in CSF glucose levels depend on the problems the patient presents and the underlying pathology, when identified.

12

Description
PROTEIN

Protein found in CSF comes from protein in serum. Albumin is predominant, but some globulin is also present. Albumin is a small molecule able to pass through the endothelium.

N O R M A L R A N G E	
Adults	15–40 mg/dl
Children	14–45 mg/dl
Newborns	30–200 mg/dl

Specimen Required
A 5–10-ml tube of CSF is required for the analysis.

Preparation of the Patient
There are no food or fluid restrictions before the lumbar puncture.

Causes of Deviation from Normal
Increases in CSF protein levels may be derived from several proteins, such as albumin, globulin, and fibrinogen, as well as combined with intact and disintegrating bacteria.

Infections of the meninges result in increased CSF protein levels. These conditions include purulent meningitis, tuberculous meningitis, and syphilis. Increased CSF protein without the presence of cells is associated with Guillian-Barré syndrome. Patients with multiple sclerosis may show increases, primarily in the gamma globulin component.

Decreases in cerebrospinal fluid protein are associated with leakage of fluid, hyperthyroidism, increased intracranial pressure, and removal of a large volume of cerebrospinal fluid.

Nursing Implications of Abnormal Findings
Assessment and Interventions. Patients with increases or decreases in CSF protein levels should be assessed for other neurological problems and deficits; interventions should be planned accordingly. Nursing care depends on the patient's underlying pathology.

Description
MICROORGANISMS

Normally, no microorganisms are found in CSF. Examination of smears of centrifuged fluid can be used to identify bacteria, fungi, or protozoa. Cultures on various media may be done to reveal specific bacteria.

N O R M A L   R A N G E

Negative.

Specimen Required

A specimen of CSF is collected in a sterile container and used for microscopic examination and culture. Care should be taken to retrieve the specimen without contamination.

Preparation of the Patient

There are no food or fluid restrictions before lumbar puncture.

Causes of Deviation from Normal

A number of bacteria and fungi may be identified in CSF. They are associated with infections of the meninges. Table 12.4 lists the more commonly identified pathogens.

Nursing Implications of Abnormal Findings

Assessment and Interventions. The assessment and interventions planned for a patient with a positive CSF culture depend on the microorganism that is identified. While the nurse is awaiting results of the culture, precautions should be instituted to protect the patient, other patients, and staff from exposure to the pathogens.

Description

CHLORIDE

Chloride is the primary anion found in the extracellular fluid. It is present in higher concentrations in the CSF than in the serum.

N O R M A L   R A N G E

Adults	118–132 mEq/l
Children	120–128 mEq/l
Newborns	110–122 mEq/l

12

Specimen Required

A 5–10-ml tube of CSF is required for analysis.

TABLE 12.4. Pathogenic Microorganisms Found in CSF

Organism	Disease	Other CSF Findings
Neisseria meningitidis	Meningococcal meningitis	Increased pressure, decreased glucose, increased protein, turbid color
Mycobacteria tuberculosis	Tuberculous meningitis	Increased pressure, decreased glucose, increased protein, clear to slightly cloudy appearance
Hemophilus influenzae	Influenza	Increased pressure, decreased glucose, increased protein, purulent appearance
Escherichia coli	E. coli meningitis	Increased pressure, decreased glucose, increased protein purulent appearance
Treponema pallidum	Syphilitic meningitis	Normal pressure, normal or decreased glucose, increased protein, clear or turbid appearance
Cryptococcus (Torula)—a yeast	Cryptococcal meningitis	Normal pressure, normal glucose, increased protein, clear or cloudy appearance
Streptococcus (Diplococcus) pneumoniae	Pneumococcal meningitis	Increased pressure, decreased glucose, increased protein, purulent appearance

Preparation of the Patient
There are no food or fluid restrictions before lumbar puncture.

Causes of Deviation from Normal
Spinal fluid chloride determination is used primarily to determine the presence of tuberculous meningitis, in which a significant depression in CSF chloride occurs. A moderate depression occurs with syphilis, tumors, encephalitis, and brain abscesses.

Nursing Implications of Abnormal Findings
Assessment and Interventions. If the chloride level of the CSF is depressed, the patient is likely to have an infectious process, most likely tuberculous meningitis. The nurse should assess the patient for other signs of tuberculosis

and should prepare for other diagnostic tests. Interventions should be related to the presenting manifestations of the disease and should include protection of staff members and other patients from the spread of infection.

Description
UREA

Urea is an end product of protein metabolism that is generally eliminated from the body via the kidneys and gastrointestinal tract. Urea in the CSF is derived from serum urea and is approximately equal in concentration to that in the serum.

NORMAL RANGE	
Adults	7–15 mg/dl
Children	Consult laboratory for reference values.

Specimen Required
A 5–10-ml tube of CSF is required.

Preparation of the Patient
There are no food or fluid restrictions before lumbar puncture.

Causes of Deviation from Normal
Increased CSF urea levels are associated with uremia. Levels rise in proportion to the rise in serum urea.

Nursing Implications of Abnormal Findings
Assessment and Interventions. If increased CSF urea is found, the nursing assessment should include observation of manifestations of uremia. Interventions should be planned in relation to the individual patient's needs.

Description
CALCIUM

Calcium is a cation found primarily in the bones and teeth combined with phosphate and carbonate. The cerebrospinal fluid contains calcium diffused from the blood plasma. Since approximately one-half the serum calcium is bound to protein, and protein does not diffuse into CSF, calcium levels in CSF are approximately one-half those in serum. If protein content of the CSF rises, the calcium level rises as well.

12

N O R M A L   R A N G E

Adults	2. 1–2.7 mEq/l
Children	Consult laboratory for reference values.

Specimen Required
A 5–10-ml tube of spinal fluid is needed for analysis.

Preparation of the Patient
There are no food or fluid restrictions before lumbar puncture.

Causes of Deviation from Normal
Increases in CSF calcium levels occur with increases in CSF protein levels. These abnormalities are associated with infectious processes. Increases in CSF calcium levels occur in tuberculous meningitis. This complication of pulmonary tuberculosis occurs when an infectious lesion erodes the subarachnoid space.

Nursing Implications of Abnormal Findings
Assessment and Interventions. When increased CSF calcium levels occur in association with tuberculous meningitis, the patient is critically ill. The nursing actions should include a baseline neurological examination and an assessment of the clinical manifestations of meningitis such as nuchal rigidity (neck stiffness), increasing head circumference, and bulging fontanels in infants. Changes in consciousness should be noted, and the nurse should be alert to the possibility of seizures. Monitoring of vital signs is important, and neurological observations should be repeated at least every hour. The nurse should monitor the patient for beginning signs of fluid and electrolyte imbalance. Interventions should be based on problems identified, but may include administration of muscle relaxants and analgesics to control seizures, measures to prevent respiratory complications, and appropriate body positioning and range-of-motion exercises.

Description
LACTIC ACID
Severe systemic lactic acidosis can cause elevated lactic acid in CSF. In the absence of systemic lactic acidosis, the presence of *lactic acid* in CSF is a result of increased glucose metabolism in the central nervous system.

N O R M A L R A N G E	
Adults	10–20 mg/dl
Children	Consult laboratory for reference values.

Specimen Required

A 5–10-ml tube of cerebrospinal fluid is required. Two or three tubes should be obtained to minimize blood contamination.

Preparation of the Patient

There are no food or fluid restrictions before lumbar puncture.

Causes of Deviation from Normal

Severe lactic acidosis will cause a parallel rise in CSF levels. Isolated increases due to glucose metabolism occur in the presence of bacterial or fungal meningitis. It is useful in distinguishing these disorders from viral meningitis.

Nursing Care of Deviations from Normal

Assessment and Interventions. If elevated levels of lactic acid in CSF is caused by systemic lactic acidosis, nursing care will be similar to that discussed in Chapter 6 for metabolic lactic acidosis.

When the elevation is a result of bacterial or fungal meningitis, nursing assessment should include a baseline neurological examination and the clinical manifestations of meningitis such as nuchal rigidity (neck stiffness), increasing head circumference, and bulging fontanels in infants. Changes in consciousness should be noted and the nurse should be alert to the possibility of seizures. Monitoring of vital signs is important and neurological observations should be repeated at least every hour. The nurse should monitor the patient for beginning signs of fluid and electrolyte imbalance. Interventions should be based on problems identified, but may include administration of muscle relaxants and analgesics to control seizures, measures to prevent respiratory complications, and appropriate body positioning and range-of-motion exercises.

CRYOGLOBINS

12

Description

Cryoglobulins are protein globulins that precipitate at low temperatures and re-dissolve when warmed.

NORMAL RANGE	
Adults	<5 mg/dl
Children	negative

Specimen Required

A 5–10-ml sample of venous blood is collected in a plain collecting tube or syringe.

Preparation of the Patient

There are no food or fluid restrictions before venipuncture.

Causes of Deviation from Normal

Cryoglobins are present in the blood of patients with multiple myeloma, chronic leukemia, connective tissue diseases, autoimmune diseases, mononucleosis, hepatitis, infected endocarditis, leprosy, and syphilis.

Nursing Implications of Abnormal Findings

Assessment and Interventions. If the presence of cryoglobins is associated with a specific disease, a medical-surgical nursing textbook should be consulted for related nursing care.

Cryoglobins can precipitate in the fingers when exposed to cold temperatures. Therefore, patients should be taught to prevent pain, cyanosis, and cold fingers by wearing warm gloves or mittens during the winter and other cold periods.

SPUTUM CULTURE, SMEAR, AND CYTOLOGY EXAMINATION

Description

Sputum is produced by the mucous glands and goblet cells of the tracheobronchial tree and brought up by coughing. It is composed of 95% water and 5% solids that include carbohydrates, proteins, lipids, deoxyribonucleic acid (DNA), and discarded cells from the lining of the respiratory tract. Mucus production and the action of the cilia that line the tracheobronchial tree provide a normal mechanism for cleansing the respiratory system of inhaled organisms. The secretions within the mucus also have antimicrobial properties.

N O R M A L   R A N G E

The contents of the lower respiratory tract are normally sterile. However, when sputum is raised and expectorated, it may be contaminated with organisms from the upper respiratory structures.

Specimen Required
SPUTUM CULTURE

When a sputum culture is ordered, a covered specimen cup is used. The patient expectorates the sputum raised into this container, which is immediately sent to the laboratory or refrigerated until it can be delivered to the laboratory.

Preparation of the Patient

There are no food or fluid restrictions. Specific instructions for the collection of sputum specimens are discussed in Chapter 1.

Causes of Deviation from Normal

Many pathogenic microorganisms are found in the sputum. Some of the more common ones that cause disease are listed in Table 12.5.

Nursing Implications of Abnormal Findings

Assessment. When a sputum culture indicates that the patient has a bacterial infection of the respiratory tract, the following areas should be included in the nursing assessment:

1. The presence of the clinical manifestations that usually accompany the disease;
2. The patient's ability to participate actively in pulmonary care;
3. The patient's psychological response to the diagnosis;
4. The amount of patient education that will be needed.

Interventions. The nursing interventions planned for a patient with a bacterial pulmonary disease depend upon the data gathered during the nursing assessment. When a patient has a severe infection with respiratory signs and symptoms such as dyspnea, cyanosis, and thick, voluminous bronchopulmonary secretions, nursing care should include activities that will help mobilize and remove secretions, such as intensive breathing exercises, chest percussion and vibration, postural drainage, and frequent position changes. In addition, fluids should be encouraged (if not contraindicated) to maintain hydration. The inspired air should be humidified, and suctioning should be used when coughing is ineffective. Care of the mucous membranes in the oropharyngeal area, maintenance of adequate physical and mental rest, and observation of side or

12

TABLE 12.5. Pathogenic Microorganisms Found in Sputum

Organism	Gram Stain	Morphology	Disease
Pneumococci	+	Cocci single or in pairs	Pneumococcal pneumonia
Staphylococci	+	Cocci in clusters	Staphylococcal pneumonia
Streptococci	+	Cocci in chains	Hemolytic streptococcal pneumonia
Klebsiella	−	Bacilli	Friedländer's (Klebsiella) pneumonia
Enterobacteria (Escherichia coli proteus species)	−	Bacilli	Bacterial pneumonias secondary to respiratory contamination
Pseudomonas aeruginosa	−	Bacilli	Pneumonia secondary to respiratory contamination
Corynebacterium diphtheriae	+	Bacilli	Diphtheria
Mycobacterium tuberculosis	+	Bacilli	Tuberculosis
Diplococcus pneumoniae	+	Diplococci	Pneumonia
Haemophilus influenzae	−	Bacilli	Pneumonia, laryngo-tracheobronchitis

toxic effects of medications administered are also aspects of the nursing care of patients with respiratory disease.

A plan to provide continuous emotional support and reassurance should be made when fear, anxiety, or panic accompany respiratory distress. The psychological impact that newly diagnosed tuberculosis may have on a patient and family should also be considered when planning emotional support. When a patient has a respiratory disease that is communicable, precautions should be instituted to prevent transmission of the organisms to the nursing staff and to other patients. The patient and family must also be educated about the transmission of the disease, how it may be prevented from spreading, and the necessity of taking medications when they are prescribed prophylactically.

Prevention should be a focus of the teaching plan. This plan should include information about nutrition and a well-balanced diet, the prompt treatment of colds and flu in persons susceptible to pneumonia, oral hygiene (especially for persons who are mouth breathers), the importance of frequent coughing and expectoration when sputum production is increased, and the safe disposal of the secretions. More detailed discussions of the nursing responsibilities for patients with infectious respiratory diseases can be found in medical-surgical nursing tests.

Specimen Required
SPUTUM SMEAR

When a sputum smear is ordered, a special covered specimen cup is used. The patient expectorates the sputum raised into this container, which is immediately sent to the laboratory or refrigerated until it can be delivered to the laboratory.

Preparation of the Patient

There are no food or fluid restrictions. Specific instructions for the collection of sputum specimens are provided in Chapter 1.

Causes of Deviation from Normal

The microorganisms that may be found in the sputum of carefully stained smears are the same ones that may be grown in a sputum culture (see Table 12.5). In addition, the sputum smear may be examined for the presence of materials such as eosinophils, epithelial cells, and many other substances that are not present in normal sputum. When a person has bronchial asthma, the sputum smear will contain eosinophils which help confirm the diagnosis of this disease. Some fungus infections may also be diagnosed by means of a sputum smear.

Nursing Implications of Abnormal Findings

Assessment and Interventions. When a sputum smear indicates that the patient has a bacterial infection, the nursing assessment and interventions are the same as those discussed in the section on sputum culture. When bronchial asthma is present, the severity of the clinical manifestations the patient is experiencing must be assessed along with the acute or chronic nature of the illness and the psychological reactions of the patient. There is a broad range of nursing interventions that may be performed for a patient who has bronchial asthma. Those chosen depend upon the patient's status. For example, if the patient has had a mild asthma attack, nursing interventions are related to comfort measures and prevention, with patient education as the primary focus. If the patient has chronic asthma and is suffering from an acute attack, nursing care focuses on maintaining a patent airway, providing adequate ventilation, and attempting to prevent vascular collapse. In any case, when a person is having difficulty breathing, anxiety and apprehension occur. When this happens, the

12

patient may be comforted by a nurse who can maintain a quiet, calm approach while giving nursing care quickly and efficiently. The amount of patient teaching that should be provided depends on the type of asthma present (intrinsic or extrinsic), the severity of the attack, and when the original diagnosis was made.

When a fungus infection has been diagnosed by means of a sputum smear, nursing assessment and interventions depend on the fungus that has been identified and the severity of the patient's illness. For discussion of the many fungus infections, consult a medical-surgical nursing textbook.

Specimen Required
SPUTUM FOR CYTOLOGY

Various methods of specimen collection and preparation are used for cytological examination of sputum; therefore, it is best to consult the pathology laboratory personnel for instructions before collecting the specimen.

Preparation of the Patient

The most common specimen used is the single, early-morning specimen collected after a deep cough. When this is the case, the patient should be instructed to save the sputum collected with the first cough of the morning and to notify the nurse as soon as it is collected. Specific instructions for the collection of sputum specimens are provided in Chapter 1.

Causes of Deviation from Normal

The cytological examination of sputum is done for the diagnosis of cancer of the lung. This laboratory test is positive in approximately 50% of the cases of early pulmonary carcinoma, compared with 25% positive results when bronchoscopy and bronchial biopsy are performed.

Nursing Implications of Abnormal Findings

Assessment. Since the cytological examination of sputum is part of the diagnostic workup for lung cancer, the nursing assessment should focus on the psychological impact that the possible diagnosis of cancer has on the patient. It is important to assess the patient's interpretation of the meaning of the diagnosis of cancer and what it may mean for the patient's family and for the future. The local and systemic effects of cancer that the patient experiences must also be identified.

Interventions. The nursing interventions planned for a patient with an abnormal cytological sputum sample depend on the level of awareness the patient has about the diagnosis and the results of the tests performed. Fear of death, fear of the unknown, and fear of changes in body image must be dealt with in the care plan, in addition to loneliness and depression. Physical care depends on the extent of the tumor and its local and systemic effects. Anemia, hemorrhage, infection, pain, and malnutrition are some of the primary problems that must be considered.

THROAT CULTURE

Description

Throat cultures are used to identify the presence of bacteria in the throat. They are ordered when a patient has a sore throat accompanied by the signs and symptoms of a bacterial infection. These include white patches, exudate or ulcerations on the throat, an elevated white blood count, and a high temperature.

N O R M A L R A N G E	
Adults and children	Negative

Specimen Required

The throat is swabbed with a sterile applicator and the specimen is placed in a sterile container or tube of culture medium. The detailed procedure is outlined in Chapter 1.

Preparation of the Patient

Food and fluids are not restricted prior to collection of the specimen. The patient should be told the reason for the culture and how the specimen will be obtained. It is important to explain to children that the procedure will be uncomfortable but that it will be done quickly.

The tongue should be depressed with a tongue blade, and the throat exposed and illuminated. The swab should be wiped firmly, gently, and quickly over the back of the throat, both tonsils, and any areas of inflammation, exudate, or ulceration that are in the back of the throat. Care should be taken not to contaminate the swab with secretions from the lips and forward part of the tongue. Precautions for the health professional collecting the swab include mask and goggles, as the motion of the swab over the back of the throat generally causes the patient to gag and cough.

Causes of Deviation from Normal

Positive throat cultures are generally caused by group A beta-hemolytic streptococci or *Corynebacterium diphtheriae* (diphtheria). *Neisseria gonorrhoeae* may be found in persons who have engaged in oral sex with a partner who had gonorrhea.

Thrush (candidal infection of the mouth) can also be identified. Several carrier states can be detected through positive throat cultures, and include Beta hemolytic streptococcus, *Neisseria meningitidis*, *Corynebacterium diphtheriae*, and *Staphylococcus aureus*.

12

Nursing Implications of Abnormal Findings

Assessment and Interventions. When a positive culture is suspected or has been reported by the laboratory, the nurse should assess the patient for any other signs and symptoms of infection. The nurse should also determine what the patient knows about the organism identified and its effect on the body.

Since patients with a positive throat culture are usually placed on antibiotics, the nurse must assess the patient, or the parents if the patient is a child, to determine if the reasons for antibiotic therapy are understood. The importance of continuing antibiotic therapy even after symptoms are relieved should be stressed. The nurse must explain that discontinuing the course of therapy may result in a recurrence of the infection or future complications such as rheumatic fever.

Follow-up of people with whom the patient has been in contact is an important aspect of nursing care. The parents and siblings of a child with a streptococcal infection should be evaluated. When *Neisseria gonorrhoeae* is the infecting organism, the patient should be instructed to refer sex partners for examination.

ALCOHOL

Description

This test measures blood levels of *ethyl alcohol,* a substance that is ingested rather than produced by the body. Blood alcohol levels are measured when a semiconscious or unconscious patient is admitted to the hospital and the cause for this condition is unknown. The test is also performed for medicolegal purposes when a traffic accident has occurred in a state where there are laws related to driving while intoxicated.

NORMAL RANGE	
Normally, there is no alcohol in the blood.	
<50 mg/dl (<0.05%)	Not usually considered to be legally under the influence of alcohol
50–100 mg/dl (0.05–0.1%)	Vision and reaction time may be adversely affected
100 mg/dl (0.1%)	Legally intoxicated
100–150 mg/dl (0.1–0.15%)	Prolonged reaction time
150–200 mg/dl (0.15–0.2%)	Reaction time severely affected, equilibrium and coordination disturbed
200–250 mg/dl (0.2–0.25%)	Marked intoxication and stupor
350–400 mg/dl (0.25–0.4%)	Coma occurs; death may result

Specimen Required

A 5–10-ml specimen of venous or arterial blood should be collected using a closed system and completely filling the collecting tube. The laboratory personnel should be consulted regarding the type of tube required. Capillary blood may be used if it is collected using a closed system.

Preparation of the Patient

Alcohol or tinctures that contain alcohol must not be used to cleanse the patient's skin. Studies have shown that when alcohol is used, ethanol levels are falsely elevated if alcohol is inadvertently aspirated into the blood collection tube. Patient education about the procedure depends on the circumstances requiring the test. Emotional support may be needed, especially if there has been an accident or if police are present. There are no food or fluid restrictions before venipuncture.

Causes of Deviation from Normal

The cause of the presence of alcohol in the blood is the ingestion of alcohol.

Nursing Implications of Abnormal Findings

Assessment. There are three main areas to be assessed: (1) the medical status of the patient at the time of admission and whether surgery is required; (2) the physiological ability of the patient to detoxify alcohol; and (3) the psychosocial aspects of the patient's immediate situation. A complete, in-depth assessment in this area cannot be done in emergency settings. The assessment should include the patient's immediate situation and the events surrounding the patient's present status.

Interventions. If the patient needs emergency surgery, the operating- and recovery-room staffs should be informed of the patient's condition. The possible occurrence of delirium tremens should also be considered and plans made by the nursing staff to deal with the problem postoperatively. If the patient has liver disease, the nursing staff should all be informed and the patient watched closely for increasing signs of toxicity. Plans should not be made for the patient's release until there is evidence that blood alcohol levels have returned to low levels.

Emotional support must be provided with a nonjudgmental attitude. The patient should be supported and protected from individuals who show a curious but non-helpful interest in the patient and the circumstances surrounding the need for blood alcohol determinations. If the patient is admitted to the hospital, the nursing assessment and interventions begun on admission should be sent to the nursing unit.

12

BARBITURATES

Description

This test is used to measure blood levels of barbiturates when there has been an accidental or intentional ingestion of an overdose of these drugs. Barbiturates reversibly depress the excitable tissue of the central nervous system. Absorption of short-acting barbiturates is more rapid and elimination slower than that of the long-acting barbiturates.

N O R M A L   R A N G E

Normally, there are no barbiturates in the blood. Therapeutic and toxic levels are as follows:

Therapeutic levels of phenobarbital for
patients with seizure disorders   10–40 g/ml
Toxic levels
  Short-acting
    Secobarbital   20–30 μg/ml
  Intermediate-acting
    Amobarbital   30–50 μg/ml
  Long-acting
    Phenobarbital   50–80 μg/ml

Specimen Required

A 5–10-ml specimen of venous blood is collected in a plain collecting tube or syringe.

Preparation of the Patient

There are no food or fluid restrictions before venipuncture.

Causes of Deviation from Normal

The presence of barbiturates in the blood is caused by ingestion of barbiturates. Therapeutic levels may be prescribed for persons receiving long-term treatment for chronic problems such as seizure disorders. Toxic levels are caused by accidental or intentional overdose. The physiological reaction to high serum barbiturate levels varies depending on the amount of time the patient has been using these drugs. People who are addicted may tolerate larger doses than those who are not habitual users. In general, short-acting barbiturates have more serious consequences and may be more lethal in smaller doses than the long-acting variety.

Nursing Implications of Abnormal Findings

Assessment. The patient's level of consciousness should be noted on admission and continually monitored until full consciousness has returned and blood levels have begun to diminish rapidly. The identity of the agent used should be recorded in the nurse's notes, and the frequency of physiological assessment should be based on whether the patient has ingested a short- or long-acting drug, as well as on the amount of the drug present in the serum. Since respiratory problems are the major cause of death in these patients, respiratory status must be closely observed, particularly in unconscious patients. The nurse should try to determine if the patient is a habitual user demonstrated by the associated increase in tolerance. The psychosocial assessment should begin when the patient is admitted and should continue throughout the patient's hospitalization. Family and friends should be included in the data-gathering process when possible.

Interventions. Routine nursing care for an unconscious patient should be planned. Objectives of care include maintenance of normal body functions and prevention of pulmonary complications, contractures, and other problems that may result. A medical-surgical nursing textbook should be consulted for specific details. Information gathered during continuous monitoring should be reported to the physician and the nursing care altered based on these assessments.

If the patient's overdose of barbiturates was accidental, the nurse should develop a teaching plan to help the patient understand the normal use of these drugs and the harmful results that can occur when they are taken with other drugs or with alcohol. If the overdose was intentional, psychological care is needed. Consultation should be made with the psychiatric nursing staff or a clinical specialist as needed.

DIGITOXIN AND DIGOXIN LEVELS

Description

Laboratory measurement of *digitoxin* and *digoxin* (cardiac glycoside) levels is done to determine whether blood levels are within therapeutic or toxic ranges. There is a very slim margin of safety between therapeutic and toxic doses and between toxic and lethal doses. The safe blood level of digitoxin is higher than that of digoxin.

NORMAL RANGE

Normally, there is no digitoxin or digoxin in the blood. Therapeutic and toxic levels are as follows:

Adults		
Digitoxin		
	Therapeutic	11–23 ng/ml
	Toxic	26–35 ng/ml
Digoxin		
	Therapeutic	0.8–2.1 ng/ml
	Toxic	>2.4 ng/ml

12

Children
   Digitoxin
      Therapeutic   11–23 ng/ml
      Toxic   26–35 ng/ml
   Digoxin
      Therapeutic   0.8–2.1 ng/ml
      Toxic   >2.4 ng/ml
Infants
   Digitoxin
      Therapeutic   11–23 ng/ml
      Toxic   26–35 ng/ml
   Digoxin
      Therapeutic   2–4 ng/ml
      Toxic   >3 ng/ml

Specimen Required

A 5-ml sample of venous blood is collected in a plain collecting tube or syringe. *The spelling of the drug on the label should be checked carefully*, because different antibodies are used for digitoxin and digoxin analysis.

Preparation of the Patient

There are no food or fluid restrictions before venipuncture.

Causes of Deviation from Normal

Most often, the cause of toxicity is a response to attempts to reach a therapeutic level of the drug. This occurs because the margin of safety is so narrow. When the desired therapeutic response is attained, an estimated 60% of the toxic dose has been administered; when the patient has toxic symptoms, approximately 50% of the lethal dose has been given.

Another common cause of toxicity is a fall in serum potassium levels, which enhances the effect of digitalis preparations. This often occurs when a patient is also receiving diuretic therapy and the potassium being lost in the urine is not adequately replaced. Older people tend to become toxic on lower drug levels than younger adults or children.

Nursing Implications of Abnormal Findings

Assessment and Interventions. When a patient has a toxic reaction to a digitalis preparation, the nurse should observe for clinical manifestations of the toxicity (see Table 12.6). Any symptoms that might signal a toxic reaction should be reported, no matter how innocuous they seem.

Teaching is an important aspect of nursing care for all patients receiving digitalis therapy and should be re-emphasized if a patient has become toxic to the therapy. The patient should be taught the name, dosage, and action of the drug and the importance of not missing a dose or taking extra doses. Written, as well as verbal instructions should be used, and a record-keeping system should be developed with the patient. If the patient is also taking a diuretic and potassium, the relationship of these medications should be explained and the patient reminded not to stop or alter the dose of a medication without consulting a physician. Symptoms of toxicity should be described. If an episode of toxicity has already occurred, the patient should be reminded to call the physician if any of the same signs and symptoms recur. A digoxin antibody derived from sheep serum, digoxin immune fabovine (digibind), may be administered to diminish the signs and symptoms of digitalis toxicity. Patients should be assessed for allergies to sheep proteins prior to administration. Following administration of digibind, patients should be assessed for hypokalemia, dysrhythmias, and an exacerbation of congestive heart failure.

PHENYTOIN (DILANTIN)

Description

This test is used to measure the blood levels of *phenytoin* (diphenylhydantoin, Dilantin) to determine if they are within therapeutic or toxic ranges. Phenytoin inhibits the spread of seizure activity in the motor cortex by stabilizing neurons against hyperexcitability. It also exerts stabilizing effects on cell membranes.

NORMAL RANGE
Normally, there is no phenytoin in the blood. Therapeutic and toxic levels are as follows:

Adults
  Therapeutic level   10–20 μg/ml
  Toxic level   >20 μg/ml
Children   Consult laboratory for reference values.

12

Specimen Required

A 3–5-ml specimen of venous blood is collected in a plain collecting tube or syringe.

TABLE 12.6. Clinical Manifestations of Digitalis

Cardiovascular Effects	Neurological Symptoms
Every cardiac arrhythmia can be produced	Confusion
	Delirium
Irregularities in cardiac rhythm	Drowsiness
Rapid or slow pulse rate	Fatigue
Regularization of a chronic irregular pulse	Headache
	Insomnia
	Vertigo
Visual Disturbances	**Gastrointestinal Manifestations**
Blind spots	Anorexia
Difficulties in reading	Diarrhea
Disturbances of color vision, especially green or yellow	Nausea
Halos around dark objects	Vomiting
Hazy or shimmering vision	

Preparation of the Patient

There are no food or fluid restrictions before venipuncture.

Causes of Deviation from Normal

The presence of phenytoin in the blood is caused by ingestion or injection of the drug. Toxic levels may occur when the correct maintenance dose is being established or if an overdose of the drug has been taken.

Nursing Implications of Abnormal Findings

Assessment and Interventions. When the therapeutic levels of phenytoin are being established, the nurse must assess the patient for any signs and symptoms of the clinical disorder being treated, as well as any toxic effects of the drug. Assessment of a patient who suddenly develops a toxic reaction to the drug should include information about how and when the patient takes the drug and any changes in life-style that might have affected this pattern.

The nurse should be prepared to treat clinical manifestations of toxicity of phenytoin when toxic levels are present. If the toxic levels occur because of an accidental overdose, a teaching plan should be developed to help the patient understand how the drug is to be taken and the harmful results that can occur when this regimen is not followed.

LEAD

Description

Lead is a toxic substance that enters the body through the gastrointestinal and respiratory systems. It has a slow excretion rate through the kidneys. It is stored in the bones and may also be deposited at the base of teeth in small children.

The test for lead is performed when there is a possible diagnosis of acute lead poisoning or an acute episode superimposed on a case of chronic lead poisoning. The lead content of both blood and urine may be measured.

N O R M A L R A N G E	
Adults and children	
Whole blood	<25 μg/dl
Urine	<80 μg/dl

Specimen Required

Blood Test. A 5-ml sample of venous blood is collected and placed in a tube containing an oxalate fluoride mixture, heparin, or EDTA.

Urine Test. The total urine excreted by the patient over a 24-hour period is collected.

Preparation of the Patient

There are no food or fluid restrictions before venipuncture or urine collection.

Causes of Deviation from Normal

Lead toxicity occurs in children who eat lead-based paint that peels from the surfaces of toys or furniture. It is also seen in adults who inhale fumes from burning battery casings, battery fumes, and fumes from acetylene torches. It may also occur in people who drink alcoholic beverages that have been distilled in lead-contaminated equipment.

Nursing Implications of Abnormal Findings

Assessment. When a patient has a positive test for lead toxicity, the nursing assessment should focus on the presence of clinical manifestations. These include anorexia, weight loss, constipation, abdominal colic, muscle pains, weakness, pallor, and anemia. In addition, children should be observed for clumsiness, irritability, hyperactivity, and progressive neuromuscular excitement. Altered hearing, difficulty processing language, and disruptive classroom behavior may also be present. Children's teeth should also be examined for the

12

presence of a lead line, which is a bluish-black deposit of lead compounds at the base of the teeth.

Interventions. Specific nursing interventions depend on the signs and symptoms exhibited by the patient. A teaching plan should be developed for all patients with lead toxicity. The parents of children should be told that paint containing lead should not be used on children's toys and furniture. They should also be reminded to sand old paint off of furniture to be repainted to prevent a child from chewing through the new paint and eating the old. They should also be advised to have their home inspected for sources of lead contamination. Some states have a lead department that will perform the inspection free of charge. Adults should be advised to avoid fumes from lead-containing products. If lead is an industrial hazard, they should request that the company take appropriate measures to protect its employees.

LITHIUM

Description
Lithium in the form of lithium carbonate is a medication used for control of the manic phase of a manic-depressive psychiatric state.

NORMAL RANGE

Normally, there is no lithium in the blood. The desired therapeutic range during lithium therapy is 0.6–1.4 mEq/l, which is reached 8–12 hours after administration of the drug.

Specimen Required
A 5-ml sample of venous blood should be obtained in a plain collecting tube or syringe.

Preparation of the Patient
No special preparation of the patient is necessary if suspected toxic levels are being assessed. For patients just beginning to receive lithium therapy, the specimen should be drawn 8–12 hours after medication administration to ensure that the therapeutic level has been achieved.

Causes of Deviation from Normal
An abnormal increase in serum lithium levels is attributable to toxic administration of lithium carbonate. Because lithium levels can vary at different times of the day, a lithium tolerance test may be performed to determine how an individual handles the dose and how the drug may be best administered.

Nursing Implications of Abnormal Findings

Assessment and Interventions. When patients are put on lithium therapy, the nurse should make sure that the medication is administered at the specified time. This makes it possible to determine the exact time specimens should be drawn to determine if therapeutic levels have been achieved. Patients should be taught the importance of this exact timing. If toxic effects occur, the nurse should assess the patient for transient nausea, fine tremors, anorexia, vomiting, diarrhea, thirst, and polyuria. Patients should be encouraged to have adequate fluid and sodium intakes as lithium limits antidiuretic hormone (ADH) secretion causing fluid loss. Patients should be observed for signs and symptoms of dehydration and advised not to take diuretics.

SALICYLATES

Description

This test is used to measure blood levels of *salicylates* when there has been an accidental or intentional overdose of acetylsalicylic acid (aspirin), and to determine blood salicylate levels when large doses are being used for therapy.

NORMAL RANGE

Normally, there are no salicylates in the blood.

Adults
    Therapeutic levels   20–25 mg/dl
    Toxic level   >30–35 mg/dl
    Lethal level   >60 mg/dl
Children   Consult laboratory for therapeutic level norms.
    Toxic levels   >5–25 mg/dl, depending on age of child.

Specimen Required

A 5-ml sample of venous blood is collected in a plain collecting tube or syringe.

Preparation of the Patient

There are no food or fluid restrictions before venipuncture.

12

Causes of Deviation from Normal

Salicylates are present in the blood when drugs containing aspirin are ingested. Therapeutic levels may be prescribed for persons receiving long-term treatment for chronic problems such as rheumatoid arthritis. Toxic levels are caused by accidental or intentional overdose.

Nursing Implications of Abnormal Findings

Assessment. When patients receiving therapeutic doses of salicylates have a rise or drop in serum levels, the method of administration should be reviewed with the patient. All other medications the patient is taking should be included in the nursing assessment. If an overdose has been taken accidentally by a child, the way medications have been handled and stored should be discussed with the parents. When an adult has taken an intentional overdose, the psychosocial assessment should include an attempt to determine the reasons for the overdose.

Interventions. When the patient receiving long-term therapy is unable to maintain therapeutic salicylate levels, a plan should be developed to establish a consistent method of administration of medications. The patient's life-style should be considered when planning the times at which the drug is to be taken. The patient should be told that antacids containing aluminum hydroxide and magnesium hydroxide have been found to interfere with the action of salicylates. If these substances are taken to relieve gastric distress, the patient's physician should be consulted about altering the dose or type of medication prescribed.

When a child has taken an accidental overdose of salicylates, better methods of storage should be discussed with the parents in a non-judgmental way. The use of safety containers should be encouraged; however, the fact that they are not child-proof should be stressed.

If an intentional overdose of salicylates has been taken, nursing care should include a long-term evaluation of the patient's psychological status and plans should be made with the health team to provide counseling or psychiatric care as needed.

BIBLIOGRAPHY

Barker, P.O., and D.A. Lewis. "The Management of Lead Exposure in Pediatric Populations." *Nurse Practitioner,* 15:8–16 (December 1990).

Byrne, C.J., D.F. Saxton, P.K. Pelikan, and P.M. Nugent. *Laboratory Tests: Implications for Nursing Care.* Menlo Park: Addison-Wesley, 1986.

Connelly, C.E. "Compliance with Outpatient Lithium Therapy." *Perspectives in Psychiatric Care,* 22:44–50 (April–June 1984).

Corbett, J.V. *Laboratory Tests and Diagnostic Procedures with Nursing Diagnoses.* Norwalk, Connecticut: Appleton and Lange, 1992.

Fischbach, F.T. *A Manual of Laboratory and Diagnostic Tests.* Philadelphia: J.B. Lippincott Company, 1992.

Giannini, A.J., and A.E. Slaby. *Handbook of Overdose and Detoxification Emergencies.* New Hyde Park, New York: Medical Examination Publishing Company, 1983.

Ignatavicius, D.D., and M.V. Bayne. *Medical-Surgical Nursing: A Nursing Process Approach.* Philadelphia: W.B. Saunders, 1991.

Lee, W.R. "Low Level Exposure to Lead." *British Medical Journal*, 301:504–505 (September 15, 1990).

Levine, E.R. "Complications of Emphysema . . . Hypoxia." *Respiratory Therapy*, 15:11, 17 (January–February 1985).

Lewis, S.M., and I.C. Collier. *Medical-Surgical Nursing: Assessment and Management of Clinical Problems*. St. Louis: Mosby Yearbook, 1992.

Longren, E. "Barbiturates." *Emergency*, 171:18–19 (July 1985).

Longren, K. "Barbiturates." *Emergency*, 17:18–19 (July 1985).

Luckman, J., and K.C. Sorensen. *Medical-Surgical Nursing: A Psychophysiological Approach*. Philadelphia: Saunders, 1987.

Matson, C. "Streptococcal Pharyngitis." *Consultant*, 28(12):87, 90 (December, 1988).

Neu, H.C. "CNS Infection: First Things First." *Hospital Practice*, 20:69, 70, 72, 74 (November 30, 1985).

Nythan, L.S. "Clinical Management of the Lead Poisoned Child." *Journal of Community Health Nursing*, 2:135–144 (1985).

Olsen, E., *et al*. "Recognition, General Considerations and Techniques in the Management of Drug Intoxications." *Heart and Lung*, 12:110–114 (March 1983).

Phipps, W.S., B.C. Long, N.F. Woods, and V. Cossmeyer. *Medical-Surgical Nursing*. St. Louis: Mosby Yearbook, 1991.

Price, M.B., *et al*. "A Quick and Easy Guide to Neurological Assessment." *Journal of Neurosurgical Nursing*, 17:313–320 (October 1985).

Pritchard, R.C. "Clinching the Diagnosis—Sputum and Other Specimens in Respiratory Tract Infection." *Pathology*, 16:345–349 (July 1984).

Ravel, R. *Clinical Laboratory Medicine*. Chicago: Year Book Medical Publishers, 1989.

Sacher, R.A., and R.A. McPherson. *Widmann's Clinical Interpretation of Laboratory Tests*. Philadelphia: F.A. Davis, 1991.

Schaken, B.L, and P. Arft. "Digoxin Toxicity Treated with Digibind." *Critical Care Nurse*, 9:16–17, 20, 22 (May 1989).

Smetzer, S.C., and B.G. Ball. *Brunner and Sudarth's Medical-Surgical Nursing*. New York: J.B. Lippincott, 1992.

Squires, S., *et al*. "Sensory Alterations in Alcohol Abuse." *Topics in Clinical Nursing*, 6:51–63 (January 1986).

"To Stop Lithium, Taper the Dose." *Nurses Drug Alert*, 8:54 (July 1984).

Wallach, J. *Interpretation of Diagnostic Tests*. Boston: Little, Brown, and Company, 1992.

Wasley, G. "Laboratory Tests: Detecting Sexually Transmitted Diseases." *Nursing Times*, 84 (39):59–61 (September 28–October 4, 1988).

Wilson, J.D., *et al*. *Harrison's Principles of Internal Medicine*. New York: McGraw-Hill, 1991.

12

13

Diagnostic Tests

Angiography
Arteriography
Digital Subtraction Angiography
Lymphangiography
Venography

Electrodiagnostic Studies
Electrocardiography
Vectorcardiography
Electrophysiologic Study
Electroencephalography
Electromyography

Computed Tomography

Magnetic Resonance Imaging

Nuclear Scans
Radionuclide Imaging
Positron Emission Tomography

Radiography
Arthrography
Bronchography
Barium Enema
Barium Swallow (Esophagram,
Esophagography)

Chest Radiography
(Chest X-Ray)
Cholangiography
Cholecystography
Cystography (Voiding, Retrograde,
Urethrography)
Intravenous Pyelography (Excretory
Urography)
KUB (Kidney-Ureter-Bladder)
Mammography
Myelography
Upper Gastrointestinal (Small Bowel)
Series

Ultrasonography
(Ultrasound)

Endoscopy
Arthroscopy
Bronchoscopy
Colonoscopy
Cystoscopy/Cystourethroscopy
Gastroscopy,
Esophagogastroduodenoscopy

Nursing Implications for Diagnostic Studies

In caring for patients having diagnostic studies, it is important to consider several nursing diagnoses that are common to a variety of studies. These nursing diagnoses and nursing implications are outlined in Table 13.1.

TABLE 13.1. Nursing Diagnoses and Implications

Nursing Diagnosis	Nursing Implications
Knowledge deficit related to experiencing an unfamiliar diagnostic test.	Provide a clear explanation of the purpose of the study to the patients/significant others and what they can expect to occur preprocedurally, intraprocedurally, and postprocedurally. Include information regarding the duration of the procedure and teach patients about sensations they may experience: patients may have fewer negative emotional responses during the procedure than if they receive only procedural information. Inform patients that they do not need to talk during the procedure except for answering the few questions asked by the physician. This may minimize the increases in heart rate and blood pressure that occur during speech. The educational approach will be determined by the patient's age, educational background, perceptual-cognitive function, anxiety level, and coping style. Select educational materials that are appropriate to meet the individual patient's specific needs. These may be in the form of audiovisual or preprinted materials. Standardized materials should be previewed by the nurse and tailored to address the individual patient's needs.
Fear/anxiety related to unknown, unfamiliar experience, the meaning of the event, unfavorable results, risks of complication or injury, or actual or anticipated discomfort.	Teach patients what to expect. When the expected experience is congruent with the actual experience, there is a decrease in the state of anxiety. The type of information given to patients should be determined by their individual coping style. Patients who attempt to minimize the impact of threatening events by avoidance should be provided with procedural information only. This approach allows them to use their usual coping mechanisms for dealing with anxiety-provoking experiences. Individuals who cope with stressful events by actively seeking out information should be provided with procedural and sensation informa-

(Continued)

13

TABLE 13.1. (*Continued*)

Nursing Diagnosis	Nursing Implications
	tion. This allows them to be more prepared for the experience. Tailoring the educational approach to coping styles may decrease the level of anxiety, the psychophysiological arousal, the heart rate, and the blood pressure. The coping style should also be considered in determining the approach to obtaining informed consent. The nurse should tailor the approach to the individual's coping style.
	Teach relaxation techniques, imagery, or both to patients to offer distraction from the external stimuli of the equipment and the activities of the personnel during the procedure. Suggest that they listen to relaxation tapes or relaxing music tapes during the procedure, if appropriate. Inform the patients that comfort measures will be employed and that their feedback will be helpful and incorporated into the care.
	Assure the patients of the expertise of the personnel performing the study, which minimizes the risks involved. Inform patients that test results will be discussed by the physician at the earliest possible time. Encourage the patients to focus on other components of their lives instead of on unknown test results.
Alteration in comfort related to techniques of invasive procedures, prolonged positioning, or restricted movement.	Teach patients progressive muscle relaxation exercises to relax tense muscles during prolonged positioning and offer distraction from discomfort. Instruct the patients to inform laboratory personnel about their comfort level. This may facilitate patient comfort by allowing for more effective administration of local anesthetics or other pharmacological agents. Encourage patients to participate actively in determining the most comfortable position possible within the constraints of procedural positioning.

General Nursing Considerations

Nurses have a responsibility to patients to influence the variables that have an impact on the reliability and the cost-effectiveness of the diagnostic study being performed. If patients are psychologically prepared, it increases the likelihood of active and cooperative participation. This may increase the quality of the test results and decrease the length of time for the study, thus increasing the cost-effectiveness.

Patients may also need to be physically prepared for diagnostic studies. Meticulous attention should be directed to the physical preparation of patients to ensure reliable results and efficient time utilization. This may involve dietary, bowel, or skin site preparation or administration of pharmacotherapeutic agents, depending on the specific study. The nurse's role may be to instruct the patient in self-preparation, assist them with the preparation, or perform components of it.

Nurses also have a role in minimizing patient risks associated with diagnostic studies. It is important to make sure that all allergies are documented on the health record and that an appropriate allergy-identification wristband is in place. Other pertinent information that should be documented includes current drug therapy, physical limitations, communication considerations, and underlying medical conditions.

The nurse should perform and document a patient assessment that is focused on mental, emotional, and physical status related to the physical function of the body system being studied and the procedural risks. This allows for postprocedural comparison of assessment findings in order to detect subtle changes in the patient's condition.

Prior to the diagnostic procedure, the nurse should clarify with the primary physician whether or not regularly scheduled medications should be administered. If possible, diagnostic studies should be scheduled to avoid missing doses of medication. Particular attention and arrangements may be necessary to ensure maintenance of therapeutic blood levels for such drugs as antihypertensives, antiarrhythmics, antibiotics, and bronchodilators. Management of the diabetic patient may include special scheduling of medications, dietary intake, and the diagnostic study.

The geriatric and pediatric patient populations are a high risk for fluid and electrolyte imbalances as a result of the physical preparation for diagnostic studies that require bowel preparation, NPO status or use of radio-contrast medium. It is very important for the nurse to assess fluid volume and electrolyte status prior to the diagnostic study and to provide adequate hydration.

The use of radio-contrast material including non-ionic, low-osmolality contrast agents can cause contrast nephrotoxicity. Contrast agents can cause powerful, transient renal vasoconstriction resulting in diminished renal blood flow. They are also toxic to renal medullary cells. Patient categories with the greatest risks include patients with pre-existing renal insufficiency including diabetic

13

nephropathy, conditions causing low cardiac output with diminished renal blood flow including congestive heart failure, conditions characterized by sclerosis of renal vasculature, liver impairment, and any condition characterized by dehydration.

Another procedural risk of diagnostic studies using iodinated contrast media is allergic reactions. The nurse needs to facilitate the screening of high-risk patient populations. Patients with a history of allergic reactions to contrast dye and those who have a history of allergic reactions to various substances may be at risk for an allergic reaction. Any history of allergic reaction to any type of agent should be reported to the radiologist. Historically, seafood allergies were believed to identify patients at risk for allergic reactions to contrast medium; however, more recent evidence suggests there is no significant correlation.

Allergic reactions can vary from being very mild to very severe. Mild reactions are characterized by nausea, vomiting, flushing, erythema, coughing, sneezing, diaphoresis, dizziness, headache, or tachycardia. They are usually treated with administration of an antihistamine. Moderate reactions are characterized by abdominal cramps, diarrhea, urticaria, pruritus, asthma attack, wheezing, palpitations, hypotension, bradycardia, agitation, vertigo, or oliguria. Moderate reactions may be treated with antihistamines, epinephrine, or steroids. Severe reactions are characterized by anaphylactic shock. Symptoms include tingling and itching of soles and palms, dysphagia, laryngospasm, expiratory wheezes, laryngeal edema, a feeling of doom, disorientation progressing to coma, acute pulmonary edema, and shock. This is a medical emergency and the patient may need to be medically treated for shock, respiratory arrest, and cardiac arrest. Allergic reactions usually occur immediately but can occur one hour or longer after administration of the contrast medium. Therefore, it is important for the nurse to monitor the patient postprocedurally for signs of an allergic reaction. This includes cardiovascular, respiratory, neurological, gastrointestinal, and integumentary assessment.

A procedural risk of diagnostic studies using radiographic techniques of X-rays or radionuclides includes that of radiation exposure. It is the responsibility of the radiologist to minimize patient exposure to ionizing radiation during diagnostic procedures; however, the nurse has the responsibility to facilitate patient protection. This can be done by identifying patients who have a history of repeated exposure and women of childbearing age who could be pregnant. A menstrual history should be obtained to determine if the patient could be pregnant. Because of embryo and fetal susceptibility to defects caused by ionizing radiation, pregnant women should not have diagnostic studies using these modalities.

Patients who have a history of exposure to X-rays or radionuclides may be at risk for the cumulative effects of small doses over a period of time. The nurse can facilitate obtaining "old films" or studies done at other health-care institutions. Access to these studies may negate the necessity of having a repeat study, enhance diagnostic analysis, or influence the type of study indicated, thus minimizing radiation exposure. Exposure may also be influenced by patient participation and cooperation as well as physical preparation, as discussed previously.

Before transporting the patient to the diagnostic study area, secure and label all tubing and tape all connection sites to prevent disconnection during transportation and positioning of the patient. To minimize the risk of interrupted therapy, the nurse may need to advocate educational sessions for transportation and radiological personnel so that proper precautions can be taken to maintain the integrity of intravenous therapy, nutritional therapy, and drainage systems.

The following sections present a general description of specific diagnostic studies that should allow the nurse to administer patient care prior to and following these studies. The sections are organized by general categories of diagnostic studies, including angiography, electrodiagnostic studies, endoscopy, magnetic resonance imaging, nuclear scans, radiography, computed tomography, and ultrasound. Specific studies are presented to address special considerations.

The format for the presentations of the diagnostic studies is as follows:

Description

Duration

Normal findings

Causes of deviation from normal

Nursing implications

> *Preprocedural*

> *Postprocedural*

Diagnostic procedures, patient preparation, and postprocedural care may vary according to institutional procedures, physician preference, and patient situation. The intent of this discussion of these diagnostic studies is to serve as a guide.

ANGIOGRAPHY

This diagnostic category includes studies of vascular structures by visualization using fluoroscopy following injection of contrast medium. It includes arteriography, cardiac catheterization, digital subtraction angiography, lymphangiography, and venography.

Description

ARTERIOGRAPHY

Arteriography is a radiographic study of the vascular system following injection of a radiopaque dye through a catheter. The patient is usually placed in a supine position and cardiac monitoring leads are applied. Vital signs are taken for baseline data. The catheter insertion site is selected, shaved, cleansed, and

13

draped. A local anesthetic is administered at the insertion site. An incision is made and the catheter is inserted into the peripheral artery. The catheter is threaded into the arterial vascular structure being studied using fluoroscopy to guide placement. A contrast medium is injected through the catheter and a rapid-sequence series of films are taken until adequate visualization of the vasculature is accomplished.

Specific structures that are commonly studied include the aorta, cerebral arteries, coronary arteries, pulmonary artery, renal arteries, and iliac, femoral, and popliteal arteries. The mammary, pancreatic, and splenic arteries can also be studied.

Cardiac catheterization can also be done, which includes injection of dye into the heart, coronary arteries, and pulmonary vessels. With right cardiac catheterization, a catheter is inserted into a peripheral vein and threaded into the right atrium, right ventricle, and into the pulmonary artery. Pressures within each structure are measured and blood gas studies are done. The function of the tricuspid and pulmonary heart valves can be observed and cardiac output measured. During left cardiac catheterization, the catheter is inserted into a peripheral artery and advanced retrograde into the aorta to the coronary arteries or the left ventricle. The coronary arteries, the function of the aortic and mitral valves, and left ventricular wall motion can be studied. Pressures and blood gas studies are also done.

Duration

1–1.5 hours.

NORMAL FINDINGS

Normal, symmetrical, unobstructed blood flow in the vascular structures being studied
Normal vascular pressure and blood gas values

Causes of Deviation from Normal

Angiography may reveal one or more of the following:

Aneurysms	Malformations of vascular structures
Thromboemboli	Arteriosclerosis
Tumors	Collagenous vascular disease
Trauma	Hemorrhage
Hematoma	Congenital anomalies
Arteriovenous fistula	Vascular spasms

Valvular heart disease   Altered contractility of the heart

Coronary artery disease

Nursing Implications

Preprocedural. A consent form must be signed. Explain the purpose and the procedure of the study. Patients should be told that they may experience a warm, flushed, or hot, burning sensation during injection of the dye. This sensation should last only 30–90 seconds. Patients may also experience unusual sensations while the catheter is being threaded through the vessels or heart. Patients should be instructed to alert the physician if they experience chest pain, shortness of breath, or any other unusual sensations. They may also be taught relaxation techniques or imagery.

Patients may have nothing by mouth for 4–8 hours prior to the test depending on hospital policy or physician's orders. This is to minimize the risk of aspiration. Usually a clear-liquid or full-liquid dinner is given on the evening before the procedure. Intravenous therapy is instituted to ensure adequate hydration preprocedurally, intraprocedurally, and postprocedurally. Vital signs and nursing assessment are documented for baseline data. History of allergies and allergic reactions to iodine or dye studies should be noted. Nursing assessment should focus on neurological status, circulatory status of the peripheral arteries, and the status of underlying conditions. Clarification should be made with the physician regarding administration of the patient's usual medications. Administration of medication that may alter sensorium for 4 hours prior to the study should be avoided unless specifically ordered. Jewelry should be removed and placed in a secure area. Patients should wear a hospital gown and may wear dentures. They should void before leaving for the procedure.

Premedications are administered as ordered and patient safety is enhanced by having the patient in bed with the siderails up. Other preprocedural drugs that may be administered include steroids, antihistamines, antibiotics, or mannitol. Special preparations may be required for visualization of abdominal vascular structures. These may include laxatives or enemas prior to the test to minimize interference of bowel contents.

Postprocedural. Direct pressure is applied to the catheter insertion site for 5–20 minutes or longer and a pressure dressing is applied. The catheter insertion site should be assessed for bleeding and hematoma formation every 15 minutes for 1 hour, every 30 minutes for 2 hours, and then every hour for 4 hours. Patients should be instructed to inform the nurse if they feel a trickling, warm sensation or a damp dressing. Vital signs should be taken and documented using the same schedule. Peripheral pulses should be assessed for presence, quality, and character. Any changes should be reported immediately to the physician. The color, temperature, and tactile sensation of the extremity should also be assessed. It is important to monitor for procedural complications,

13

including allergic reactions, neurological changes, cardiovascular changes, pulmonary changes, changes in fluid volume status, and elevated serum creatinine levels. The patient is kept on bed rest in a recumbent position with the leg or arm straight for 6–24 hours as ordered. The patient may use 1 or 2 pillows to minimize stress on the puncture site. Unless contraindicated, fluids are given to rehydrate and to facilitate excretion of the contrast medium. The patient's normal diet is usually resumed unless otherwise ordered.

Description
DIGITAL SUBTRACTION ANGIOGRAPHY

Digital subtraction angiography is a computerized imaging technique by which the vasculature can be visualized on a monitor screen following intravenous injection of iodinated contrast medium. Images are recorded by a computer and can be manipulated to isolate and enhance iodine contrast and visually eliminate superimposing structures. These images can be stored for future reference.

The advantage of digital angiography is that the procedure can be performed on an outpatient basis because there is less risk of complications with venous access. Less contrast medium may be used, which is especially beneficial to renal, cardiac, and diabetic patients who may not tolerate hyperosmolar contrast agents.

A local anesthetic is administered following preparation of the catheter insertion site. The catheter is inserted into the antecubital or femoral vein and threaded into the superior vena cava with the tip entering the right atrium. Contrast medium is injected through a power injector and images are recorded on tapes or discs. Following adequate imaging, the catheter is removed and a sterile dressing is applied over the insertion site.

Duration
30–60 minutes.

NORMAL FINDINGS

The normal findings are normal blood flow in the vascular structure studied; this includes normal aortic arch and aorta; normal renal, iliac, and femoral arterial systems; normal carotid and vertebral arteries; normal coronary arteries, cardiac motion and contractility; normal brachiocephalic arteries; normal abdominal aorta; and normal femoral/popliteal arteries.

Causes of Deviation from Normal
Digital subtraction angiography may reveal one or more of the following:

Stenosis	Obstruction
Emboli	Ulcerative plaques
Aneurysms	Tumors and other masses
Atherosclerotic occlusive disease	Vascular malformations

Nursing Implications

Preprocedural. An informed consent must be signed. The purpose and the procedure should be explained to patients. They should be told that it will be important to stay motionless at times during the procedure. Patients should be assessed for history of allergies or allergic reactions to iodine or contrast medium. Vital signs and assessment data should be recorded for baseline information. Assessment data should include blood urea nitrogen and serum creatinine levels.

Postprocedural. Vital signs should be monitored including cardiac rhythm. Patients should be assessed for signs of allergic reactions and changes in renal function. Catheter insertion site should be assessed for bleeding and hematoma formation. Patients should be told to observe for any signs of infection at the catheter insertion site following discharge and to report this to the physician. They should be instructed that they may remove the dressing after 24 hours. They should also be instructed to drink plenty of fluids to rehydrate and to facilitate excretion of the contrast medium.

Description

LYMPHANGIOGRAPHY

Lymphangiography is a radiographic study of the lymphatic system following injection of an oil-based contrast medium into a lymphatic vessel. Following location of lymphatic vessels by the intradermal injection of blue contrast medium, a local anesthetic is injected at the catheter insertion site. An incision is made, the vessel is cannulated, and the contrast medium is injected over 1–2 hours. Radiographic films are taken. When adequate visualization of the lymphatic system is accomplished, the catheter is removed, the incision is closed, and a sterile dressing is applied. Radiographic films are repeated in 24 hours for visualization of the lymph nodes.

The contrast medium is injected into the lymphatic vessels in the foot for visualization of lymph structures of the leg, inguinal, iliac, retroperitoneum, and thoracic duct. The contrast medium is injected into the hand for visualization of the axillary, supraclavicular, and cervical lymph structures.

Duration

3 hours.

13

N O R M A L   F I N D I N G S

Normal filling of the lymphatic vessels and normal size and placement of lymph nodes with regular, uniform opacity are normal findings.

Causes of Deviation from Normal

Lymphangiography may reveal one or more of the following:

Lymphoma

Metastatic disease

Lymphedema

Nursing Implications

Preprocedural. An informed consent must be signed. The purpose and the procedure of the diagnostic study should be explained to patients. They should be told about the normal urine and stool discoloration from the blue dye, which may last several days. The skin may also have a bluish tinge. Patients should be taught relaxation techniques since they will have to remain still during the prolonged injection of the contrast medium. No food or fluid restrictions are necessary. Patients should be instructed to cleanse their feet or hands with an antiseptic soap prior to the procedure. Vital signs and baseline assessment data including allergies or allergic reactions to iodine or contrast medium should be recorded. Patients should void before leaving for the procedure. Preprocedural medications, such as sedatives, should be administered if ordered.

Postprocedural. Vital signs should be monitored and recorded every 4 hours for 48 hours. Patients should be observed for signs of pulmonary embolization including shortness of breath, chest pain, cough, hypotension, and low-grade fever. Patients are placed on bed rest for 24 hours with the extremity elevated to minimize peripheral edema. Incision sites may be painful requiring the administration of analgesics; they should be assessed for signs of hematoma formation and infection. Patients should be instructed in the care of the incision sites. The sterile dressing should be kept in place for 2 days and the site kept dry. Tub baths should not be taken until the sutures are removed in approximately 7 days. Signs of infection should be reported to the physician immediately.

Description

VENOGRAPHY

Venography is a radiographic study of the venous system following injection of an iodine contrast substance. The patient is positioned on a tilt table angled at 40–60 degrees so there is no weight bearing on the tested leg. A vein is located on the dorsum of the foot and a needle inserted. Intravenous normal saline is injected before and after injection of the contrast medium. Contrast dye is injected over several minutes and visualized using fluoroscopy. Radiographic films are taken of the lower extremity including the groin area. Following adequate visualization, the needle is removed and a sterile dressing is applied.

Duration
30–60 minutes.

N O R M A L   F I N D I N G S

Normal venous blood flow

Causes of Deviation from Normal
Venography may reveal one or more of the following:

Thrombi

Soft tissue compression

Trauma

Nursing Implications
Preprocedural. An informed consent must be signed. The purpose and the procedure should be explained to patients. Patients must be told that it is necessary to keep the leg very still during fluoroscopy and the radiographic exposures. Patients should also be told that there may be a temporary burning sensation during injection of the dye. Vital signs, including peripheral pulse, and risks from allergic reaction to the iodine contrast medium should be assessed. Patients should be instructed to keep the leg elevated prior to the study to reduce edema. Patients will usually have nothing by mouth for 4 hours prior to testing; they should also void before leaving for the procedure.

Postprocedural. Vital signs, including peripheral pulse, and signs of an allergic reaction should be assessed every 15 minutes for 1 hour and then every 2 hours until stable. The needle site should be assessed for signs of bleeding or hematoma formation. Patients should be instructed to observe for signs of infection after discharge. Medical therapy should be given as ordered if deep venous thrombosis is present.

ELECTRODIAGNOSTIC STUDIES

This category of diagnostic studies includes electrocardiography, vectorcardiography, electroencephalography, electromyography, and electrophysiologic study. These studies measure and record electrical activity or nerve impulse conduction of various body structures.

13

Description

ELECTROCARDIOGRAPHY

An electrocardiogram (EKG) is a graphic representation of the electrical activity, impulse formation, and conduction in the heart. The electrical activity produces electrical currents that can be measured by applying electrodes to the skin and amplifying them through an EKG apparatus to produce a graphic readout or display.

Patients are placed in a recumbent, supine position. If they are unable to assume a recumbent position, the exact body position should be documented for future reference and for consideration in the interpretation of the EKG. Electrodes are applied to the extremities or anterior trunk of the body, equidistant from the heart and precordium, using electrode conducting gel or pads. Patients are instructed to remain still to minimize skeletal muscle motion artifact. The EKG is recorded in the frontal and horizontal planes of the body through the EKG machine.

Variations of this procedure may occur if there is continuous monitoring of the EKG using a continuous recording device. A Holter monitor is an example of such a device. Continuous monitoring may be done to analyze the occurrence of dysrhythmias during exercise or activities of daily living or the effectiveness of pharmacotherapeutic agents.

Duration

15 minutes or continuous.

NORMAL FINDINGS

Normal anatomical position of the heart
Normal-size heart chambers
Normal rhythm and conduction
Normal electrical axis
Normal EKG wave size, deflection, and duration

Causes of Deviation from Normal

Electrocardiography may reveal one or more of the following:

Coronary artery spasm
(Prinzmetal's angina)
Cardiac dysrhythmias
Cardiac tamponade
Myocarditis

Myocardial infarction and ischemia
Conduction disturbances
Cardiomyopathy
Myocardial hypertrophy
Pulmonary hypertension

Cor pulmonale

Pulmonary emboli

Drug toxicity (digoxin, quinidine)

Electrolyte imbalances
(hypokalemia, hyperkalemia,
hypocalcemia, hypercalcemia)

Implications

Preprocedural. The purpose and the procedure should be explained to the patient, emphasizing that the procedure will not cause discomfort. It is important for the patient to understand that the test is electrically safe and does not administer any electrical current. This test is usually done at the bedside or in an outpatient setting. The nurse should provide for privacy during the test since the precordial area will be exposed for electrode placement. Clothing should be selected to allow easy access to the arms, legs, and chest for electrode placement.

Patients with excessive chest hair may need small areas shaved for lead placement to prevent electrical interference from poor electrode contact. Adhesive pads should only be used if the patient is not allergic to adhesive. In case of allergy to adhesive, an alternative approach to electrode connection may be necessary.

Vital signs and the current medications that the patient is taking should be recorded. In addition, any chest pain the patient is experiencing should also be recorded.

Postprocedural. Conducting gel should be removed from the skin. Patients should be told how to receive results of the test.

Description
VECTORCARDIOGRAPHY

Vectorcardiography is a graphic representation of the direction and magnitude of the action potential during the cardiac cycle. Electrodes are applied to the skin and transmit impulses to a machine that displays the vector loops. The vector loops represent the electrical potentials as measured along the vertical, horizontal, and sagittal axes of the heart. The procedure is similar to an electrocardiogram.

Duration
15–30 minutes.

NORMAL FINDINGS

Three distinct loops representing normal electrical activity of the heart

13

Causes of Deviation from Normal
Vectorcardiography may reveal one or more of the following:

Ventricular hypertrophy

Posterior and anterior fascicular blocks

Atrial enlargement

Bundle branch block

Myocardial infarction

Myocardial ischemia

Atrial septal defects

Nursing Implications
Preprocedural. Same as for electrocardiography.
Postprocedural. Same as for electrocardiography.

Description
ELECTROPHYSIOLOGIC STUDY
An electrophysiologic study (EPS) is an intracardiac electrogram where electrode catheters are placed within the heart to record electrical activity. EPS can enhance evaluation of the cardiac conduction system, locate the origin of impulse formation or site of impulse block, identify the risks of developing life-threatening dysrhythmias, and evaluate the effectiveness of medical treatment of dysrhythmias (pacing, medications, or electrosurgery).

The patient is attached to an EKG monitor. The catheter access site (femoral area) is shaved, cleansed, and draped. A local anesthetic is administered. An electrode catheter is inserted into the femoral vein through an introducer. A total of 3–6 electrode catheters may be inserted. Electrode catheter insertion sites may include the femoral (most common), brachial, subclavian, and/or jugular vein. The catheters are advanced one at a time through the inferior vena cava into the right atrium and right ventricle using fluoroscopy. The catheters are placed at different locations in the right atrium and right ventricle.

Following electrode catheter placement, an intracardiac electrocardiogram is recorded. Atrial or ventricular pacing through the catheters can be used to induce dysrhythmias or assess the conduction system. Drugs can be administered through the intravenous line to assess the efficacy of specific drug therapy for the treatment of dysrhythmias. Defibrillation equipment and emergency cardiac drugs are available to treat life-threatening dysrhythmias. At completion of the test, the catheters are removed, direct pressure is applied for 10 minutes, and a sterile dressing is applied.

Duration
2–4 hours.

N O R M A L   F I N D I N G S

Normal electrical conduction of the heart

Causes of Deviation from Normal

Electrophysiological studies may reveal one or more of the following:

Sinus node dysfunction	Sick sinus syndrome
Bradyarrhythmias	Atrioventricular conduction delays
Ventricular dysrhythmias	Supraventricular tachycardia
Wide-complex tachycardia	

Nursing Implications

Preprocedural. The purpose and the procedure should be explained to the patient and an informed consent form signed. The importance of lying still during the procedure in order to minimize electrical artifact, minimize changes in the heart rate, and prevent catheter position change should be included.

To minimize interference with study findings, antiarrhythmic drugs may be discontinued by the physician. Reassure the patients that they will be continuously monitored in order to identify and treat any rhythm disturbance that might occur when they are not receiving their usual medications. If serial studies are being conducted to evaluate the effectiveness of the drug treatment program, antiarrhythmics will be continued. The patient's heart rate, rhythm, and blood pressure should be recorded. Patients are given nothing by mouth after midnight on the day of the test to minimize the risk of aspiration. If they are scheduled to have the procedure late in the day, a clear-liquid breakfast may be ordered. Intravenous therapy is initiated to provide access for emergency drug therapy. Patients should void before leaving for the procedure. A sedative should be administered prior to the procedure, if ordered. Patients are transported by stretcher with cardiac monitoring and emergency cardiac equipment available.

Postprocedural. The heart rate and rhythm should be monitored continuously for 24 hours to detect the occurrence of dysrhythmias. Vital signs should be recorded every 15 minutes until stable. The catheter insertion site should be observed for signs of bleeding, hematoma formation, or infection. Patients should be observed for signs of pulmonary emboli, pneumothorax, and neurological changes. Patients should remain on bed-rest with the leg kept straight for 6–12 hours to decrease the risk of bleeding from the catheter insertion site(s). The head of the bed can be elevated 15°. Patients should avoid bending at the hip for a total of 24 hours. Their regular diet can be resumed following the procedure.

13

Description
ELECTROENCEPHALOGRAPHY

An electroencephalogram (EEG) is a recording of the electrical activity of the cerebral cortex of the brain. The procedure may be performed during wakefulness, drowsiness, exposure to external stimuli, or sleep. There are approximately 20 electrodes placed on the scalp with skin glue or paste at predetermined positions that correlate with anatomical structures of the brain. The electrical waveforms are recorded on graph paper.

The study is performed in a quiet environment with the patient in a sitting, relaxed position or in a lying position. A baseline recording is taken while the patient is relaxed, with eyes closed. Recordings are made during phases of various activities. The patient may be asked to hyperventilate to initiate seizure activity. The patient may also be subjected to photic stimulation, such as flickering lights. A mild sedative may be administered to promote the drowsiness and sleep required for the last phase of recording.

Duration
1.5–2 hours or longer.

NORMAL FINDINGS

Normal symmetrical pattern of regular, short alpha waves in an awake, relaxed state with eyes closed

Causes of Deviation from Normal
Electroencephalography may reveal one or more of the following:

Brain tumors	Abscesses
Subdural hematomas	Cerebrovascular disease
Narcolepsy	Alzheimer's disease
Cerebral death	Epilepsy
Head injury	Metabolic disorders
Drug overdose	Sleep disorders
Depression	

Nursing Implications
Preprocedural. The purpose and the procedure should be explained to patients, emphasizing that the procedure will not cause discomfort and that the test only records electrical activity and not thoughts or intelligence. Patients should be told that the test does not administer electrical shocks and is electrically safe.

In order to collect reliable data, it is important that patients are calm and relaxed during the procedure. Anxiety can interfere with alpha-wave activity and can also generate electrical artifact from skeletal muscle tension.

There are no food or fluid restrictions except coffee, tea, cola drinks, alcohol, and other stimulants or depressants. Anticonvulsants, sedatives, and tranquilizers may be withheld for 48 hours prior to the EEG and specific orders should be written by the physician.

If a sleep phase is ordered, it is best if the patient goes to sleep 3 hours later than usual and arises early, allowing for approximately 5 hours of sleep. The patient should not nap before the recording. Hair is shampooed prior to the test, and sprays, oils, or conditioners should not be applied in order to maximize electrode contact and minimize interference with test results.

Since anticonvulsants are usually withheld for the study, patients may be at risk for seizure activity. Safety should be provided by following seizure precautions and recording and reporting any seizure activity. Preprocedural assessment data including vital signs and neurological signs, sleep patterns, and behavior should also be recorded.

Postprocedural. The patient's hair should be washed to remove the electrode paste. Use of acetone may be necessary. Drug therapy should be resumed per physician's orders and postprocedural assessment data recorded. Rest periods should be provided following the procedure.

Description
ELECTROMYOGRAPHY

Electromyography (EMG) is a graphic recording of the electrical activity of peripheral nerves and skeletal muscles. The patient is positioned in a recumbent, relaxed position. Following skin preparation, needle electrodes are inserted into the skeletal muscle or muscles being studied. The electrical activity of muscle nerve impulses is recorded on graph paper, viewed on an oscilloscope, or audioamplified and tape-recorded. The amplitude and duration of muscle contraction are recorded. The patient may be requested to relax or contract certain muscles during the test. The patient may experience pain if the electrode is placed near a terminal nerve. When this occurs, the needle is usually repositioned since pain can yield unreliable results.

For nerve conduction studies, electrical current is passed through the patient and the amplitude wave is recorded. This, too, can cause a painful sensation.

Duration
Approximately 1 hour.

N O R M A L   F I N D I N G S

Normal muscle action potential
Normal nerve conduction

13

Causes of Deviation from Normal

Electromyography may reveal one or more of the following:

Neuromuscular disorders affecting the lower motor neuron, the neuromuscular function, skeletal muscle fibers, and sensory neurons

Denervation of a muscle

Injury to peripheral nerves

Peripheral neuropathies secondary to diabetes, alcoholism, metabolic and nutritional disorders

Muscle disease causing decreased amplitude and duration of conduction

Nursing Implications

Preprocedural. A consent form must be signed following an explanation of the purpose and the procedure. The patient should be told that there may be some discomfort with needle electrode placement and nerve stimulation. Food and fluids are not restricted except coffee, tea, and cola drinks, and smoking is restricted for several hours prior to the test.

Medications that may interfere with the results should be withheld before the test per physician's orders. These include muscle relaxants, anticholinergics, and cholinergics. If ordered, enzyme studies of serum glutamic oxaloacetic transaminase (SGOT), lactate dehydrogenase (LDH), and creatinine phosphokinase (CPK) should be done prior to the study, as these enzymes will be released and result in misleading levels for up to 10 days.

Postprocedural. Pain relief should be provided by administering analgesics ordered by the physician. The needle insertion site should be observed for hematoma formation.

COMPUTED TOMOGRAPHY

Description

Computed tomography (CT) is an imaging technique that makes precise multidimensional images by scanning a cross-section of the body with X-ray beams and radiation detectors. A computer transcribes these quantitative measurements and reconstructs internal structures into images.

The patient is placed on the scanning table and the position is secured. The scanner ring produces X-ray beams in a rotating pattern around the body area being studied. The computer calculates the density of the body area based on the energy absorbed and an image is displayed on a viewing screen.

This scan can be performed with or without contrast medium. Use of contrast medium allows for enhancement of tissue absorption and increases tissue density for better imaging. It may be administered orally or intravenously.

Duration

30–90 minutes.

N O R M A L   F I N D I N G S

Normal tissue density, size, location, shape, and symmetry of the body
structures studied

Causes of Deviation from Normal

CT may reveal one or more of the following:

Tumors	Cysts
Enlarged lymph nodes	Abscesses
Trauma	Fractures
Spinal cord stenosis	Enlarged body organs
Thrombus	Hematoma
Infection	Infarction
Calcification	Degenerative disease
Renal calculi	Aneurysm and other vascular
Abnormal collection of body fluid or blood	abnormalities

Nursing Implications

Preprocedural. An informed consent must be obtained. Women should be
screened for possible pregnancy as this test is contraindicated during pregnancy
because of risks to the fetus. History of allergies to contrast medium or other
substances should be obtained and the radiologist should be informed. The purpose and the procedure should be explained to the patient. An explanation of
the importance of remaining motionless during the procedure should be included. Patients may be asked to hold their breath several times during the procedure. Inform patients that the machine emits a subtle clicking-whirl sound.
They should also be informed that an intravenous contrast medium may be
used and that they may experience a warm, flushed, or hot burning sensation
and a salty taste from the injection. They may be asked to drink a thick, chalky
contrast substance. Other contrast-enhancement methods may be used depending on the anatomical structures being studied and should be explained to each
patient.

If the abdomen and pelvis are being studied, a contrast medium is given.
Female patients may require vaginal tampon placement in order to distend the
vagina and allow for easier identification of the cervix of the uterus.

13

The nurse should emphasize that this procedure is not painful. Patients should be taught relaxation techniques or imagery in an attempt to minimize reactions to confinement. Patients may have nothing by mouth for 2–4 hours prior to the test if it is likely that contrast medium is to be used. Jewelry, hair pins, and other metal objects should be removed. Patients should be dressed in a hospital gown.

A sedative or analgesic may be administered prior to the procedure to enhance relaxation and motionlessness during the procedure. The patient should be asked to void before the procedure unless the pelvis is being studied. The radiologist may request that the patient have a full bladder for better visualization.

Postprocedural. If iodine contrast medium was given intravenously, patients should be observed for an allergic reaction. If signs of a reaction occur, the nurse should report them to the physician immediately and be prepared to administer medical therapy as ordered. In addition, the nurse should observe for signs of inflammation or hematoma formation at the intravenous insertion site and encourage oral fluid intake and frequent voiding to facilitate elimination of contrast medium. Preprocedural diet and activity can be resumed unless otherwise ordered.

MAGNETIC RESONANCE IMAGING

Description

Magnetic resonance imaging (MRI) is a noninvasive imaging technique using a strong magnetic field and radiowaves to make contiguous cross-sectional images of the body. This technique allows the detection of differences in total water content of body tissues and other physiochemical constituents.

The MRI machine creates a strong magnetic field that causes the nuclei of elements with an odd number of protons and neutrons to align themselves in relation to this electromagnetic field. Radiowaves are then applied perpendicular across these aligned nuclei and the nuclei absorb the energy and change the direction of their spin to align against the field. When the radiowaves are switched off, the nuclei spontaneously return to their original direction of spin and they emit the energy they absorbed from the radiowaves. This energy is detected and converted to a well-defined visual image by computer.

Earphones may be placed on the patient to allow for communication with the technician. The patient is positioned on a pallet that is guided into a cylindrically shaped, tunnel-like machine. The patient is instructed to lie motionless during the procedure. The machine makes a clanging sound during cross-sectional imaging. The patient is removed from the cylinder following adequate imaging.

An advantage of this procedure is that contrast medium may not be required. Intravenous paramagnetic contrast media may be used; however, since these agents do not contain iodine, there is less risk of reaction. An allergic reaction is uncommon and usually consists of a headache. There are no risks of radiation to the patient because there is no exposure to ionizing radiation.

Duration

15–90 minutes.

N O R M A L   F I N D I N G S

Normal body tissues and structures

Causes of Deviation from Normal

MRI may reveal one or more of the following:

Atherosclerosis

Ischemia

Muscle disease

Thrombus

Hemorrhage

Hematoma

Trauma

Skeletal abnormalities

Bone marrow disease

Edema

Infiltrative breast cancer

Pathology of the posterior fossa

Metastatic carcinoma of the brain

Cysts

Lymphadenopathy

Infarction

Valvular heart disease

Aneurysms and other vascular abnormalities

Demyelinating disease

Atropy

Intervertebral disc disease

Infection

Dementia

Compression of the spinal cord

Neuropathy

Tumors or masses (differentiate malignant versus benign)

Soft-tissue abnormalities of the pelvis

Upper airway and pulmonary abnormalities

Nursing Implications

Preprocedural. An informed consent must be obtained. The purpose and the procedure should be explained to the patient. Patients should be told that they will be completely inside a cylindrically shaped machine headfirst and the space in the machine only allows several inches of clearance above their body. They will need to lie completely still and they may feel unusual sensations from fillings in their teeth.

13

Imagery may be taught to patients in an attempt to minimize reactions to confinement and feelings of claustrophobia. If a patient is at high risk of experiencing claustrophobia, a sedative may be administered without interfering with test results.

Patients should be instructed to remove their jewelry, hair pins, glasses, removable prostheses, and any other metal objects. Patients who have metal prostheses such as total joints, orthopedic screws, and heart valves should not have this test because the magnetic field can move these objects within the body. Also, patients with pacemakers should not have this procedure because the MRI machine deactivates pacemakers. Critically ill patients cannot be monitored adequately during this procedure.

There are no food or fluid restrictions. Patients should be encouraged to void prior to the test for comfort reasons. Patients must wear a hospital gown without metal fasteners.

Postprocedural. No procedural follow-up care is necessary. If sedation was used, the patient should be observed for 1–2 hours to evaluate and provide for safety.

NUCLEAR SCANS

Description
RADIONUCLIDE IMAGING

Nuclear scans are diagnostic studies that use *radionuclides* or radiopharmaceuticals to image morphological and functional abnormalities in various body areas. The radiopharmaceutical is administered intravenously, inhalationally, or orally and distributed with blood flow, air flow, or enteral flow to the body tissues being studied. There is a time delay to allow for distribution. The radiation that is emitted is detected by a scintigraphic scanner that is positioned over the area being studied and a visual image is produced and displayed or recorded on film. The image is compared to normal distribution for either an area of increased uptake or an area of decreased uptake depending on the type of imaging. There are specific radiopharmaceutical "tracers" that are specific for different organs and body tissues and/or processes that are studied.

Duration
Duration and delay time between administration of radiopharmaceutical and scanning vary depending on the specific radiopharmaceutical used and the body area being studied. Consult the institution's department of nuclear medicine for this information.

Normal size, shape, location, structure, and function of organ(s) or tissue(s) being studied
Normal blood flow

Causes of Deviation from Normal

Radionuclide imaging may reveal one or more of the following:

Tumors	Infarction
Ischemia	Abscesses
Cysts	Metastatic disease
Degenerative diseases	Fractures
Bone disease	Abnormal cardiac output
Trauma	Thyroid gland disease
Parenchymal renal disease	Abnormal renal function
Abnormal thyroid function	Cirrhosis
Emboli	Atelectasis
Hepatitis	Enlarged organs and glands (cardiomegaly, hepatomegaly, splenomegaly)
Pneumonia	
Congenital abnormalities	

Nursing Implications

Preprocedural. An informed consent must be obtained with thorough explanation of the radiation hazard explained to the patient by the physician. The purpose and the procedure should be explained to the patient. A delay follows administration of the radiopharmaceutical depending on the agent and study; multiple imaging may also be done at different time intervals. The department of nuclear medicine should be consulted for specific information for these time intervals.

Patients should be told they may be asked to change body position for imaging of different sections of the body and that they will need to lie still during imaging except for the necessary repositioning.

A patient history must be obtained, including allergies that may have an impact on the selection of the radiopharmaceutical agent, recent radionuclide procedures, presence of internal prostheses, and current medications. Antihypertensives may affect test results. If a thyroid scan is scheduled, diet and drugs containing iodine should be avoided for 3–7 days prior to the study

13

as ordered. These include thyroid replacement hormones, multivitamins, phe-
nothiazines, aspirin, over-the-counter drugs with iodine, seafood, and iodized
salt. If this is not possible, the nurse should note the agent and dose on the
health record so that the nuclear medicine physician can consider this information during interpretation of test results. Patients who could possibly be pregnant or who are breast-feeding should be identified and special precautions
taken by the physician.

There are usually no food or fluid restrictions except for thyroid scans, as previously mentioned, and for stress thallium tests and pancreas scans. Fluids
should be encouraged unless contraindicated. Specific fluid intake volume may
be ordered for specific procedures.

Patients should remove all jewelry, hair pins, removable metal prostheses,
and any other metal objects. Patients should be asked to void prior to the procedure. Sedatives or other medications are administered as ordered. Blocking
agents specific to the radiopharmaceutical agents and specific procedures may
be ordered. The specified time schedules should be followed very closely to help
maximize the reliability of the test results. The scanning time is specified
according to the radiopharmaceutical used and the area of the body being
studied.

Postprocedural. The intravenous site should be assessed for inflammation
and hematoma formation. No special precautions are followed for patient's ex-
creta at this time unless large volumes of blood are lost closely following the
administration of the radiopharmaceutical agent. If this occurs, the department
of nuclear medicine should be consulted.

Description
POSITRON EMISSION TOMOGRAPHY

Positron emission tomography (PET) is a nuclear scan technique that is capable
of registering blood flow, glucose metabolism, and physiologic or biochemical
processes in cross-sections of the brain and other body tissues. The radiopharmaceutical is administered and the electromagnetic radiation that is emitted by
positron-electron interaction is detected and transformed into a computer-
generated visual display.

The patient is positioned and secured in a comfortable, reclining chair. Two
intravenous lines are placed, one to infuse the radiopharmaceutical and one to
draw blood-gas samples. Comparison is made between blood samples and the
computer image of the organ or tissue.

If the brain is being studied, the patient may be asked to perform different
cognitive activities, such as memory or reasoning, in order to measure metabolic activities of the local brain areas performing these functions. Extraneous
auditory and visual stimuli are minimized with placement of a blindfold and ear
plugs. Upon completion of the imaging, the intravenous lines are discontinued.

Duration

60–90 minutes.

N O R M A L   F I N D I N G S

Normal glucose metabolism and other metabolic processes in the brain and other body organs

Normal blood flow to the brain and other body organs

Causes of Deviation from Normal

Positron emission tomography may reveal processes associated with one or more of the following:

Tumors	Epilepsy
Migraine headaches	Parkinson's disease
Schizophrenia	Depression
Alzheimer's disease	Ischemia in any body part
Infarction in any body part	Tissue water or density measurement
Infection	Pulmonary ventilation/perfusion abnormalities
Renal function	Amyloid deposits

Nursing Implications

Preprocedural. An informed consent must be obtained. The purpose and the procedure should be explained to the patient including the fact that the machine will be making a clinking sound and the patient must be as still as possible. Imagery as a relaxation technique is not taught as this mental activity may interfere with test results.

Patients are instructed to abstain from alcohol, caffeine, and tobacco for 24 hours prior to the study. They should be told to eat a meal 3–4 hours before the test. Diabetic patients should take their pretest dose of insulin before this meal as ordered by the physician. Consult with the physician regarding other drugs that may alter metabolic processes in order to minimize interference of test results.

Postprocedural. Patients are instructed to slowly move into an upright position to minimize postural hypotension. They should be instructed to urinate frequently following the test to empty the radiopharmaceutical from the bladder. Preprocedural diet and activity can be resumed unless otherwise ordered.

13

RADIOGRAPHY

Radiography is the study of X-ray- or gamma ray-exposed film demonstrating radiopaque internal body parts either as they exist or with the enhancement of contrast medium. While in many instances radiography is being superseded by the use of computed tomography, ultrasonography, fiberoptic endoscopy, and newer imaging techniques, the radiograph still has an invaluable role as a diagnostic study.

Frequently used terms in radiography are fluoroscopy and "spot" films. *Fluoroscopy* is a continuous visualization of x-ray images that can demonstrate motion of organs and contrast medium. Fluoroscopy can be used to guide the timing of actual radiographic film recording, which is called the "spot" film.

There are general nursing considerations in caring for patients having a radiographic study. Female patients of childbearing age should be screened for pregnancy or possible pregnancy. Patients who are pregnant should not undergo radiographic studies because of the risks to the fetus. Patients who will receive iodine contrast medium should be screened for a history of allergies, allergic reactions to iodine or other contrast medium, and a history of asthma. This patient population may receive a test dose of the contrast medium to be used or may receive medication prior to, during, or following the procedure to prevent or minimize an allergic response.

It is important to sequence radiographic examinations. All other radiographic studies, computed tomography, or fiberoptic endoscopic studies should precede any radiographic techniques that require barium administration. Similarly, laboratory tests or nuclear scanning that relies on the measurement of radioactive labels should precede any radiographic study requiring the administration of iodine contrast. Finally, within the abdominal group of radiographs, an intravenous pyelogram should precede a cholecystogram.

Description
ARTHROGRAPHY

Arthrography is a radiographic examination of a joint to determine whether or not cartilage and membrane capsule or the articular surfaces of the joint are intact or damaged. The patient is positioned to allow access to the joint. The skin site is cleansed and a local anesthetic may be injected. Fluoroscopy is used to ensure correct needle placement. Synovial fluid is aspirated prior to injection of the contrast medium. Following iodine or other contrast injection, the joint may be manipulated to facilitate distribution of the contrast medium. Radiographic films are taken.

Duration
30–45 minutes.

Causes of Deviation from Normal

Arthrography may reveal one or more of the following:

Synovial cyst	Fracture
Joint dislocation	Erosion of cartilage
Torn menisci, ligaments, or tendons	Inflammation of the joint

Nursing Implications

Preprocedural. An informed consent must be obtained. The purpose and the procedure should be explained to the patient. Patients should be told that there may be immobilization of the joint and application of an elastic wrap to the involved joint following the procedure.

Patients should provide information about allergies and allergic reactions to iodine or other contrast medium prior to the study. Female patients should be screened to determine possible pregnancy as this procedure is contraindicated during pregnancy because of risks to the fetus. Joints should be assessed for signs of infection. Patients should be instructed to scrub the site with soap prior to the procedure.

Postprocedural. The nurse should observe and report signs of an allergic reaction to contrast medium. Necessary analgesics are administered and ice applied to the joint, if ordered. If air contrast was used, patients should be told to refrain from resuming normal activities for 3–4 days to allow for reabsorption of all the air.

Patients should be told that crepitus is normal for 1–2 days; however, the physician should be notified if it persists or returns. Patients should be assessed for swelling, excessive pain, hematoma formation, or inflammation at needle puncture site. They should be instructed in proper application of elastic wrap.

Description
BRONCHOGRAPHY

Bronchography is a radiographic contrast study of the trachea and bronchi. There are several methods of instilling the contrast medium into the tracheobronchial tree, one of which is by placement of a catheter. Most methods require suppression of the gag and cough reflex. This may be accomplished by

13

administration of a topical anesthetic agent to the internal throat. The patient is placed in a sitting position and instructed to take rapid, shallow breaths, and to avoid coughing during the procedure. Following instillation of the contrast, the patient's position may be changed several times to facilitate distribution of the contrast medium. Fluoroscopy is used for visualization of the flow of the radiopaque liquid, and chest films are taken. The patient may be placed in postural drainage position and instructed to cough to remove the contrast substance.

Duration

45–60 minutes.

NORMAL FINDINGS

Normal anatomical integrity of the tracheobronchial tree

Causes of Deviation from Normal

Bronchography may reveal one or more of the following:

Obstruction   Stenosis

Tumors   Cysts

Bronchiectasis

Nursing Implications

Preprocedural. An informed consent must be signed. The purpose and the procedure should be explained to the patient. Instruction includes breathing technique, coughing considerations during the procedure, and postural drainage following the procedure.

Female patients of childbearing age should be screened to determine possible pregnancy as the procedure is contraindicated because of risk to the fetus. The patient should be assessed for allergies to contrast medium, iodine, and local anesthetic agents, and these should be reported to the physician. Aggressive pulmonary hygiene may be indicated to remove secretions from the airway to maximize visualization. Food and fluid restrictions are recommended for 6–12 hours prior to the test to reduce the risk of aspiration. Patients should be instructed to remove dental prostheses.

Preprocedural medication should be administered, which may include a sedative and a medication to reduce secretions.

Postprocedural. NPO status is continued until return of the gag and cough reflexes and the patient is alert. Patients should be assessed for signs of respiratory distress including stridor, dyspnea, wheezing, and allergic reaction to the iodine contrast. The nurse should assist with gentle coughing and postural drainage, as ordered. Warm saline gargle or lozenges may be provided for throat discomfort following return of gag and cough reflexes.

Description

BARIUM ENEMA

The *barium enema* is a radiographic contrast study of the large intestine that allows visualization of its shape, location, and patency. A contrast medium is instilled into the rectum and distributed throughout the colon by patient positioning until the entire lining of the large intestine has been coated or filled. This process is followed fluoroscopically and may be interrupted for spot films. A double-contrast effect may be obtained by instilling air along with a thicker barium preparation.

Duration

60–90 minutes.

N O R M A L   F I N D I N G S

Normal contour, filling, and patency of the colon without distention, overlapping, or torsion

---

Causes of Deviation from Normal

A barium enema may reveal one or more of the following:

Crohn's disease	Tumors
Intussusception	Diverticulosis
Polyps	Fistula
Stenosis	Hernias
Obstructions	Inflammation

Nursing Implications

Preprocedural. The purpose and the procedure should be explained to the patient including specific instructions for bowel preparation; this may include a low-residue diet for 2–3 days prior to the X-ray series. A clear-liquid diet is given the evening before the examination. Oral or rectal laxatives or cathartics may be prescribed 12 hours before the examination, culminating in 1–3 tap-water enemas until clear on the morning of the examination or 1 hour preprocedurally. Unless contraindicated, liberal fluid intake should be encouraged prior to NPO status to avoid dehydration. Other abdominal diagnostic studies should be scheduled prior to the barium enema. If stool specimens are to be collected, these should be obtained before the bowel preparation is initiated.

13

Postprocedural. Dietary and fluid intake may be resumed as ordered. The nurse should administer or instruct the patient to take a laxative for 2 days or until stools have returned to normal, as ordered. Patients should be told that the color of their stools will be chalky white to light until all of the barium is eliminated. Rest periods should be provided after this examination, as this can be an exhausting study.

Description

BARIUM SWALLOW (ESOPHAGRAM, ESOPHAGOGRAPHY)

A *barium swallow* is a radiographic contrast technique performed to visualize the esophageal portion of the upper gastrointestinal tract. Contrast medium is taken orally and the lumen of the esophagus is fluoroscopically visualized. Standard X-ray films are usually taken prior to administration of the contrast medium and follow-up films may be taken 24 hours following the initial films.

Duration

45–60 minutes.

NORMAL FINDINGS

Normal size and contour with concentric movement of the esophageal musculature
Unobstructed flow through the cardiac sphincter
Lumen free of strictures

Causes of Deviation from Normal

A barium swallow may reveal one or more of the following:

Esophageal varices	Tracheoesophageal fistulas
Tumor or masses	Congenital abnormalities
Polyps	Esophageal reflux
Foreign bodies	Fibrosis
Inflammation	Stricture
Spasm	

Nursing Implications

Preprocedural. The purpose and the procedure should be explained to the patient. Patients should be told that they will be NPO after midnight. Any metal objects should be removed that may interfere with the field of examination.

Postprocedural. Fluid intake should be encouraged following the procedure. The nurse should administer a laxative following the examination, if ordered. Patients should be instructed to observe the color of the stool and to expect chalky white stools for several days. Patients should report constipation to their physician.

Description
CHEST RADIOGRAPHY (CHEST X-RAY)

One of the most common radiographic tests is that of the plain, non-contrasted chest X-ray. The best view is obtained with the patient erect and the film exposed in a posterior-anterior (PA) fashion. Patient mobility limitations may require the less desirable anterior-posterior (AP) film. Either of these approaches may be accompanied by a lateral view, and all are exposed on full inspiration.

Duration
15 minutes.

NORMAL FINDINGS

Normal vasculature including the aortic arch, pulmonary vasculature, and abdominal arteries
Normal lung fields
Normal body structures including symmetrically displayed clavicles and ribs
Sharp, clear cardiophrenic and costaphrenic angles with intact diaphragm
Normal structures of mediastinum
Normal heart shadow to the left of the sternum

Causes of Deviation from Normal
Chest radiography may reveal one or more of the following:

Cysts	Tumors
Masses	Pneumonia
Abscesses	Pleural effusion
Pneumothorax	Hemothorax
Atelectasis	Sarcoidosis
Tuberculosis	Emphysema
Skeletal deformities	Trauma
Sarcoma	Adult respiratory distress syndrome
Pulmonary edema	

13

Nursing Implications

Preprocedural. Female patients of childbearing age should be assessed for the possibility of pregnancy as radiographic studies would be contraindicated. Patients are instructed to remove metal objects, such as clothing with metal fasteners, necklaces, and pins.

Postprocedural. There are no specific nursing implications following chest radiography.

Description
CHOLANGIOGRAPHY

Cholangiography is a radiographic study of the integrity of biliary ducts. There are several approaches that can be used depending on the mode of administration of contrast medium including intravenous, percutaneous, and T-tube cholangiography.

Intravenous cholangiography involves administration of Cholografin meglumine, which is selectively removed from the blood by the liver and is eliminated via the biliary ducts and the gallbladder. Using fluoroscopy and tomography, the ducts can be visualized 20 minutes after contrast medium has been administered.

Percutaneous cholangiography bypasses the liver and the gallbladder, with contrast medium instilled directly into the biliary tree through a catheter introduced percutaneously into the liver during fluoroscopy. This method is selected instead of the intravenous approach if bilirubin levels are elevated. Bilirubin levels greater than 1.5–4 mg/dl indicate hepatic dysfunction too profound to allow uptake and excretion as described for the intravenous route.

T-tube cholangiography involves administration of iodine contrast medium through an external, artificial drain tube placed in the common bile duct during gallbladder surgery. This approach allows visualization of the patency of the hepatic and common bile duct prior to removing the T-tube drainage system.

Duration

Intravenous cholangiogram	2–4 hours
Percutaneous cholangiogram	1–2 hours
T-tube cholangiogram	30 minutes

NORMAL FINDINGS

Unobstructed biliary, cystic, and hepatic ducts
Normal gallbladder function

Causes of Deviation from Normal

Cholangiography may reveal obstruction or strictures of the biliary tree.

Nursing Implications

Preprocedural. All three forms of cholangiography require that patients have nothing by mouth for 8–12 hours prior to the procedure. Patients are also given a laxative the evening before the test or a cleansing enema the morning of the test, or both. This minimizes the interference of bowel contents during the visualization of the biliary system.

Patients should be given individualized explanation of the test based on the type of approach to be used. The percutaneous approach requires that the prothrombin time and the platelet count are clearly documented in the health record.

A patient history of allergies and allergic reactions to iodine should be documented and reported to the physician. The nurse should also verify that a consent form has been signed and included in the health record.

Postprocedural. If the percutaneous transhepatic cholangiography approach is performed, the vital signs should be monitored and recorded every 15 minutes for 1 hour, then every 30 minutes over the next 2 hours. Patients should also be assessed for signs of peritonitis and bleeding at the catheter insertion site. Patients' activity levels are limited to bed rest for 6–8 hours following the procedure to decrease the risk of bleeding.

If the intravenous approach has been used, the nurse should assess for signs of phlebitis and a delayed allergic reaction to the contrast medium. Patients should be encouraged to take oral fluids.

If the T-tube approach has been performed, the nurse should observe the drainage from the T-tube and maintain the integrity of the drainage system. This facilitates removal of any residual contrast medium from the bile duct and prevents skin irritation at the T-tube site.

Description

CHOLECYSTOGRAPHY

Oral cholecystography is a contrast radiographic study that visualizes the gallbladder and any stones that may be contained within it by using a contrast medium that is ingested in the form of tablets or powder. The pathway for the radiopaque medium is through the small intestine to the liver where it will be processed and excreted with bile into the gallbladder for concentration and storage. Bile and the contrast medium are released from the gallbladder when fats are ingested. The test may be divided into stages to reflect the filling and subsequent emptying of the gallbladder as two separate events.

The oral contrast medium is administered, taking approximately 12 hours to reach the gallbladder. A series of X-ray films are taken with the patient assuming sitting or standing, prone, and right-side-lying positions. Agents that stimu-

13

late contraction of the gallbladder may be administered, demonstrating empty-ing of the gallbladder. X-ray films are also taken during this phase.

Duration

1 hour.

N O R M A L   F I N D I N G S

Normal filling, contraction, and emptying of the gallbladder
No stones present in the gallbladder or connecting ducts

Causes of Deviation from Normal

Cholecystography may reveal one or more of the following:

Cholelithiasis	Inflammation of the gallbladder
Liver disease	Obstruction of the cystic duct
Tumors of the gallbladder	

Nursing Implications

Preprocedural. Jaundice or bilirubin levels of greater than 1.5 mg% may indicate hepatic dysfunction sufficient to interfere with manufacturing of bile in the liver. The nurse should alert the physician to these test results, because the procedure may be canceled. The purpose and the procedure should be explained to the patient.

In acute situations, a nasogastric tube may be placed to evacuate the stomach and instill contrast medium. Typically, however, a patient is prepared for this test in the following manner. The first meal on the day preceding the examina-tion may contain fatty foods to promote emptying of the gallbladder. Subsequent meals are low fat, progressing to limited clear liquids after dinner. Two hours after dinner, contrast tablets or capsules are administered. They are usually swallowed one at a time every 5 minutes with a full glass of water. No food is permitted after the contrast has been administered. An oral laxative or stool softener may be ordered to be administered following the evening meal.

On the morning of the examination, a cleansing enema may be ordered to minimize the interference of bowel contents during visualization. Patients should be screened for a history of allergies to iodine contrast medium.

Postprocedural. Patients should be provided with rest periods. Food or fluids should be resumed as ordered. If an iodine-based contrast medium was used, the nurse should assess for signs of an allergic reaction.

Description

CYSTOGRAPHY (VOIDING, RETROGRADE, URETHROGRAPHY)

Cystography is a contrast radiographic study of the bladder, urethra, and ureteral openings. An aqueous iodine contrast is instilled into the bladder through a urinary catheter, and X-ray films are taken. A kidney, ureter, and bladder (KUB) "scout" film may be taken to allow distinction of other contents of the abdomen from the contrast-filled bladder. Air may also be instilled in the bladder following elimination of contrast-urine to allow double-contrast films. Voiding cystography may be visualized fluoroscopically during voiding of contrast-urine following removal of the catheter.

Duration

60 minutes.

N O R M A L   F I N D I N G S

A smooth, thin-walled, suprapubic, midline bladder with the vesicoureteral sphincters competent to prevent reflux

Normal bladder emptying and patent, intact urethral structure

---

Causes of Deviation from Normal

Cystography may reveal one or more of the following:

Tumors	Urinary retention
Renal stones	Urinary strictures
Vesicoureteral reflux	Hemorrhage or clots

Nursing Implications

Preprocedural. Female patients of childbearing age who are or could be pregnant should not undergo this diagnostic study because of the risks to the fetus. A recent history of pelvic trauma is also a contraindication for this procedure because of possible urethral tears or transection; therefore, it is important for the nurse to screen for this patient population. A patient history of allergies and allergic reactions to iodine should be documented and reported to the physician.

The purpose and the procedure should be explained to patients, emphasizing that they may experience minor discomfort during insertion of the catheter and from a distended bladder. Further explanation should include that repositioning during the procedure may be necessary to allow for various X-ray exposures.

13

Inclusion of the informed consent in the health record should be verified. A nursing assessment should be documented, including characteristics of the urine, urinary patterns, and urinary sensations.

Specific fluid intake should be administered as ordered. A gentle enema may be ordered to allow for minimizing interference of bowel contents during visualization of the urinary structures.

If a urinary catheter is to be placed prior to sending the patient for this diagnostic study, the nurse should follow strict aseptic technique as included in the hospital's procedure manual.

Patients should wear a hospital gown and may wear their dentures.

Postprocedural. Urinary output and characteristics should be monitored and documented every 2 hours for 24 hours unless otherwise ordered. Any abnormal findings should be reported to the physician, including signs of urinary infection. Food and fluids should be resumed as ordered.

Description

INTRAVENOUS PYELOGRAPHY (EXCRETORY UROGRAPHY)

Intravenous pyelography (IVP) is a contrast radiographic study of the kidneys, ureters, and bladder. The patient is placed in a supine position on the X-ray table. Following an intravenous injection of iodine contrast, a series of X-rays are taken at specific time intervals over a 30-minute period to visualize the kidney, ureters, and bladder. The patient is then asked to void and a final X-ray is taken to visualize bladder emptying. Tomography studies may also be included during this procedure.

Duration

45 minutes.

NORMAL FINDINGS

Normal structure and function of the kidneys, ureters, and bladder

---

Causes of Deviation from Normal

Intravenous pyelography may reveal one or more of the following:

Renal calculi	Acute renal failure
Tumors	Polycystic kidney disease
Hydronephrosis	Chronic pyelonephritis
Congenital abnormalities	Ureteral calculi
Urinary retention	Trauma

Nursing Implications

Preprocedural. A history of allergies and allergic reactions to iodine should be assessed and reported to the physician. An explanation of the purpose and the procedure should be reviewed with patients, emphasizing that they may experience a warm, flushed, or hot, burning sensation during injection of the dye.

Patients are given nothing by mouth for 8–12 hours prior to the test. This is to minimize the risk of aspiration and to achieve a certain amount of dehydration. Patients with renal dysfunction may be given small amounts of water as ordered by the physician.

Administration of steroids, antihistamines, or other drugs may be ordered for patients who have a history of allergies to iodine or contrast dye, asthma, and any other severe allergies.

Administration of a laxative is usually ordered on the evening before the study and a cleansing enema may be ordered the morning of the study to minimize interference of bowel contents during visualization of the renal and urinary structures. Verification of the inclusion of the signed informed consent form in the health record should be done prior to the procedure.

A baseline nursing assessment should be documented to include vital signs, characteristics of the urinary output, urinary patterns, and urinary sensations. This allows for postprocedural comparison. The most recent blood urea nitrogen (BUN) and other indices of renal function should be noted. If the BUN is over 40 mg/dl, the test may not be performed.

Postprocedural. Vital signs should be monitored and documented every 30 minutes for 1 hour, including signs of an allergic reaction. Routine vital signs can be resumed unless otherwise indicated.

The intravenous infusion site should be assessed for signs of inflammation and hematoma formation and this should be reported to the physician. Urinary output should be monitored for detection of the renal response to the preprocedural dehydration.

Food and fluids should be administered as ordered by the physician to facilitate rehydration. Explanation of the importance of fluid intake may enhance patient cooperation. Patients may be placed on activity restrictions if they are elderly and weakened by the procedure.

Description

KUB (KIDNEY-URETER-BLADDER)

The *KUB* is a radiographic study of an anterior–posterior exposure of the flat, supine abdomen to visualize the kidney, ureters, and bladder. It can also be done to visualize the gastrointestinal tract, including the gallbladder, liver, and spleen. This X-ray film is sometimes referred to as a "scout" film.

Patients are first placed in a supine recumbent position, then a sitting or standing position as several X-ray films are taken. Patients may be asked to

13

hold their breath after exhaling to enhance the flatness of the abdomen during exposure.

Duration
15 minutes.

N O R M A L   F I N D I N G S

Normal gross structure of the kidney, ureter, bladder, spleen, liver, gall-bladder, and gastrointestinal tract.

Causes of Deviation from Normal
KUB may reveal one or more of the following:

Intestinal obstructions	Congenital abnormalities
Soft-tissue masses	Abnormal kidneys
Enlarged abdominal organs	Ascites

Nursing Implications
Preprocedural. Women of childbearing age should be screened for possible pregnancy as exposure to radiation is contraindicated because of risks to the fetus. An explanation of the purpose and the procedure should be given to patients. They should be dressed in a hospital gown without metal fasteners.

Postprocedural. There are no specific nursing implications following KUB.

Description
MAMMOGRAPHY
Mammography is a radiographic study using a low-dose X-ray technique to examine breast tissue. The patient is placed in a sitting or standing position with her breasts flattened in a plastic compressor. Care is taken to smooth the surface free of skin folds or air pockets. The patient is instructed to hold her breath during the X-ray exposure.

Duration
15–30 minutes.

N O R M A L   F I N D I N G S

Normal breast tissue

Causes of Deviation from Normal

Mammography may reveal one or more of the following:

Tumors

Cysts

Congenital abnormalities

Nursing Implications

Preprocedural. Women of childbearing age should be screened for possible pregnancy as radiographic studies are contraindicated during pregnancy because of risks to the fetus.

Explanation of the purpose and the procedure should be reviewed with patients, emphasizing that there is minimal discomfort during compression of the breast tissue.

Psychologically, patients should be prepared for at least 2 X-rays of each breast. They should know that the radiographer may need to palpate or reposition the breast and retake certain films without inferring that an abnormality exists. A nursing history should elicit patient concerns and any specific areas where masses have been palpated on breast self-examination.

All jewelry, metal objects and fasteners, powders, and deodorants should be removed and patients should wear a gown with the opening in the front.

Food and fluids are not restricted.

Postprocedural. Patients should be taught and encouraged to perform breast self-examination.

Description

MYELOGRAPHY

Myelography is a contrast radiographic technique used to outline the spinal cord and the surrounding subarachnoid space. Using the posterior lumbar puncture to gain access to the subarachnoid space, cerebrospinal fluid is withdrawn after recording opening pressures and sent for laboratory analysis. When 6–12 ml has been collected or drained, the X-ray contrast is instilled. The specific gravity of the contrast agent is greater than that of cerebrospinal fluid, so the direction of flow after injection will depend on the tilt of the X-ray table and patient position. This flow is followed fluoroscopically with spot X-ray films taken as indicated. If an oil-based contrast medium is used, the spinal needle will remain in place throughout the test to allow for removal of the contrast at the end of the procedure. This is accomplished by positioning the patient so the medium will flow toward the needle where it can be aspirated and removed. If a water-based contrast medium is used, it will be absorbed from the subarachnoid space and does not have to be aspirated; therefore, the spinal needle is removed immediately after administration of the contrast.

Myelography is contraindicated in patients with multiple sclerosis and increased intracranial pressure.

13

Duration

60–90 minutes.

```
N O R M A L    F I N D I N G S
```

Unobstructed gravitational flow of contrast within the spinal subarachnoid space outlining a spinal cord of normal anatomy throughout the
cervico-thorico-lumbar region

Causes of Deviation from Normal

Myelography may reveal one or more of the following:

Tumors	Compression of the spinal cord
Cysts	Herniated intervertebral discs
Spinal nerve root injury	

Nursing Implications

Preprocedural. The purpose and the procedure should be reviewed with
patients. Teaching should include the following:

1. Patients may feel some discomfort during the lumbar puncture.
2. They will be secured on the table in a prone position.
3. The table will be tilted in a variety of positions during the study.

It is recommended that patients ingest nothing by mouth for 4–8 hours prior
to the test and that a cleansing enema be administered the evening before or
the morning of the study.

The physician may order a sedative and an anticholinergic agent to be
administered to the patient prior to being transported to the procedure.

The nurse should determine if any premedications ordered are contraindicated by choice of the contrast medium. The radiologist should be contacted
for this information.

Inclusion of the signed consent form in the health record should be verified
prior to administration of any sedatives.

A nursing assessment focusing on the patient's neurological status should be
documented on the health record for postprocedural comparison.

Postprocedural. At this stage, the nurse must know the type of contrast
medium that was used for the test. Oil-based contrast will have been removed
from the spinal subarachnoid space, leaving a depleted volume of cerebrospinal
fluid. These patients should be kept on bed rest with the head of the bed flat for
6–24 hours and should have increased fluid intake to decrease the likelihood of
headache and to replenish the cerebrospinal fluid. If water-based contrast is

used, patients should be positioned so as to prevent the contrast from traveling to the middle fossa or reaching the hypothalamus. Untoward side effects of this occurrence may include severe headache, nausea, vomiting, and seizure activity. To prevent these side effects, patients should be kept on bed rest with the head of the bed elevated 30°–60° at all times for the first 8–24 hours. This position should also be used if an oil-based contrast was used but was not entirely removed. This important information is available from the radiologist, and specific positioning should be ordered by the physician. Fluid intake should be encouraged to restore cerebrospinal fluid.

Vital signs including neurological status should be monitored and recorded every 30 minutes for 2 hours, every hour for 4 hours or until stable, and then every 4 hours for 24 hours. The nurse should also observe for signs of meningeal irritation, which include severe headache, stiff neck, irritability, photophobia, fever, changes in level of consciousness, and seizures. The nurse should monitor patients for bladder distention and record urinary output every 4 hours.

Description

UPPER GASTROINTESTINAL (SMALL BOWEL) SERIES

The *upper gastrointestinal* (GI) or *small bowel series* is an oral contrast radiographic study of the stomach and small bowel often done in conjunction with the barium swallow. While using fluoroscopy, the patient swallows 2–3 cups of a barium sulfate mixture. The path of the contrast medium is followed through the cardiac sphincter into the stomach, through the pyloric sphincter into the duodenum. If the entire small intestine is studied, spot films are taken every 30 minutes to 1 hour until the contrast reaches the cecum. If double contrast is desired, the patient may swallow air with the barium by using a perforated straw or may be given a carbon dioxide-producing beverage or tablet.

Duration

Stomach	45–60 minutes
Small bowel	2–6 hours

NORMAL FINDINGS

Normal structure and motility of the upper digestive tract with competent sphincters

Causes of Deviation from Normal

An upper GI series may reveal one or more of the following:

13

Congenital abnormalities	Polyps
Pyloric stenosis	Diverticula

Gastric reflux	Tumors
Volvulus of the stomach	Gastrointestinal filling defects
Foreign bodies	Intussusception
Malabsorption syndrome	Ulceration of gastric or duodenal mucosa
Hiatal hernia	Inflammation of gastric or intestinal mucosa

Nursing Implications

Preprocedural. Patients may be ordered to follow a low-residue diet for 2–3 days prior to the study. Patients should have nothing by mouth and should not smoke or chew gum for at least 8 hours prior to the study.

Physician's orders may include instructions to hold narcotics or anticholinergics to avoid suppression of gastrointestinal motility. If any oral medication must be administered within 8 hours before the test, the radiographer should be informed. A cleansing enema may be ordered to evacuate the large intestine.

Patients should void, remove all jewelry and other metal objects, and be dressed in a hospital gown before being transported to the radiology department.

Vital signs and a baseline nursing assessment should be documented on the health record, focusing on the gastrointestinal status.

Postprocedural. A cathartic or enema should be administered to facilitate evacuation of the barium. Verification of completion of the X-ray series should be done prior to allowing the patients to resume dietary intake. Patients should be instructed in recognizing barium stools and reporting constipation. (Stools should be light in color for several days.)

ULTRASONOGRAPHY (ULTRASOUND)

Description

Ultrasonography is a safe, noninvasive diagnostic technique that enables visualization of the structure and function of organs within the body. A short, high-frequency pulse of sound is discharged into the body by a transducer held over the body surface. This wave travels through body tissue, encountering reflecting surfaces. The waves are reflected back toward the source, producing echoes. These reflected waves or echoes are received and processed by an ultrasound scanner. Images are produced and displayed on an oscilloscope, video monitor, or X-ray film.

The patient is placed in a supine or other position depending on the structures of the body being studied. A lubricant is applied to the skin area or the transducer to provide acoustic coupling over the surface of the skin and prevents air from interfering with sound transmission. The materials used can be aqueous gels or mineral oil. The transducer is applied to the skin by the examiner and is moved in a sweeping motion; images are produced and recorded. The only sensation is a gentle pressure from application of the transducer on the skin.

Ultrasound can be used to study the abdominal aorta, brain, vascular structures, gallbladder, heart, kidney, liver, pelvis, pancreas, spleen, and thyroid.

Duration

30–60 minutes.

NORMAL FINDINGS

Normal pattern image of the structure being studied

Causes of Deviation from Normal

Ultrasonography may reveal one or more of the following:

Aneurysms	Placental abnormalities
Liver disease	Vascular and valvular stenosis
Vascular occlusion	Gallbladder disease
Hemorrhage	Hydrocephalus
Cysts	Meningomyelocele
Tumors	Abscesses
Trauma	Infection
Inflammation	Pregnancy
Enlarged organs	Fluid in body spaces (pleural effusion,
Congenital abnormalities	pericardial effusion)

Nursing Implications

Preprocedural. The purpose and the procedure should be explained to patients, emphasizing that the procedure is safe and will not cause discomfort. This procedure is safe for pregnant women and the fetus. Patients will not be exposed to radiation. The nurse should also emphasize that patients will need to remain still during imaging.

Food and drink restrictions will vary according to the body area being studied. For pelvic and obstetric studies, patients should have a full bladder to facilitate transmission of the ultrasound beam and to displace bowel structures for

13

better visualization. This requires that the patient drink 3–4 glasses of water prior to the test and refrain from voiding until after the test.

Patients having ultrasonography of structures in the abdomen should have nothing by mouth for 8–12 hours prior to the test. Patients having a gallbladder study may need a low-fat meal the evening before the test.

Postprocedural. Patients will need to void to relieve the discomfort of a distended bladder following pelvic studies. They can resume preprocedural dietary intake and activities unless otherwise ordered. The nurse may need to remove the lubricant from the skin and replace any soiled hospital gowns.

ENDOSCOPY

This category of diagnostic studies includes arthroscopy, bronchoscopy, colonoscopy, cystoscopy and cystourethroscopy, gastroscopy and esophagogastroduodenoscopy, and laparoscopy. These studies allow for direct visualization of internal body structures through a flexible fiberoptic instrument.

Description
ARTHROSCOPY

Arthroscopy is the direct visualization of a joint, usually the knee, through a fiberoptic endoscope. This diagnostic procedure is usually done under general anesthesia; however, a local anesthesia can be used. Using careful aseptic technique and a surgically draped field, a small incision is made and a cannula is advanced into the joint capsule for aspiration of synovial fluid and subsequent instillation of saline. The fiberoptic arthroscope is inserted and the joint is visually explored. Visualization may be sufficient for diagnostic purposes or may be combined with biopsies, arthrostomies, or therapeutic procedures. When the fiberoptic scope is removed, the wound is copiously irrigated to remove residual debris or blood. The incision is closed with sutures and a sterile pressure dressing is applied.

Duration
20 minutes.

NORMAL FINDINGS

Normal joint structures
Smooth joint surfaces free of loose bodies, and all ligaments and tendons are competent
Normal synovial fluid

Causes of Deviation from Normal

Arthroscopy may reveal one or more of the following:

Degenerative joint disease   Bone fracture fragments

Inflammatory changes   Ruptured or torn ligaments or tendons

Arthritis

Nursing Implications

Preprocedural. The purpose and the procedure should be reviewed with patients, including the type of anesthesia that will be used. Patients should be prepared with an explanation and demonstration of leg exercises and crutch-walking techniques if the knee is studied.

Patients should have nothing by mouth after midnight prior to the study if general anesthesia is scheduled. The joint should be cleansed and shaved or a depilatory cream used on the surrounding surfaces.

A history of allergies should be documented on the health record and an allergy wristband placed. A nursing assessment should be documented, including vital signs, cardiopulmonary status, and involved joint status. Verification of inclusion of the signed consent form in the health record should be done by the nurse.

If general anesthesia is scheduled, the general nursing considerations for care prior to general anesthesia should be instituted. Patients should be encouraged to void before the procedure. They should be dressed in a hospital gown.

Postprocedural. Following return of a gag reflex and alertness, dietary and fluid intake should be resumed as ordered. The pressure dressing should be observed for signs of bleeding and proper application and ice applied, if ordered. Vital signs should be taken as ordered. Circulatory status and sensation should be assessed distal to the dressing in order to detect undue constriction.

Patients may need to be instructed or reinforced in progressive exercises of the involved joint to increase strength and decrease swelling, as ordered by the physician. Crutch-walking may be ordered for patients with arthroscopy of the knee. This aid is time-limited until the patient can ambulate without a limp. Physical therapy should be consulted, if necessary.

Analgesics should be administered for joint pain, as ordered. If general anesthesia was used, standard postanesthesia care should be instituted. Prior to discharge, patients should be instructed to observe and report any signs of infection.

Description

BRONCHOSCOPY

Bronchoscopy is the direct visualization of the trachea and bronchi through a flexible fiberoptic bronchoscope. A local anesthetic is applied to the oropharynx and epiglottis and the scope is inserted into the trachea through the

13

mouth. Nasal access may be used. The structures are visualized, cytologic washings or biopsies may be obtained, and the scope is removed. Suctioning equipment may be used during the procedure to remove secretions and to maintain a patent airway.

Duration

30–60 minutes.

N O R M A L F I N D I N G S

Normal tracheal and bronchial structures

Causes of Deviation from Normal

Bronchoscopy may reveal one or more of the following:

Tumors	Inflammation
Foreign objects	Mucous plugs
Granulomatous regions	Mucosal swelling or bleeding
Burned epithelium	Stenosis

Nursing Implications

Preprocedural. The purpose and the procedure should be reviewed with patients, including the possibility of experiencing the sensations of dyspnea and airway obstruction during the insertion of the scope. Patients should be reassured that their pulmonary status will be closely monitored and that they will receive an adequate air supply. Relaxation techniques should be taught to patients in order to enhance a relaxed posture during the procedure. They should be informed that the throat will feel numb and that swallowing may be difficult but that these sensations last for a very short time following the procedure.

Patients should have nothing by mouth for 4–6 hours prior to the study to minimize the risk of aspiration. A sedative or analgesic and anticholinergic agent may be administered 30 minutes prior to transporting patients to the procedure room.

A nursing assessment should include cardiovascular and pulmonary assessments for postprocedural comparison. Allergies should be documented and reported accordingly. Verification of inclusion of the signed consent form in the health record should be done by the nurse.

Patients should remove dentures, glasses, jewelry, and contact lenses and wear a hospital gown for the procedure. Patients should be encouraged to void before the procedure.

Postprocedural. Verification of the return of the gag and swallow reflex should be done before resuming foods or fluids, as ordered. The nurse should assess for signs of procedural complications, including dyspnea, hoarseness, coughing, wheezing, tachycardia, cardiac dysrhythmias, bloody mucus production, noisy respiration, subcutaneous emphysema, unequal chest wall expansion, unequal breath sounds, and other signs of hypoxia. Warm, saline gargles are recommended for throat discomfort, following the return of the gag reflex.

Description
COLONOSCOPY

Colonoscopy is an endoscopic examination to visualize the large intestines. It may be used for diagnostic purposes when the results of a barium enema or shorter proctosigmoidoscopy of the colon are inconclusive. The patient is positioned in Sims' position, the rectum is dilated, and the colonoscope is inserted anally. The scope is maneuvered through the rectum, sigmoid colon, and large intestine to the ileocecal valve. Air may be used to distend the intestine for better visualization. The scope is then slowly removed and careful visualization is done. Biopsies and cytologic brushings can be performed, and polyps can be removed during this procedure.

This procedure is contraindicated for patients with acute myocardial infarctions, third-trimester pregnancies, or acute inflammatory bowel disease.

Duration
30 minutes–3 hours.

N O R M A L   F I N D I N G S

Normal structure and mucosa of the large intestine

Causes of Deviation from Normal
Colonoscopy may reveal one or more of the following:

Polyps	Inflammation of the mucosa
Foreign bodies	Intestinal bleeding
Tumors	

Nursing Implications
Preprocedural. The purpose and the procedure should be reviewed with patients, including explanation that parts of this procedure may be uncomfortable or embarrassing. Patients should be prepared to experience the sensations of a bowel movement or gas expulsion during the procedure and reassured that

13

their intestine will have been thoroughly cleansed prior to the study. Relaxation techniques should be taught to ease the insertion of the colonoscope. Bowel preparation for visualization is very important and may vary depending on individual patients, physician preference, or institution procedures.

Patients may be placed on a clear-liquid diet and given laxatives for up to 3 days prior to the study and given nothing by mouth for 8 hours prior to the study. A strong laxative, such as magnesium citrate or castor oil, may be administered the evening before and the morning of the procedure followed by a tap-water enema until clear return 1–2 hours before the study. Whole-gut preparation, with slight dietary restrictions, and use of a mild laxative on the preceding day may be another approach to bowel preparation. Patients may become fatigued during the procedure or as a result of the bowel preparation and the nurse should provide for safety and assistance with activities. Iron preparations are discontinued 4 days prior to the study to facilitate bowel preparation.

The nurse should check to be sure a consent form has been signed and is included in the health record. A sedative may be ordered intramuscularly or the physician may order an intravenous line placed to allow for administration of sedatives, analgesics, anticholinergics, or glucagon during the procedure. The nurse should ensure that allergies, hemoglobin, hematocrit, and coagulation studies are documented on the health record. A baseline pulse oximetry reading should be taken as these patients may experience arterial oxygen desaturation during the procedure.

Postprocedural. Patients should be allowed to rest as this is an exhausting preparation and procedure. Fluids should be resumed as soon as the patient is fully awake, and fluid volume and electrolyte status should be assessed. Vital signs should be taken every 30 minutes for 2 hours, then less frequently as sedation abates and there are no signs of bleeding or perforation. Gross bleeding, mucopurulent drainage, abdominal cramps, severe pain, or fever should be reported to the physician immediately. Hemoglobin, hematocrit, and pulse oximetry should be monitored for comparison and changes.

Description

CYSTOSCOPY/CYSTOURETHROSCOPY

Cystoscopy allows direct visualization of the bladder walls, ureteral openings, bladder neck, and urethra with the aid of two fiberoptic instruments, the *urethroscope* and the *cystoscope*. An anesthetic lubricant may be used to insert a sheath. Once the sheath for instrument passage is in place in the urethra, collection of urine from individual ureters can be achieved or ureteral catheters can be passed if retrograde pyelography is desired. The procedure may be performed under local or general anesthesia.

Duration

45–60 minutes.

N O R M A L   F I N D I N G S

Normal structure of the urethra, prostatic urethra, bladder, and ureteral orifices

---

Causes of Deviation from Normal

Cystoscopy may reveal one or more of the following:

Tumors	Polyps
Urethritis	Multiple ureteral orifices
Renal calculi	Strictures
Enlarged prostate	

Nursing Implications

Preprocedural. The purpose and the procedure should be reviewed with the patient, including that there is minor discomfort during the procedure. Patients should be taught deep-breathing exercises to allow for relaxation during insertion of the urethral sheath. When the procedure is done using a local anesthetic instilled into the urethra, patients are not fluid restricted and may have fluids encouraged to provide dilute sterile urine for expansion of the bladder wall and flushing of the urinary tract. Patients usually receive a full-liquid breakfast on the morning of the study. A nursing assessment should include vital signs, urinary patterns, urinary sensations, and urine characteristics. The nurse should also verify that the consent form is included in the health record. Sedatives or analgesics should be administered as ordered. Patients should be dressed in a hospital gown.

Postprocedural. Vital signs should be monitored every 15 minutes for 1 hour, every 30 minutes for the next hour, and every hour for the following 4 hours. Itemized urine output should be monitored, including assessment of urinary sensations and urine characteristics. Patients may experience slight burning with urination, blood-tinged urine, and difficulty initiating urination for 24 hours following the study. Heavy bleeding, inability to urinate, urinary retention, and decreased urine output should be reported to the physician. Patients should also be assessed for signs of infection even though antibiotics are usually ordered prophylactically for several days surrounding the study. Fluids should be encouraged, unless contraindicated.

13

An indwelling urinary catheter may be needed to drain the bladder until edema subsides or to reestablish urinary patency related to clot formation. Patients may also experience relief of pain and spasms with a sitz bath, as ordered.

Description
GASTROSCOPY, ESOPHAGOGASTRODUODENOSCOPY

An endoscopic examination of the upper gastrointestinal tract may include direct visualization of the internal structure of the esophagus (*esophagoscopy*), stomach (*gastroscopy*), or the duodenum (*duodenoscopy*) through a fiberoptic endoscope. A local anesthetic is usually applied to the posterior pharynx. The patient is placed in a left lateral decubitus position. A sedative may be administered intravenously to facilitate patient relaxation and the endoscope is inserted into the esophagus, stomach, or duodenum. Air may be introduced through the scope to facilitate visualization. Biopsies and cytology brushings may be performed during the study and foreign objects and secretion can be removed with suction.

Duration
30 minutes.

N O R M A L   F I N D I N G S

Normal internal structures of the esophagus, stomach, and duodenum

Causes of Deviation from Normal
Endoscopy of the gastrointestinal tract may reveal one or more of the following:

Esophageal varices	Gastric lesion
Achalasia	Strictures
Duodenal ulcers	Esophagitis
Duodenitis	Tumors
Hiatal hernia	

Nursing Implications
Preprocedural. The nurse should verify that the signed consent form is included in the health record. The purpose and the procedure should be

reviewed with the patient. Patients should have nothing by mouth for 8–12 hours prior to the study. A nursing assessment should include vital signs and history of any allergies. Intravenous fluids may be initiated to allow for an access for medications during the study.

Patients should remove all dental prostheses, eyeglasses, and jewelry and should be clothed in a hospital gown. They should have oral hygiene care and void prior to the study. A sedative, analgesic, or atropine may be administered 30 minutes to 1 hour prior to the study, as ordered.

Postprocedural. Vital signs should be recorded every 30 minutes for 2 hours and then every 4 hours. Patients should be assessed for a gag reflex prior to initiating food and fluids, as ordered. Patients should be in a side-lying position until they are alert and the gag reflex is intact. The nursing assessment should include monitoring for signs of bleeding or perforation. These include pain, fever, difficulty swallowing, subcutaneous emphysema, hematemesis, or melena. Referred pain to the shoulder or pain with respiration or neck movement may suggest visceral perforation. Warm saline gargle may provide relief from throat discomfort. This is offered after the return of the gag reflex. Patients may experience a bloated feeling and "belching" should be encouraged.

Description

LAPAROSCOPY

Laparoscopy is the visualization of the peritoneal cavity using a laparoscope. A fiberoptic laparoscope is inserted through a small surgical incision in the abdominal wall and allows direct visualization of the uterus, ovaries, fallopian tubes, diaphragm, liver, peritoneal gutters, and serosal surfaces of the intestines. This procedure may be done using general anesthesia if complete abdominal relaxation is required or more extensive surgery is anticipated. If a local anesthetic is used, it is frequently supplemented by sedatives or analgesics to reduce the discomfort of bowel insufflation.

The patient is placed in a supine recumbent position. The abdominal insertion site is cleansed and a general or local anesthesia is initiated. A trocar is introduced through a small incision at the umbilicus and the laparoscope is inserted. Carbon dioxide or nitrous oxide is introduced into the peritoneal cavity, which moves the abdominal wall away from the viscera to decrease the potential for visceral penetration with the initial insertion of the trocar. The structures are visualized and biopsies may be taken. Most of the air is removed and the scope is withdrawn. The incision is sutured and a sterile dressing is applied.

Duration

30–60 minutes.

13

N O R M A L F I N D I N G S

Normal uterus, fallopian tubes, ovaries, liver, and diaphragm

Causes of Deviation from Normal

Laparoscopy may reveal one or more of the following:

Ovarian cysts	Tumors
Uterine fibroids	Adhesions
Liver lacerations	Liver nodules
Inflammation	Ectopic pregnancies
Liver cirrhosis	Ascites
Fallopian strictures	Abscesses
Endometriosis	

Nursing Implications

Preprocedural. The purpose of the procedure should be reviewed with patients. The abdominal incision should not leave a disfiguring scar. Patients usually have nothing by mouth for 8–12 hours prior to the study. Intravenous fluids may be initiated for medication administration, as ordered. The nursing assessment should be documented, including vital signs and allergies. Verification of inclusion of the signed consent form in the health record is done by the nurse. Patients should be dressed in a hospital gown and should void before administration of sedatives or analgesics, as ordered.

Postprocedural. Vital signs should be documented every 30 minutes for 2 hours and every hour for the following 2 hours. Intravenous fluids should be administered as ordered and food and fluid intake should be progressed as tolerated following return of alert level of consciousness and protective reflexes. If general anesthesia was used, administer postanesthesia care, as ordered. The nurse should assess for signs of infection and bleeding. Patients should be instructed to report pain and signs of infection to their physician. It is not uncommon for patients to experience back or shoulder pain related to air in the abdominal cavity; however, it is important to differentiate pain caused by irritation from the presence of air versus pulmonary emboli.

BIBLIOGRAPHY

Bandyk, D.F. "Preoperative Imaging of Aortic Aneurysms." *Surgical Clinics of North America*, 69(4):721–735 (1989).

Barkin, J., B. Krieger, Z. Blinder, L. Bosch-Blinder, R. Goldberg, and R. Phillips. "Oxygen Desaturation and Changes in Breathing Pattern in Patients Undergoing Colonoscopy and Gastroscopy." *Gastrointestinal Endoscopy*, 35(6):526–530 (June 1989).

Baxter, G.M., W. Kincaid, R.F. Jeffrey, G.M. Millar, C. Portenteous, and P. Morley. "Comparison of Colour Doppler Ultrasound with Venography in the Diagnosis of Axillary and Subclavian Vein Thrombosis." *The British Journal of Radiology*, 64(765):771–781 (1991).

Beare, P.G., V.A. Rahr, and C.A. Ronshausen. *Quick Reference to Nursing Implications of Diagnostic Tests*. Philadelphia: Lippincott, 1983.

Boonstra, P.W., W.J. Boeve, E.L. Mooyaart, and A. Eijgelaar. "Intra-arterial Digital Subtraction Angiography (DSA) as an Outpatient Screening Method for the Follow-Up of Graft Patency in Coronary Surgery." *Journal of Cardiovascular Surgery*, 30:764–767 (1989).

Brezis, M., and F. Epstein. "A Closer Look at Radiocontrast-Induced Nephropathy." *New England Journal of Medicine*, 320(2): 179–181 (1989).

Bury, B. "Warning—Medical Imaging Can Damage Your Health." *The Practitioner*, 231:323–326 (March 8, 1987).

Chandraratna, P.A.N. "Echocardiography and Doppler Ultrasound in the Evaluation of Pericardial Disease." *Circulation*, 84(3):Suppl. 1, 303–310 (1991).

Collins, J., M. Shaver, P. Batra, K. Brown, and A. Disher. "Magnetic Resonance Imaging of Chest Wall Lesions." *Journal of the National Medical Association*, 83(4): 352–360 (1991).

Corbett, J. *Laboratory Tests and Diagnostic Procedures With Nursing Diagnoses*. Norwalk, CT: Appleton and Lange, 1992.

Dawson, P. "Digital Subtraction Angiography—A Critical Analysis." *Clinical Radiology*, 34:474–477 (1988).

Gamsu, G., and D. Sostman. "Magnetic Resonance Imaging of the Thorax." *American Review of Respiratory Disease*, 139:254–257 (1989).

Gibb, S., J. Laney, and A. Tarshis. "Use of Fiberoptic Endoscopy in Diagnosis and Therapy of Upper Gastrointestinal Disorders." *Medical Clinics of North America*, 70 (6):1307–1314 (1986).

Goin, J., and G. Hermann. "The Clinical Efficacy of Diagnostic Imaging Evaluation Studies: Program, Paradigms, and Prescriptions." *Investigative Radiology*, 26(5):507–511 (1991).

Hammill, S. "Overview of the Clinical Electrophysiology Study." *Journal of Electrocardiology*, 22 (Suppl.):209–217.

Henig, I., S. Prough, M. Cheatwood, and E. DeLong. "Hysterosalpingography, Laparoscopy and Hysteroscopy in Infertility: A Comparative Study." *Journal of Reproductive Medicine*, 36(8):573–575 (1991).

Hershman, W.Y., and G.J. Balady. "Echocardiographic Evaluation of Mitral Valve Prolapse." *Hospital Practice*, 93–100 (October 30, 1989).

13

Holder, L. "Clinical Radionuclide Bone Imaging." *Radiology*, 176(8):607–613 (1990).

Hunt, A.H. "Digital Subtraction Angiography: Patient Preparation and Care." *Journal of Neuroscience Nursing*, 19(4):222–225 (1987).

Jaquith, S. "Chest X-Ray Interpretation: Implications for Nursing Intervention." *Dimensions of Critical Care Nursing*, 5(1):9–19 (January–February 1986).

Kee, J. *Laboratory and Diagnostic Tests With Nursing Implications*. Norwalk, CT: Appleton & Lange (1991).

Lancaster, J., D. Gotley, D. Bartolo, and D. Leaper. "Hypoxia and Hypotension During Endoscopy and Colonoscopy." *Australian and New Zealand Journal of Surgery*, 60:271–273 (1990).

Leeds, N.E. "The Clinical Application of Radiopharmaceuticals." *Drugs*, 40(5):713–721 (1990).

March, K. "Transcranial Doppler Sonography—Non-Invasive Monitoring of Intracranial Vasculature." *Journal of Neuroscience Nursing*, 22(2):113–116 (1990).

McDonagh, A. "Getting the Patient Ready for a Nuclear Medicine Scan." *Nursing*, 91(2):53–57 (February 1991).

Mercer, M. "The Electrophysiology Study: A Nursing Concern." *Critical Care Nurse*, 7(2):58–65 (1987).

Monroe, D. "Patient Teaching for X-Ray and Other Diagnostics." *RN*, 44–46 (February 1989).

Monroe, D. "Patient Teaching for X-Ray and Other Diagnostics." *RN*, 36–40 (September 1989).

Monroe, D. "Patient Teaching for X-Ray and Other Diagnostics." *RN*, 50–56 (December 1989).

Montico, L., and K. Hill. "EP Studies: When They're Called For, What They Reveal." *RN*, 54–58 (February 1989).

Pagana, K., and J. Pagana. *Diagnostic Testing and Nursing Implications*. St. Louis: The C.V. Mosby Company (1990).

Peters, A. "Recent Advances and Future Projections In Clinical Radionuclide Imaging." *The British Journal of Nursing*, 90(1):27–28.

Plankey, E., and J. Knauf. "What Patients Need to Know about Magnetic Resonance Imaging." *American Journal of Nursing*, 90(1):27–28 (1990).

Polak, J. "Doppler Ultrasound of the Deep Leg Veins: A Revolution in the Diagnosis of Deep Vein Thrombosis and Monitoring of Thrombosis." *Chest*, 99(4)Suppl: 165S–172S (1991).

Robin, E., and C. Burke. "Risk Benefit Analysis in Chest Medicine: Routine Chest X-Ray Examinations." *Chest*, 90(2):258–262 (1986).

Sahn, D., and J. Kisslo. "Report of the Council on Scientific Affairs: Ultrasonic Imaging of the Heart: Report of the Ultrasonography Task Force." *Archives of Internal Medicine*, 151(1):1288–1294.

Scholz, F. "Digital Subtraction Angiography." *Medical Clinics of North America,* 70(6):1253–1265 (1986).

Schuster, D. "Positron Emission Tomography: Theory and Its Application to the Study of Lung Disease." *American Review of Respiratory Disease,* 139:818–840 (1989).

Schwab, S., M. Hlatky, K. Pieper, C. Davidson, K. Morris, T. Skelton, and T. Bashore. "Contrast Nephrotoxicity: A Randomized Controlled Trial of a Nonionic and an Ionic Radiographic Contrast Agent." *New England Journal of Medicine,* 320(3):149–153 (1989).

Scott, D., and L. Christenson. "Complications of Imaging Procedures in Six Elderly Patients." *Postgraduate Medicine,* 85(4):145–148 (1989).

Soulen, R. "Magnetic Resonance Imaging of Great Vessels, Myocardial and Pericardial Disease." *Circulation,* 84(3):1–311; 1–321 (1991).

Steinke, W., C. Kloetzsch, and M. Hennerici. "Carotid Artery Disease Assessed by Color Doppler Flow Imaging: Correlation with Standard Doppler Sonography and Angiography." *American Journal of Neuroradiology,* 11(2):259–266 (1990).

Stevens, L., and R. Redd. "Bedside Electrophysiology Study." *Critical Care Nurse* 7(4):35–41 (1987).

Treseler, K. *Clinical Laboratory and Diagnostic Tests: Significance and Nursing Implications.* Norwalk, CT: Appleton & Lange (1989).

13

Abbreviations

cc	cubic centimeters
g	gram
mg	milligram
kg	kilogram
ng	nanogram
pg	picogram
μ	micron
μg	microgram
μmol	micromol
l	liter
ml	milliliter
dl	deciliter
mm	millimeter
cu mm	cubic millimeter
U	unit
IU	international unit
μIU	micro international unit
mIU	milli international unit
mol	mole
mM	millimole
mOsm	milliosmole
μEq	micro equivalent
mEq	milliequivalent
MUU	mouse uterine units
Hg	mercury

B

Minimum Barrier Precautions for Common Patient Care Procedures

Procedure	Gloves	Gown/Apron	Mask	Eye Protect	Oral Airway
Administration Blood Products	X				
Administration PO, IV (indirect) Meds					
Angiography	X	X	X	X	
Arterial Puncture	X		X	X	
Arthrocentesis	X				
Arthrogram	X				
Autopsy	X	X	X	X	
Bedbath (non-intact skin)	X				
Body Cavity Irrigations	X				

(continued)

439

Procedure	Gloves	Gown/Apron	Mask	Eye Protect	Oral Airway
Bronchoscopy	X	X	X	X	
Cardiac Catheterization	X	X	X	X	
Cardiopulmonary Resuscitation					X
Central Line Care and Manipulation	X				
Central Line Insertion	X		X	X	
Cystoscopy	X				
Decubitus Care	X				
Dental Procedures	X		X	X	
Drainage Tubes Care and Manipulation	X				
EKG Lead Placement					
Emptying Bedpans	X				
Endoscopy	X	X	X	X	
Enemas	X				
Eye Clinic Ophthalmologic	X				
Feeding Tube Care and Manipulation	X				
Finger Stick	X				
Hemodialysis	X				
HIS Bundle Studies	X	X	X	X	
Hysterosalpingogram	X				
Injections IM/ID/Sc	X				
Interstitial/Intercavitary Procedures	X	X	X	X	

Procedure				
Intubation	X	X	X	X
Laryngoscopy	X	X	X	X
Linen (soiled with blood/body fluids)	X	X		
Lumbar Puncture	X			
Lymphangiogram	X			
Myelogram	X			
Nasogastric Tube Placement	X			
Nasotracheal Suctioning	X			
Needle Aspirations/Biopsies	X			
Opthalmologic Procedures	X			
Oral Examination and Care	X			
Paracentesis	X			
Pacemaker Placement	X	X	X	X
Percutaneous Drain/Catheter Placement	X	X	X	X
Pelvic Exam	X			
Perineal Care	X			
Peripheral IV Insertion/Care/Manipulation	X			
Pheresis	X			
Port-A-Cath Care (vascular/intraperitoneal)	X			
Post Mortem Care	X	X		
Power Sprays	X	X	X	X
Rectal Exam	X	X		
Removal Fecal Impaction	X	X		
Sialogram	X	X	X	X

(continued)

Procedure	Gloves	Gown/Apron	Mask	Eye Protect	Oral Airway
Sitz Bath	X	X			
Skin Care (non-intact skin)	X	X			
Specimen Collection	X				
Specimen Handling (if not double/bagged)	X				
Spirometry	X				
Stoma Care & Manipulation	X				
Tattooing	X	X	X	X	
Tenckhoff Cath Care & Manipulation	X				
Thoracentesis	X				
Trach Care	X	X			
Trach Change	X	X	X	X	
Tracheal Suctioning (closed)	X				
Tracheal Suctioning (open)	X	X	X	X	
Urinary Catheters	X				
Vascular Shunts	X				
Venipuncture (including direct IV push admin)	X				
Vital Signs					
Wound Care—Dressing Changes (major)	X	X			
Wound Care—Dressing Changes (minor)	X				

(Adapted from the *Manual on Infectious Diseases*, City of Hope National Medical Center, 1992)

Index

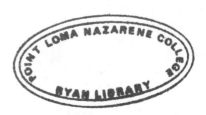

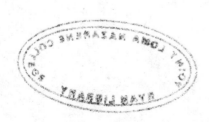